Living with a Chronic Condition:
the practitioner's guide to providing care

Senior commissioning editor: Mary Seager
Development editor: Carrie Savage
Production controller: Anthony Read
Desk editor: Jackie Holding
Cover designer: Gregory Harris

Living with a Chronic Condition: a practitioner's guide to providing care

Edited by

Alison Crumbie MSN, BSc, RGN, DipNP, Dip App, ScN, PGCE
Senior Lecturer and Nurse Practitioner, St Martin's College, Lancaster, UK

Judith Lawrence MSc, BSc, DB, RGN
Senior Lecturer and Nurse Practitioner, St Martin's College, Carlisle, UK

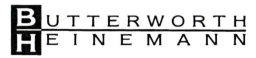

OXFORD AUCKLAND BOSTON JOHANNESBURG MELBOURNE NEW DELHI

Butterworth-Heinemann
Linacre House, Jordan Hill, Oxford OX2 8DP
225 Wildwood Avenue, Woburn, MA 01801-2041
A division of Reed Educational and Professional Publishing Ltd

 A member of the Reed Elsevier plc group

First published 2002

British Library Cataloguing in Publication Data
Living with a chronic condition: a practitioner's guide
   to providing care
   1. Chronically ill – Care
   I. Crumbie, Alison
   616'.044

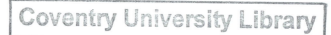

ISBN 0 7506 4808 2

For information on all of our Butterworth-Heinemann publications visit our web site at www.bh.com

Transferred to digital printing in 2006

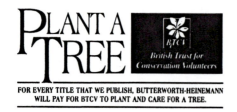

FOR EVERY TITLE THAT WE PUBLISH, BUTTERWORTH-HEINEMANN
WILL PAY FOR BTCV TO PLANT AND CARE FOR A TREE.

Contents

Contributors

Fiona Allan MA, BSc (Hons), Dip COT
Senior Lecturer, St Martin's College, Lancaster
Fiona is a senior lecturer in the Department of Occupational Therapy Studies at St Martin's College, Lancaster. She has worked for many years as an Occupational Therapist in a variety of areas, including rheumatology, orthopaedics and general medicine, but with the bulk of her clinical experience has been in the mental health field.

Gillian Armitage RGN, BSc (Hons), NP
Nurse Practitioner, Ashtree House Surgery, Kirkham
Gillian commenced working as a practice nurse in 1990 and as most practice nurses at that time, learnt to advise and treat patients with chronic conditions. She pursued an interest in epilepsy and when undertaking a BSc (Hons) degree to undertake the nurse practitioner role, her dissertation examined the perceptions of general practitioners in the care of adult epilepsy. The research recommended a definite need to raise the profile of epilepsy. Gillian works in general practice as a nurse practitioner and for a primary care group as a community nurse tutor.

Wendy Colley OBE, RGN, DN Cert
Clinical Nurse Specialist – Continence Care, West Cumbria Primary Care Trust, Whitehaven, Cumbria
In 1987 Wendy was appointed District Continence Advisor in West Cumbria, following time working as a district nursing Sister. Her special interests include the assessment of bladder problems and she developed a chart 'The Colley Model' in 1990 to help nurses identify the cause of the problem and plan a treatment programme for the patient (contact Wendy at: c/o West Cumbria Primary Care Trust, Flatt Walks Health Centre, 3 Castle Meadows, Whitehaven, Cumbria, CA28 7QE, for further details of the chart). For the work which Wendy and her colleagues implemented in West Cumbria using this model, they were awarded the Sir Bernard Tomlinson Quality of Care prize in 1992. Wendy has published articles on Assessment and other aspects of Continence Care in Nursing Journals over the last 10 years. In June 2000, she was awarded the OBE for 'services to continence nursing in West Cumbria'.

Alison Crumbie MSN, BSc, RGN, DipNP, Dip App, ScN, PGCE
Nurse Practitioner, St Martin's College, Lancaster
Alison is a nurse practitioner and senior lecturer at St Martin's College, Lancaster. She has worked and studied in Australia, the United States and Britain and has a breadth of experience in both the hospital and community setting. Alison is the course leader for the Nurse Practitioner Course at St Martin's College and plays an important role in courses for nurses who work with people who live with chronic conditions.

Una Hake RGN, HV, BSc Hons, NP
Nurse Practitioner, James Cochrane Practice, Kendal, Cumbria
Qualified in the 1970s Una has worked in a variety of settings, both hospital and community. She trained as a health visitor and worked in family planning for many years. In 1997, Una qualified as a nurse practitioner at St Martin's College, Lancaster, and has worked for the past 4 years in a semi-rural practice in Kendal, Cumbria as a nurse practitioner. Una has also worked in the USA and, more recently, as a practice nurse for over 10 years.

Kay Holt RGN, MW, HV, BSc Hons NP, MA, MscDip
Nurse Practitioner
Cleveleys Group Practice, Respiratory
Co-ordinator Wyre Primary Care Group
Kay has worked as a nurse practitioner at Cleveleys Health Centre for the past four years. Prior to this she worked as a practice nurse and health visitor. Her interest in respiratory medicine has developed since undertaking the National Asthma and Respiratory Training Centre (NARTC) Asthma and then COPD diploma courses. She is now a regional trainer for the organisation and also teaches on the Nurse Practitioner Degree Programme at St. Martin's College. Kay is employed part-time by Wyre Primary Care Group to manage their COPD Health Improvement Programme and is also involved in running community based Pulmonary Rehabilitation.

Judith Lawrence MSc, BSc, DB, RGN
Senior Lecturer/Nurse Practitioner
St Martin's College, Carlisle
Judith is a senior lecturer at St Martin's College with responsibility for the Chronic Disease Management Programme. She has a background in cardio-thoracic nursing and has worked as a nursing adviser in coronary heart disease and is currently a facilitator for the Heart Save Project, Oxford. She has extensive community nursing experience, most notably within district nursing and more recently as a nurse practitioner.

Barbara Maudsley RGN, BSc Hons, NP
Nurse Practitioner
Green Close Surgery, Kirby Lonsdale, Carnforth
Barbara is a nurse practitioner in a rural general practice at Kirkby Lonsdale, a small market town situated on the edge of both the Lake District and the Yorkshire Dales. Her background is in A&E nursing. She specialised at Leicester Royal Infirmary, and was a Sister in A&E at the Cumberland Infirmary, Carlisle. During the past ten years she has worked interalia as a practice nurse, community nurse and family planning nurse, and has been involved with a research group for a project about Farmers Health and Farm Accidents. She is a founder member of the Northern Nurse Practitioner Association and is involved with clinical skills, examination which gives her the opportunity to assess nurse practitioner students at St Martin's College, of which she is a graduate.

David Morning RMN, CPN Cert, BSc (Hons), PG Dip Ed, Med
David is a senior lecturer with SMC of Higher Education, Carlisle. Having worked in the NHS for a number of years as a community mental health nurse and a community manager, he was appointed as pathway leader for the community psychiatric nursing route of the Community Specialist Practitioner Qualification. Since then, he has developed his interest in educational theory and practice and now leads a practice educator course.

Ian Pomfret RGN, PWT, NDN cert
District Continence Adviser, Chorley and South Ribble Primary Care Trust, Primary Care Services, Chorley District General Hospital, Preston Road, Chorley, Lancashire
Nursing for over 30 years, Ian's background is General Nursing, District Nursing and Community Practical Work teaching. He has been practising as a Clinical Specialist/Continence Adviser since 1985; Treasurer of the National ACA Executive from 1990 to 1996, and Chairman of the ACA North West Branch from 1987 to date. His specialist interest is in continence products, especially in all aspects of urinary catheter care, on which he has published extensively in Professional Nursing Journals. Ian is a keen believer in the need for multidisciplinary care input in regard to continence care and is currently conducting a practical study, and managing an integrated Nursing, Occupational and Physiotherapy Continence team, the findings of which have also been published.

Jean Sargeant BSc (Hons), RGN
Nurse practitioner/Lecturer, Corbridge Health Centre, Manor Court, Corbridge, Northumberland
Jean moved from a secondary care background in Occupational Health, into primary care eleven years ago, to become a practice nurse. In 1994 she took part in the EROS Research project, which was a government-funded initiative, looking at the development of the role of the nurse practitioner in primary care. Jean also successfully undertook the BSc (Hons) Nurse Practitioner Degree at St Martin's College and

is currently working as a nurse practitioner in primary care and an Associate Lecturer at St Martins College.

Gail South MSc (Abertay, Dundee), BA (Edin), RGN, RM
Chesterfield and North Derbyshire Royal
Hospital NHS Trust, Chesterfield
Gail trained as an RGN in Edinburgh, qualifying in 1982. Following midwifery training, she worked as a midwife until moving home to Chesterfield, Derbyshire in 1988. A move into primary care provided an opportunity to train and work as a nurse practitioner where she developed an interest in the care and management of patients with respiratory disease. Returning to Edinburgh in 1995, Gail was appointed to a position of Asthma Specialist Nurse at the Royal Infirmary of Edinburgh, further developing her interest and expertise in respiratory care. During this time she became a regional trainer for the National Asthma and Respiratory Training Centre (NARTC) in Warwick. Now back in Chesterfield, Gail is employed as Practice Development Adviser at the Chesterfield and North Derbyshire Royal Hospital. She has continued to promote high strandards of care for respiratory patients through her continued links with the NARTC, providing training opportunities for nurses and other health professionals throughout the health community in North Derbyshire.

Linda Ward BA Hons, BSc, RGN, HV
Specialist Practitioner (General Practice Nursing), Dip N (Lond)
Linda is a senior lecturer at St Martin's College. She commenced her NHS career in 1973 as a cadet nurse and has since practiced within primary care as a practice nurse and Health Visitor. She has developed specialist expertise in practice nursing, primary health care policy, chronic illness and women's health.

Acknowledgements

We would like to acknowledge the patients who so freely shared their experiences of living with a chronic illness with us. They provided the motivation for this book. We would also like to acknowledge the creativity of Dr Shirley Reveley in the development of chronic disease management courses for health care professionals at St Martin's College. She has contributed to the vision for this book.

Disclaimer

The world of health care is ever changing. At the time of publishing this book the editors and contributing authors believe that all information contained herein is accurate. New research is continually being conducted and clinical experiences will continue to contribute to our knowledge and understanding of the management and treatment of people with chronic illness. In view of changes in medical and nursing science and the possibility of human error readers are encouraged to cross check the information in this book with other sources before making decisions about treatment regimens. In addition readers are encouraged to check with their laboratories for the local normal values and check with their Trusts to determine local guidelines for prescribing.

Introduction

Strauss and Corbin (1988) suggest that working with people who live with chronic illness requires sensitivity, understanding, commitment, perseverance and a strong knowledge base about chronic conditions. This book aims to equip the health care practitioner with the necessary knowledge and skills to manage the impact of chronicity on patient's lives. Part One is focused on developing an understanding of what it is like to live with a chronic condition and the ways in which we as health care professionals can enhance our sensitivity to the patients we are working with. Part Two focuses on specific chronic diseases. In this part we aim to provide an overview of the epidemiology, pathophysiology, assessment and treatment options for the patient with that particular condition. We have chosen seven of the most commonly occurring chronic conditions, however, we acknowledge that there are many more that could have been included. We hope that the themes identified in Part One will provide a valuable insight into the general issues associated with living with a chronic disease and that these will be relevant to all patients living with chronicity and not just the groups we have chosen to focus on in Part Two of this book.

Disease, illness or condition

So what is chronic illness and how does this differ from a condition or disease? Often these words are used interchangeably and yet there are important, although subtle, differences between the three. Illness refers to the human experience and to the perceptions of the patient and family and their responses to the symptoms and suffering caused by the disease process. Disease, on the other hand, refers to a problem that can be viewed from the medical perspective and can be defined by alterations in the struc-

ture and function of the body. A condition is a state of being and, as such, it describes the whole experience of a person who lives with chronic illness. Chronic disease management then refers to the activities carried out in the health care setting with patients who live with diseases such as diabetes, cardiovascular disease, epilepsy and asthma. We have used all three terms throughout this book depending upon the specific context at the time.

Chronicity

Curtin and Lubkin (1998) state that it is extremely difficult to define chronicity. Many authors have attempted to capture the essence of this concept, some of which are simple statements and others are complex definitions. Kelly and Field (1996) state that chronic illness results in the physical reality of 'bad' bodies. The body changes in chronic illness and can be seen as letting the person down. Bleeker and Mulderij (1992) speak of the body losing its silence and Morse et al. (1994) describe a body in dis-ease. Lyons et al. (1995) state that a chronic illness is not a singular event rather it signifies a set of complex processes that develop and endure over time. This links with the trajectory model of chronic illness outlined by Corbin and Strauss (1992).

Corbin and Strauss refer to the journey of chronic illness as a trajectory; a course which varies over time and can be divided into subphases. The course of the chronic illness can be shaped and managed and this is where we can have an impact upon the patient's experience of their disease. Funk et al. (1993, p. 3) quote the 1956 definition of chronic illness by The Commission on Chronic Illness as 'being caused by pathological changes in the body that are non-reversible, permanent or leave residual disability; they may be characterised by periods of recurrence and remission and they generally require extended periods of supervision, observation, care and rehabilitation'.

Curtin and Lubkin (1998 p. 6) offer a further definition of chronic illness as 'the irreversible presence, accumulation, or latency of disease states or impairments that involve the total human environment for supportive care and self-care, maintenance of function and prevention of further disability'.

Cameron and Gregor (1987) argue that chronic illness is a lived experience which involves a permanent deviation from the norm caused by unalterable pathological changes. The problem with this definition is that it labels people who have chronic illness as being abnormal. Certainly one of the important aspects of defining chronicity is the notion of permanence. Chronic conditions are not curable and this has an enormous impact upon our approach to working with people who live with chronicity. An important point to note is that most people live with rather than die from a chronic condition (Verbrugge and Jette, 1994).

It is clear that, in the experience of chronic illness, the patient becomes acutely aware of his or her body. People who do not have a chronic condition usually live alongside their bodies with little awareness of daily fluctuations in response to the stressors placed upon them. A person who lives with epilepsy or chronic obstructive pulmonary disease (COPD) for example, is not able to do this as they are constantly reminded, through their use of medication or their continuous symptoms, of the fact that they have a chronic disease. The constant monitoring required in type 1 diabetes means that the patient becomes acutely aware of responses to certain foods, exercise and simple colds and infections. People who are without chronic illness do not experience this. We cannot possibly totally understand what living with the condition is like for the patient and it is this awareness that lead us to seek the views of people who live with chronic illness.

The patient's perspective

Our approach in developing this book has been to focus firmly on the patient as being central to everything we do in working in this area of clinical practice. It is our belief that we should

never lose sight of the individual. If we do, our care becomes meaningless and will be likely to fail in achieving its aims. In Part Two of this book we have started each chapter with a quote from a patient. These quotes have come from a variety of sources. We have asked patients to be interviewed and taped or to write a few words for us on their experience of living with their particular condition. In all cases the patients gave their permission for the publication of the material. We have been deeply moved by the comments from the patients and this served to reinforce our determination to advocate for working with individuals and not diseases.

It has been interesting to note that the patients' comments shared many similarities. At first glance the reader may wonder what living with incontinence has in common with living with epilepsy or heart disease. However, we have been able to identify several themes that run through the patient narratives and it has highlighted to us that there is a shared experience of living with chronic illness that goes beyond the specifics of living with a particular condition.

Cutting off from the outside world

Most of the patients we interviewed commented on their shrinking horizons and their need to retreat from the outside world. This is highlighted in a particularly powerful way in the quote at the start of the COPD chapter (Chapter 8) as the person concerned states that he is glad that he lives away from his grandchildren as he would be unable to cope with lifting them and playing with them. The quote at the start of the continence chapter (Chapter 9) is from a woman who states that she felt dirty, isolated and alone. There are ways in which we as health care professionals can address this feeling of isolation. We may be able to offer the patient a forum to share their desperate feelings and to offer sources of support in the form of self-help organizations or local services. At the end of each chapter we have identified some of the main groups which may provide support for people living with the particular condition as this is one way to address the isolation and loneliness of living with chronic illness.

Each person is an individual

The patient who wrote to us about his cardio-vascular disease emphasized the uniqueness of each person's experience of chronic disease. This patient pointed out that no experience of chronic disease could be classed as routine and this is reinforced by the patient who consented to be interviewed about her diabetes. In the UK, 1.4 million people live with diabetes mellitus and yet the patient who was interviewed about her diabetes commented that it sometimes feels like 'you're ploughing a lonely furrow'. This patient pointed out that everyone is an individual and while you might derive some support from knowing that someone is in the same predicament as yourself, you cannot be sure that he or she is having exactly the same experience as you. We have considered this individuality throughout the book acknowledging that any treatment plan or education must be tailored to the individual needs of the patient. We have considered the issue of concordance in working with people who live with chronic conditions and have acknowledged that the patient has the ultimate power in managing the treatment plan. The health care professional can only advise and support the individual in whatever decision they make.

Fear

The issue of fear is addressed in several of the narratives. The patient with epilepsy was fearful of seizures; the patient with the thyroid disorder was fearful about losing his eyesight and fearful of 'the worst'; the patient with coronary heart disease was fearful of never waking from the anaesthetic. The patient who wrote to us about her asthma highlights the fear associated with not being able to breathe. Many of the chronic diseases result in the patient experiencing symptoms that would cause fear for any human being. Gasping for breath when you experience asthma or COPD feels like a threat to life and is bound to cause increased anxiety and a sense of panic. It is possible to help reduce the level of anxiety for patients who are experiencing these symptoms. First, with a good working knowledge of the conditions, we can work towards the best possible control of symptoms for the patient so that they do not have to experience the acute exacerbations of their condition. We can hand control to them by teaching them about their condition and how to manage acute episodes such as hypoglycaemia or acute shortness of breath. Secondly, we can listen to patients when they want to explain what they have been through and what it felt like to them. We can also listen to their family members who themselves will have been fearful for the patient's life during acute episodes. This book should equip the health care professional with the necessary knowledge to provide this education for patients.

Control

Control is mentioned in several of the narratives with reference to being 'out of control' or reference to 'needing to be in control'. The patient with thyroid disease talked about the problem of being out of control and how frightening this was to him. The patient who lives with incontinence talked about being 'ruled by' her condition and she talked about the tasks in her life she needed to address each day in order to cope with the incontinence. The patient who provided the narrative for the diabetes chapter (Chapater 6) talked about the day-to-day need to be in control and about the concentration and dedication required every day to manage her condition. This patient shared with us her feelings of getting tired with the constant work of controlling the condition and the need sometimes to forget it all and to launch into foods that she knows are not helpful to her glycaemic control.

In the chapter on the patient–professional perspective (Chapter 1) we address the balance of control between the patient and the health care professional and we advocate handing the control to the patient. Indeed, as health care professionals we have very little choice other than to recognize that the patient is ultimately in control of their condition. The patient has to live with their condition on a day-to-day basis. What we can do is equip them to maintain some kind of control over it. We can assist by ensuring that we are knowledgeable about the condition and that we refer to specialized practitioners when we are unable to help the patient.

Depression/anger and denial

Both the patient with thyroid disease and the patient with diabetes specifically mention feeling depressed and the mother of the child with eczema states that she had to take antidepressant medication as she felt so miserable. The patient with epilepsy describes facing prejudice and the patient with COPD states that he felt the 'bitterness of an unjust fate'. There are elements of denial in the narrative of the COPD patient who states that he was trying to act normally and the patient with coronary heart disease convincing himself that he was merely unfit until he could no longer deny the presence of the disease. The patient with asthma told us that she does not tell too many people about her condition because she does not want to be labelled as an invalid. Not all patients with chronic illness will develop depression or experience denial. However, there is no doubt that there will be a psychological component to their disorder which we need to address at every consultation. We have referred to the complexity of identifying depression in someone who lives with a chronic illness in the first part of this book.

The narratives at the start of each of the chapters in Part Two have given us a tiny insight into the world of the person who lives with chronic illness. We feel that they have also provided us with the reason for producing this book. If in some small way we can contribute to the health care professional's understanding of the holistic approach to chronic disease management and we maintain a focus on the patient at the centre of our care, then this book will have achieved its aims.

Alison Crumbie
Judith Lawrence

References

Bleeker H, Mulderij K (1992) The experience of motor disability. *Phenomenology and Pedagogy* **10**, 1–18. Cited in: Price B (1996) Illness careers: the chronic illness experience. *Journal of Advanced Nursing* **24**, 275–279

Cameron K, Gregor F (1987) Chronic illness and compliance. *Journal of Advanced Nursing* **12**, 671–676

Corbin J M, Strauss A (1992) A nursing model for chronic illness management based upon the trajectory framework. In: (Woog P, ed.) *The Chronic Illness Trajectory Framework.* Springer, New York, pp 29–38

Curtin M, Lubkin I (1998) What is chronicity? In: (Lubkin I, ed.) *Chronic Illness Impact and Interventions,* 4th edn. Jones and Bartlett, Sudbury

Funk S, Tornquist M, Champagne M T, Wiese R (eds) (1993) *Key Aspects of Caring for the Chronically Ill.* Springer Publishing Company, New York

Kelly M P, Field D (1996) Medical sociology, chronic illness and the body. *Sociology of Health and Illness* **18**, 241–257

Lyons R F, Sullivan M J L, Ritvo P G, Coyne J C (1995) *Relationships in Chronic Illness and Disability.* Sage, California

Morse J, Borttorff J, Hutchinson S (1994) The phenomenology of comfort. *Journal of Advanced Nursing* **20**, 189–195

Strauss A, Corbin J M (1988) *Shaping a New Health Care System: the Explosion of Chronic Illness as a Cat.* Jossey-Bass, London

Verbrugge L M, Jette A M (1994) The disablement process. *Social Science and Medicine* **38**, 1, 1–14

Part One
Perspectives on chronic illness

1

Patient–professional relationships

Alison Crumbie

Introduction

The point of diagnosis for a person who has diabetes, asthma, coronary heart disease, epilepsy or one of the many other chronic illnesses is just one stage in a long journey. Corbin and Strauss (1992) refer to this journey as a trajectory; a course which varies over time and can be divided into subphases. The course of the chronic illness can be shaped and managed and one of the conditions influencing this process is the relationship between the patient and the health care professional. The patient has the most important role to play, as people who live with chronic conditions do most of the work associated with managing the illness themselves. The health care professional, however, has an immensely important role as interactions with the patient will have repercussions far beyond the immediate consultation. In our discussions with patients even the slightest intonation of voice or an omission to recognize the importance of a comment from the patient can convey subtle messages that will affect the patient's whole experience of the illness. If we convey the message that we are shocked by the patient's admission of missing a few doses of medication or if we omit to look closely at the results of home monitoring, the patient will take powerful messages away from the encounter. The patient may learn not to be honest about alterations in medications which do not comply with the medical regimen and may begin to believe that monitoring has no value and therefore will stop engaging in this process. It is therefore important for health care professionals to consider the complexity of the relationship with patients who live with a chronic condition and to explore methods of enhancing the quality of that relationship. This chapter will focus on the patient–professional relationship and will explore some elements of the nature of this relationship. The chapter will then go on to link the issues raised in this discussion to approaches that can be taken by the health care professional to enhance the quality of the patient–professional relationship.

The sick role

People who live with a chronic condition have long suffered from the inappropriate application of therapeutic approaches which were designed for use in acute episodes (Gibson and Kenrick, 1998). A person who has an acute illness is assumed to be temporarily unwell and will be treated with the aim of full recovery. It is in this situation that the person becomes an occupant of the sick role. According to Parsons (1951), when a person is the occupant of the sick role they are exempt from their normal responsibilities, they are not responsible for their own condition, they are obliged to get well and they must seek competent help. When a person lives with a chronic condition, there may be times when they experience acute exacerbations of their illness and at these times they temporarily occupy the sick role. However, for the ongoing condition it is likely that there is no cure, they are unable to get well and therefore they cannot fulfil the obligations of the sick role. As the person who lives with a chronic condition cannot occupy the sick role they also cannot be exempt from their normal responsibilities and they have to find some way of managing their condition while meeting the chores of everyday life.

Gibson and Kenrick (1998) highlighted the problem of people who live with a chronic condition being treated with interventions more commonly associated with acute illness. They interviewed a sample of nine patients who had undergone vascular surgery for peripheral vascular disease and they found that the 'acute' style management of this group of patients often resulted in unrealistic expectations on the patient's part. People who live with peripheral vascular disease often have a series of surgical procedures to relieve the pain of the ischaemia. The surgical approach is aligned with the aim to cure, however, peripheral vascular disease is a chronic condition which is likely to worsen over time regardless of the surgical intervention. This results in a mismatch of goals and expectations. The patient undergoes vascular surgery expecting the problem to be cured and this effects the patient's perceptions of their illness. When the patient expects a cure from a surgical intervention they may not adopt appropriate coping strategies. As they realize that the symptoms may return after the surgery they may become disheartened and less able to cope. In Gibson and Kenrick's (1998) study one patient commented upon this by saying 'It's just the odd pain that frightens me I say oh God I hope it's not happening again'. Several of the participants of the study feared recurrent pain and Gibson and Kenrick found that the patients' attitudes to treatment corresponded to the sick role which is appropriate in acute illness and less appropriate for people living with a chronic condition.

Power in the patient–professional relationship

Pain and powerlessness were central features in the experience of living with peripheral vascular disease in Gibson and Kenrick's (1998) study and this was associated with the use of 'acute' interventions to manage chronic illness. These authors stated that powerlessness could be seen in the context of becoming a patient.

They found that patients talked of shrinking horizons, literally due to loss of mobility, but also metaphorically due to loss of control, acceptance of the condition and changing their outlook. Gibson and Kenrick speak of powerlessness as a response to the limits of the condition and to the power which is perceived to be vested in the health care system. In their study they found that true collaboration or power sharing appeared to be rare.

The issue of powerlessness is an important aspect of living with a chronic condition. It is interesting to note that the derivation of the word power is 'to be able to' implying that to have power means to be able to do something or to be effective (Hokanson Hawks, 1991). Hokanson Hawks (1991, p. 754) defines power as 'the actual or potential ability or capacity to achieve objectives through an interpersonal process in which the goals and means to achieve the goals are mutually established and worked toward'. This definition does not imply that one person has power over another. This is therefore relevant to our work with patients who have chronic conditions as the partnership between the professional and the patient should be based on a shared understanding and should be aiming towards enabling the patient to manage his or her condition. Power can be shared between two people and is related to a sense of control over a situation.

Langer and Rodin (1980) found that providing institutionalized elderly people with some control over their lives resulted in better mental health. In our work with people who live with chronic conditions there are many ways in which we can offer a sense of control. Providing a choice of inhaler devices for people with asthma can help them to make the best choice for themselves and discussing alternative modes of treatment for people with diabetes can give them some control over the management of their condition. The health care professional then has to be prepared to accept the consequences of the patient's decision. A patient who opts for a slightly higher blood sugar level rather than commencing on insulin therapy because he does not want to lose his flying licence is making a rational choice which is appropriate for his individual situation. The health care professional, however, needs to reconcile the elevated blood sugar readings with the understanding that this is what is right for this particular patient at this particular moment in time. Monitoring and discussions clearly need to continue so that the patient remains fully informed and aware of the consequences of the decision and the health care professional has an important role to play in this ongoing relationship.

We have traditionally considered that the ownership of medical knowledge provides the health care professional with power. We have a certain amount of knowledge about a condition and its treatment and the patient needs to have some of that knowledge. When we interact with a patient who has a chronic condition, however, they have a great deal of information too. The patient has information about their life, their family, their hopes and their desires, all of which will have an impact upon their ability to adhere to medication regimens or actively to engage in lifestyle behaviour changes. Indeed it could be suggested that the patient has much more information than the health care professional. The balance of power in the patient–professional relationship is summarized in Figure 1.1.

Marland (1998) suggested that in the event of non-adherence to a medication regimen it would make more sense to speak of the non-compliant doctor rather than the non-compliant patient. If a patient has not taken the medication according to the prescribed dose and time then this may be due to the fact that the health care professional did not spend time learning about the patient's lifestyle. An elderly lady who goes to a local meeting on a particular morning may choose to omit her diuretic on that particular day, a child who has been prescribed an inhaler to be taken four times a day may miss the two in the middle of the day because he is embarrassed about his problem and does not want other children to comment in the playground. Frequently there are alternatives to be considered when prescribing a medication and some extra time spent learning about the patient's values, beliefs and expectations might result in a more effective form of treatment and enhanced quality of life for the patient.

Empowerment

The word 'empowerment' has slightly different connotations to the word 'power' as it suggests that one person gives power to another, thereby assuming that the relationship between the health care professional and the patient is unequal at the outset. Bookman and Morgan (1988) define empowerment as a process aimed at changing the nature and distribution of power in a particular cultural context. Watson and

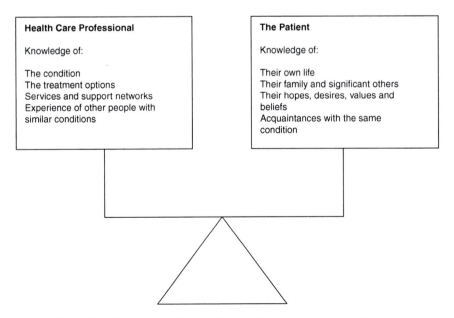

Figure 1.1 The balance of power in the patient–professional relationship

Burkholder (1990) refer to empowerment as an activity directed towards increasing a person's control over their life. Each of these definitions would imply that one person is giving power to another person, however, in our work with people who live with chronic conditions this may not always be the case. If we consider that the patient who lives with the condition has a great deal of knowledge to share with us, we can think of the process of information exchange being one of mutual empowerment, enabling both the health care professional and the patient to work together. If the patient shares information about their life with us, we will be empowered to be more effective in our recommendations for treatment. The potential exchange of information between the patient and the health care professional is summarized in Figure 1.2. We will, therefore be able to work towards the patient's goals for optimal health rather than our own assumptions about acceptable levels of well-being.

Piper and Brown (1998) describe a patient empowerment model for health education. The aim of this patient-centred model is to enhance the individual patient's control over health. This is achieved by working with the patient as an equal and facilitating patient reflection, clarification and interpretation of knowledge, attitudes and beliefs. Predetermined health issues are not imposed upon the patient, rather the health care professional raises such issues in a non-threatening way or the patient raises the issues for themselves. Social and economic determinants of health are acknowledged and patients are assisted to draw on their personal resources and strengths. Patients may then be helped to make informed choices and be in a

position to maximize their chances of moving towards what they consider health to be. It is important therefore that the health care professional has an understanding at the outset of the patient's understanding of what health is. People may decide to engage in behaviours which will not maximize their potential for positive health gain, however, this should not be seen as a failure on behalf of the health care professional.

Success or failure in the process of health education is difficult to define. Whitehead and Tones (1991) suggested the following criteria to be determinants of success for health education aimed at empowerment, control and choice:

- Acquisition of changes in knowledge and understanding
- Evidence of the development of decision-making skills
- Enhanced self-esteem and sense of personal control
- Development of various social, health and life skills.

Given that a great deal of our work with people who live with a chronic illness is focused on health education, Whitehead and Tones' determinants of success for health education can provide a useful tool to evaluate the outcome of our interventions. As we progress along the journey with the patient we can assess their level of knowledge and understanding of the condition. If this is improving as we work with them, this can be an indicator of success. In providing the patient with choices about the management of their condition we can assess whether they feel able to be engaged in the decision-making process and subsequently whether they have

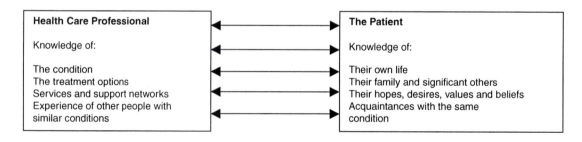

Figure 1.2 The potential exchange of information between the patient and the health care professional

an enhanced self-esteem and sense of control over the situation. We can also assess to what extent the patient is able to incorporate the management of their condition with the rest of their life and to learn to live with the condition rather than be controlled by it. Each of these areas provides us with indicators of success and progress when previously we may have tended to concentrate on blood glucose readings, numbers of seizures experienced, peak expiratory flow rate recordings or lipid levels. The four determinants of success identified by Whitehead and Tones (1991) involve working with patients to understand them and to help to educate them about their condition and this acknowledges the patient as much more than a passive recipient of care.

Participants in care

Engaging the patient as a participant in care is one method of enhancing the power of the patient. Patient participation is particularly important in the management of chronic illness. The success of treatment and management regimens relies upon the patient's willingness to be involved and to collaborate with health care professionals. There are a variety of definitions of patient participation in the literature. Holloway (1993) suggests that participation is the involvement of many people in decisions, giving them a feeling of control or sense of responsibility. Brownlea (1987, p. 605) provides a more extensive definition by stating that participation means 'getting involved or being allowed to be involved in the decision-making process or the delivery of a service or the evaluation of a service or even simply to become one of a number of people consulted on an issue or matter'. Other definitions have referred to a variety of aspects relating to the participation process, however, Cahill (1998) points out that patient participation is a complex concept and remains ill defined. In her review of the literature, Cahill found that some patients do derive security from the 'nurse knows best' stance and not all patients desire active participation in the management of their condition. She concludes, however, that in general, patients prefer to participate in their care while professionals acknowledge the potential value of patient

participation but generally prefer patients to be passive recipients of care.

A recent survey of coronary heart disease patients conducted by the Department of Health (2000) revealed that patients wanted more information about their treatment and wanted to be more involved in decisions about their care. The survey was based on 84 300 coronary heart disease patients in England who had received hospital treatment. Twenty per cent of patients surveyed had worries or fears about their condition and felt unable to enter into a discussion about their worries whenever they wanted with their doctor or nurse. Twenty-four per cent of the respondents said that there had been occasions when doctors, nurses or other hospital staff had talked about them as though they were not present. The results of this survey would suggest that patients are not always considered to be active participants in the management of their condition and this would be supported by a study carried out by Hewison (1995).

Hewison (1995) carried out a participant observational study of the use of language in nurse–patient interactions and found that the language used by nurses was powerful, with nurses telling patients what they could and could not do. Nurses placed limitations on the activities of patients and patients generally accepted that the nurse was in charge of the situation. Examples of overt power and persuasion were found and Hewison concluded that nurses exercise a great deal of power and control over patients. The power dimension in the nurse–patient relationship was found to be a barrier to patient participation in care as patients generally became submissive to the control of the nurses and agreed with their suggested course of action even if they disagreed with the plan of action at the outset. This study was based on 37.5 hours of hand-written observations and therefore may not be generalizable to all interactions between health care professionals and patients; however, it does highlight the unequal status in patients' relationships with health care professionals. If we are going to work in partnership with patients who live with chronic conditions we need to be aware of these dynamics so we can address them and minimize them at the outset. We need to examine the use of language in our interactions with patients and to be sensitive to the powerful messages we can convey.

Compliance, adherence and concordance

It has been argued that there is no place for concern over the issue of patient compliance in the management of people who live with chronic conditions. Members of an expert nurse advisory group have responded to the finding of a study into diabetes nurse specialists and their views on the changing NHS and how it will affect their ability to care, by stating that compliance is almost an obsession in chronic illness management. Nurses should be more interested in empowering patients and should be enabling people to make informed choices (Healy, 2000a). The study had found that diabetes nurse specialists say 'patient compliance' is a key issue for them and 68% of the specialist nurses believed that the patient's unwillingness to change inhibits the nurse's ability to care (Healy, 2000b). Even though the expert nurse advisory group feel that compliance should not be a focus for health care professionals who work with people who live with chronic conditions, it does become an issue simply because much of the time spent with health care professionals is directed towards improving patient compliance as is illustrated by the results of the diabetes nurse specialist study. It is worthwhile exploring this issue in order to consider the problems associated with the focus on compliance when working with patients. We will explore this issue and go on to consider alternative approaches to working with patients in practice.

There has been a great deal of literature focused on the issue of patient compliance with medication regimens (Simons, 1992; Cameron, 1996; Kyngäs and Lahdenperä, 1999; Haynes *et al.*, 2000). The research that has been carried out has estimated that the rates of non-compliance with prescribed medications are 50% (Haynes *et al.*, 2000) and ranging from 10% to 94% (Simons, 1992). Cameron and Gregor (1987) state that the rate of non-compliance in people with chronic conditions is higher than in those with acute conditions. It is clear that there is a significant problem with compliance or adherence to a treatment regimen and this problem has been present for as long as health care professionals have been prescribing medical treatments. Sackett and Snow (1979) noted that there is a distressingly wide gap between the regimen recommended by the health care professional and the patient's behaviour and Hippocrates is reported to have made reference to the fact that 'patients often lie when they state that they have taken certain medicines' (Haynes, 1979).

The results of studies into non-compliance have to be treated with caution because there seems to be no consensus over the use of the terms *compliance, adherence* or *concordance*. Buchmann (1997) points out that there is a lack of consistency in the definition of the term 'compliance' in the research. Given the difficulty with defining this term, the research that has been carried out on the rate at which patients adhere or do not adhere to the prescribed treatment regimen is problematic. If a patient is prescribed a treatment to be taken four times a day and only takes it three times a day, is he or she non-compliant? Is this the same as the patient who does not take the medication at all? If measures of compliance are used such as HbA1c results in diabetes mellitus (Chan and Molassiotis, 1999), how do we know that this represents the degree of compliance and does not reflect the fact that the patient had an infection during the time of the study which elevated the blood sugar readings temporarily?

The term 'compliance' has been defined by Haynes (1979) as 'the extent to which a person's behaviour (in terms of taking medications, following diets or executing other lifestyle changes) coincides with medical or health advice'. If patients are non-compliant they are not following our professional advice and therefore they are in the wrong. Playle and Keeley (1998) state that compliance is an ideology based on professional beliefs concerning the proper roles of patients and professionals; implicitly this requires a dependent lay person and a dominant professional. According to Hussey and Gilliland (1989) non-compliance can be described in two ways, unintentional non-compliance and intentional non-compliance. Unintentional non-compliance results from an inadequate understanding of the disease or condition being treated and intentional non-compliance is a conscious choice by the patient to find another method of treatment or not to comply (Hussey and Gilliland, 1989). Unintentional non-compliance then can be addressed by working with patients to provide information in a variety of formats. The information can be presented in written form, verbally, by video, by providing contact names and numbers for support groups and internet web site addresses. The patient's understanding can then be assessed with each interaction and this can help to address the issue of unintentional non-compliance. Intentional non-compliance can be the result of a rational decision based on the patient's own wishes and understanding of optimal health. In this situation the health care professional needs to spend more time learning about the patient's expectations, values and beliefs and to adapt treatment plans accordingly. Using the definitions outlined above the word 'compliance' has negative connotations in that it places the power with the health care professional; the health care professional makes a decision about a plan of treatment and the patient is either compliant or non-complaint with the prescribed regimen. Non-compliance is associated with judgement and blame and it is for this reason that some authors have turned to alternative words.

Adherence is a word which has been used as an alternative to compliance. Adherence is defined by Haynes *et al.* (2000) as the extent to which patients follow the instructions they are given for prescribed treatments. There is a great deal of similarity between this definition of adherence and the definition of compliance provided by Haynes in 1979 as outlined above. This term still places the power with the health care professional. The similarity in the terms is demonstrated by authors such as Buchmann (1997) who uses the terms interchangeably. Cameron (1996) points out that compliance, adherence and therapeutic alliance can be placed on a continuum based on a social control continuum developed by Barofsky (1978). Compliance can be linked with coercion, adherence suggests conformity and therapeutic alliance suggests negotiation. The continuum varies in the degree to which the patient is actively involved in the decision-making process with relative passivity at the compliance end of the continuum and relative activity in the therapeutic alliance. Madden (1990) points out that adherence and compliance are outcomes, whereas therapeutic alliance is a process and as such they cannot be compared equally in a continuum. As adherence and compliance are outcomes, they are still both associated with a judgemental approach. If the patient is non-compliant or not adhering to the treatment regimen then there is a tendency to blame them and

not the health care professional. The words we use in addressing the issue of the patient's adherence to medical treatment are powerful indicators of our perception of the problem. This in turn will shape the way we choose to address the situation and will determine our choice of a solution to the problem.

In recognition of this difficulty the Royal Pharmaceutical Society of Great Britain launched a paper in 1997 entitled 'From compliance to concordance: towards shared goals in medicine taking' (Marinker, 1997). Concordance is defined as *'a new approach to the prescribing and taking of medicines. It is an agreement reached after negotiation between a patient and a health care professional that respects the beliefs and wishes of the patient in determining whether, when and how medicines are to be taken. Although reciprocal, this is an alliance in which the health care professionals recognise the primacy of the patient's decisions about taking the recommended medications'* (Concordance Co-ordinating Group, 2000). Concordance is not a substitute for the word compliance, there are subtle differences in the approach taken when concordance with medical regimens is the focus. Concordance requires the agreement of two parties, it cannot be imposed. If concordance is being used as a framework for the development of treatment plans the patient will be encouraged to express concerns about the treatment and will be involved in decision making about their medications. If concordance is successful some patients will decide not to take their medication and the outcome may not be what the health care professional thinks is in the best interests of the patient (Dickinson *et al.*, 1999). It is important to accept this situation and review the goals of treatment which may differ with each individual patient.

The term 'concordance' does alter our perspective in the event of non-adherence with medical regimens. It is acceptable to make individualized decisions about treatment and if a patient chooses not to take the prescribed treatment this may be meeting the patient's individual expectations and wishes and therefore the result is not one of failure but one of success in meeting the goals of the patient. There are problems with this approach and Milburn and Cochrane (1997) stated that there are at least three situations where the concordance model will fail. First, according to Milburn and Cochrane, clinical trails depend upon complete compliance on the part of the patient and therefore there is no room here for concordance. Secondly, non-compliance is associated with complex human behaviour and there is a high degree of association between non-compliance and depression. Research into the human behaviour of medicine taking does not fit the concordance model as there may be important processes occurring related to non-compliance. Thirdly, they point out that in potentially life-threatening disease or in the event of disease that may infect other people there is no room for the patient to decide not to take the medication. Erratic drug taking in the use of antibiotics can result in the disease being spread to other people and the development of resistant strains of microorganisms.

If we use concordance as a framework for our interactions with patients we also risk becoming too relaxed about a patient who is not following the therapeutic dose of medication. We may feel that the patient's persistent refusal to take treatment is based on their individual expectations and wishes and therefore this is acceptable. This scenario is only acceptable if it is based on true concordance. It remains our responsibility to ensure that we have fully understood the patient and they in turn have fully understood the implications of following or not following the treatment plan.

Given the lack of consensus over the use of the words compliance, adherence and concordance and the fact that they are not synonymous with each other, the following discussion will utilize the words used by the authors of the work being presented.

Interventions to promote concordance

No study has been able to offer a universally acceptable solution to the problem of non-adherence with treatment regimens (Cameron, 1996; Haynes *et al.*, 2000), however, there has been an analysis of the issues involved and there have been suggestions of models to enhance understanding between patients and health care professionals. Chen (1999) suggests that improving the consultation and communication skills of health care professionals would enhance concordance and Mullen (1997) agrees by stating that time should be spent assessing not only the best medication for a particular

condition but also the best for the individual patient with a certain lifestyle preference. In a study of 52 Chinese people with type 2 diabetes, Chan and Molassiotis (1999) found that there was no association between diabetes knowledge and compliance. They conclude that providing knowledge is only one step in the process of facilitating patient participation and compliance. They suggest that strategies to enhance the patient's self-efficacy and confidence in self-management should be incorporated in diabetic teaching programmes.

Cameron (1996) highlighted the complexity of compliance behaviour by stating that the main social and psychological factors involved in patient compliance are: knowledge and understanding including communication; quality of interaction including the patient provider relationship and patient satisfaction; social isolation and social support including the effect of the family, health beliefs and attitudes; and illness and treatment including the duration and complexity of the regimen. Each of these factors can exert a positive or negative influence on compliance.

In an attempt to explore the issue of non-compliance further Kyngäs and Lahdenperä (1999) identified internal and external factors associated with compliance. Internal factors included patient characteristics such as age, social background, values, attitudes and emotions and external factors included the impact of health education, the relationship between the patient and the health care professional and the support from the family, health care professional and friends. Based on interviews with patients in chronic heart failure Strömberg *et al.* (1999) also identified internal and external factors associated with patient compliance. These included, internal factors, personality, the disease, the treatment and external factors, social activities, social relations and health care professionals. The internal and external factors associated with compliance identified by Kyngäs and Lahdenperä (1999) and Strömberg *et al.* (1999) are listed in Table 1.1.

As an illustration of the complexity of compliance behaviour Buchmann (1997) developed a stepwise approach to achieving compliance through addressing the relationship between self-efficacy and social power in a group of elderly patients. Self-efficacy is defined as a person's feelings and thoughts about his or her own capability of accomplishing a task. Social

Table 1.1 Internal and external factors affecting compliance

Internal factors	External factors
Age	Impact of health education
Social background	Relationships with health care professionals
Values	Relationships with friends and family
Attitudes	
Emotions	Social activities
Personality	Social relations
The disease	
Treatment	

power according to Buchmann (1997) is made up of referent power and expert power. Referent power is an individual's ability to act as a frame of reference and to serve in the role of a significant other – a person who has referent power is viewed as being benevolent and caring. Expert power is based on the knowledge and skills that a person brings into a relationship through education, knowledge, skills and experience. The theory is based on approaches to increase the patient's self-esteem and self-efficacy, thereby increasing their expert and self-referent power and this results in compliance with the treatment regimen. The steps are as follows:

Make specific enquiries

The health care professional engages in a thorough history taking process with the patient. Nolan and Nolan (1995) would agree with this as they state that, in working with people who have a chronic condition, the illness should be seen as having a past and a future which need to be taken into account when planning current care. The aim is to gather information upon which to build the best plan of action.

Be benevolent

In the information gathering process the health care professional needs to be demonstrating a sense of caring. This can be achieved through effective communication processes and will help to build the patient's self-esteem.

Encourage self-disclosure to gain insight

When the patient shares information about themselves with the health care professional they must feel that this is important and of value to the decision-making process. The health care professional can communicate this through citing the need for the information and this again will help to build the patient's self-esteem.

Determine the patient's knowledge base

Further inquiry can help to determine how much knowledge the patient has about their condition. This represents the patient's level of expert knowledge and can help the professional to guide the patient's learning.

Determine the patient's commitment to taking appropriate actions

The patient can be asked specifically how much effort they are willing to expend upon the treatment regimen. This will give the health care professional some insight into the patient's level of self-efficacy and can help determine whether the patient's self-efficacy needs to be improved as part of the treatment plan.

Maintain an attitude of positive regard

The health care professional needs to display an attitude of genuine concern for the patient. Effective communication is a necessary component to demonstrating a high level of interest for the patient. As the patient senses this genuine concern, the health care professional builds referent power and this promotes support for the subsequent recommendations on treatment.

Build a sense of personal responsibility

If the patient has built a sense of personal responsibility for the management of the condition they will have a strong desire to follow the recommendations for treatment.

Match client needs and wishes

Choosing a medication regimen that best suits the client's daily routine can help the client to feel that they are contributing to the decision-making process. This in turn enhances self-esteem and self-efficacy and therefore, according to Buchmann (1997) the likelihood of adhering to the treatment regimen.

Use selective positive feedback

Feedback should be given to promote referent power and the health care professional should remain accepting and understanding of the client's behaviour.

Attribute endorsed norms to a respected secondary group

It may be helpful to identify traditions and norms to endorse specific recommendations. This is particularly valuable in the elderly population who have developed norms and traditions over long periods of time.

Buchmann (1997) concludes that the above approach to incorporating the theory of self-efficacy and power will remedy non-compliance in the elderly population and will encourage individuals to participate fully in an agreed regimen. This would seem to be based on scant evidence and is a rather hopeful conclusion to a complex phenomenon, however, it does provide us with a framework from which we can develop an approach to working with patients who have a chronic condition.

Haynes *et al.* (2000) conducted a systematic review of available studies on the issue of compliance. These authors used the terms compliance, adherence and concordance inter-changeably. They noted that the literature concerning interventions to improve adherence with medications was surprisingly weak and they also point out that increasing adherence is not a justifiable end in itself. It cannot be assumed that measures to increase adherence do more good than harm. Interventions to increase adherence consume resources, can lead to loss of privacy and autonomy and can lead to increased adverse effects of medications. Strömberg *et al.* (1999) agree with this as they state that non-compliance can be a rational choice made on the basis of side effects or drug inefficacy or it may even be seen as a way of exerting some control over the situation and the disease process. Haynes *et al.* (2000) conclude that there are many shortcomings in the research to date, however, simpler treatment regimens can improve adherence for both short- and long-term treatments and recalling patients who miss appointments is simple and effective in enhancing adherence and treatment outcomes. Several other complex strategies including more thorough patient instructions and counselling, reminders, close follow up, supervised self-monitoring and rewards for success can have an effect on adherence and treatment outcomes, although these have not been shown to be effective in adherence with long-term treatments.

It must be stressed that the goal of our interactions with patients who live with chronic conditions is not compliance of the patient to our prescribed course of treatment. The goal is that all health care professionals interacting with the patient at any stage in the trajectory of the illness work towards the highest possible quality relationship with the patient to enhance understanding and to develop concordance. We need to acknowledge that the medical regimen is only part of the life regimen the patient must manage (Cameron, 1996). The health care professional needs to consider a variety of approaches to enhance the patient–professional relationship and also needs to be cognizant of the wealth of knowledge that the patient brings to the situation. Figure 1.3 summarizes some of the issues that have been addressed in this chapter and highlights issues for the health care professional to be aware of in the patient–professional relationship. Above all else the health care professional needs to work towards an understanding of the patient as an individual and to respect their personal goals and aims.

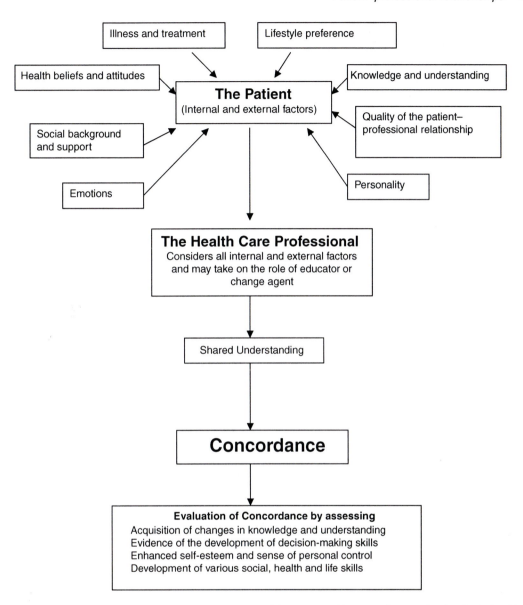

Figure 1.3 Issues which the health care professional should be aware of in the patient–professional relationship

'Let us learn when our patients want to be treated as partners, but let us also learn when they want to be in control of our actions and when they want us to assume complete control. Only then will we be able to offer the full range of support the chronically ill tell us they need to live their lives as productively and as fully as is possible within the limits of their illness' (Thorne and Paterson, 1998).

References

Barofsky I (1978) Compliance, adherence and the therapeutic alliance: steps in the development of self care. *Social Science and Medicine* **12** (5), 369–376. Cited in: Cameron C (1996) Patient compliance: recognition of factors involved and suggestions for promoting compliance with therapeutic regimens. *Journal of Advanced Nursing* **24** (2), 244–250

Bookman A, Morgan S (1988) *Women in the Politics of Empowerment.* Temple University Press, Philadelphia. Cited in: Conway-Welch C (1996) Empowerment: Activism in professional practice. In: (Hickey J, Ouimette R, Venegoni S, eds) (1996) *Advanced Practice Nursing: Changing Roles and Clinical Applications.* Lippincott, New York

Brownlea A (1987) Participation: myths realities and prognosis. *Social Science and Medicine* **25** (6), 605–616

Buchmann W F (1997) Adherence: a matter of self-efficacy and power. *Journal of Advanced Nursing* **26** (1), 132–137

Cahill J (1998) Patient participation – a review of the literature. *Journal of Clinical Nursing* **7**, 119–128

Cameron C (1996) Patient compliance: recognition of factors involved and suggestions for promoting compliance with therapeutic regimens. *Journal of Advanced Nursing* **24** (2), 244–250

Cameron K, Gregor F (1987) Chronic illness and compliance. *Journal of Advanced Nursing* **12** (6), 617–676

Chan Y M, Molassiotis A (1999) The relationship between diabetes knowledge and compliance among Chinese with non-insulin dependent diabetes mellitus in Hong Kong. *Journal of Advanced Nursing* **30** (2), 431–438

Chen J (1999) Medication concordance is best helped by improving consultation skills. *British Medical Journal* **318**, 670

Concordance Co-ordinating Group (2000) What Do We Mean By Concordance? http://www.concordance.org/ November 2000

Corbin J M, Strauss A (1992) A nursing model for chronic illness management based upon the trajectory framework. In: (Woog P, ed.) *The Chronic Illness Trajectory Framework.* Springer, New York, pp 29–38

Department of Health (2000) *Patient empowerment at the heart of the government's plan to modernise the national health service.* Press Release, Tuesday April 18th 2000

Dickinson D, Wilkie P, Harris M (1999) Taking medicines: concordance not compliance. *British Medical Journal* **319**, 787

Gibson J, Kenrick M (1998) Pain and powerlessness: the experience of living with peripheral vascular disease. *Journal of Advanced Nursing* **27**, 737–745

Haynes R B (1979) Introduction. In: (Haynes R B, Sackett D L, Taylor D W, eds) *Compliance in Health Care.* Johns Hopkins Press, Baltimore. Cited in: Playle J F, Keeley P (1998) Non-compliance and professional power. *Journal of Advanced Nursing* **27**, 304–311

Haynes R B, Montague P, Oliver P, McKibbon K A, Brouwer M C, Kanani R (2000) Interventions for helping patients to follow prescriptions for medication. *The Cochrane Database of Systematic Reviews*, Issue 1 2000. Oxford: Update Software

Healy P (2000a) Let patients with diabetes make their own decisions. *Nursing Standard* **14** (27), 8

Healy P (2000b) Whose lifestyle is it anyway? *Nursing Standard* **14** (30), 13

Hewison A (1995) Nurses' power in interaction with patients. *Journal of Advanced Nursing* **21** (1), 75–82

Hokanson Hawks J (1991) Power: a concept analysis. *Journal of Advanced Nursing* **16**, 754–762

Holloway W (1993) Work Psychology and Organisational Behaviour: managing the individual at work. Sage Publications, London. Cited in: Cahill J (1998) Patient Participation – a review of the literature. *Journal of Clinical Nursing* **7**, 119–128

Hussey L C, Gilliland K (1989) Compliance, low literacy and locus of control. *Nursing Clinics of North America* **24** (3), 605–611

Kyngäs H (1999) A theoretical model of compliance in young diabetics. *Journal of Clinical Nursing* **8** (1), 73–80

Kyngäs H, Lahdenperä T (1999) Compliance of patients with hypertension and associated features. *Journal of Advanced Nursing* **29** (4), 832–839

Langer E, Rodin J (1980) Aging labels: the decline of control and the fall of self esteem. *Journal of Social Issues* **36** (2), 19–29. Cited in: Piper S M, Brown P A (1998) The theory of health education applied to nursing: a bi-polar approach patients. *Journal of Advanced Nursing* **27** (2), 383–389

Madden B P (1990) The Hybrid Model for Concept Development: its value for the study of therapeutic alliance. *Advances in Nursing Science* **12** (3), 75–87. Cited in: Cameron C (1996) Patient Compliance: recognition of factors involved and suggestions for promoting compliance with therapeutic regimens. *Journal of Advanced Nursing* **24** (2), 244–250

Marinker M (ed.) (1997) *From Compliance to Concordance: Achieving Shared Goals in Medicine Taking.* Royal Pharmaceutical Society, London

Marland G (1998) Partnership encourages patients to comply with treatments. *Nursing Times* **94** (27), 58–59

Milburn H J, Cochrane G M (1997) Treating the patient as a decision maker is not always appropriate. *British Medical Journal* **314**, 1905

Mullen P D (1997) Compliance becomes concordance. *British Medical Journal* **314**, 391

Nolan M, Nolan J (1995) Responding to the challenge of chronic illness. *British Journal of Nursing* **4** (3), 145–147

Parsons T (1951) *The Social System.* Routledge and Kegan Paul, London

Piper S M, Brown P A (1998) The theory of health education applied to nursing: a bi-polar approach to patients. *Journal of Advanced Nursing* **27** (2), 383–389

Playle J F, Keeley P (1998) Non-compliance and professional power. *Journal of Advanced Nursing* **27**, 304–311

Sackett D L, Snow J C (1979) The magnitude of compliance and non-compliance In: (Haynes R B, Sackett D L, Taylor D W, eds) *Compliance in Health Care.* Johns Hopkins Press, Baltimore. Cited in: Playle J F, Keeley P (1998) Non-compliance and professional power. *Journal of Advanced Nursing* **27**, 304–311

Simons M R (1992) Interventions related to compliance. *Nursing Clinics of North America* **27** (2), 477–484

Strömberg A, Broström A, Dahlström U, Fridlund B (1999) Factors influencing patient compliance with therapeutic regimens in chronic heart failure: a critical incident analysis. *Heart and Lung* **28** (5), 334–341

Thorne S, Paterson B (1998) Shifting images of chronic illness. *Image: Journal of Nursing Scholarship* **30** (2), 173–178

Watson R, Burkholder J (1990) Conflict resolution: coping skills, empowerment and decision making strategies for today's nurses. *Dermatology Nursing* **2** (1), 29–37. Cited in: Conway-Welch C (1996) Empowerment: activism in professional practice In: (Hickey J, Ouimette R, Venegoni S, eds) (1996) *Advanced Practice Nursing: Changing Roles and Clinical Applications.* Lippincott, New York

Whitehead M, Tones K (1991) *Avoiding the Pitfalls.* HEA, London Cited in: Piper S M, Brown P A (1998) The theory of health education applied to nursing: a bi-polar approach patients. *Journal of Advanced Nursing* **27** (2), 383–389

2

Approaches to teamwork in chronic illness

Judith Lawrence

Introduction

A patient with a chronic condition will encounter a variety of health and social care providers, from different organizations and professional disciplines. Each patient is unique and their needs will vary depending on their personal circumstances and physical condition. The quality and consistency of the care they receive will be dependent on the ability of all those involved to work together.

Collaborative partnerships are viewed as being essential to meeting the growing demand for health and social care. However, developing effective teamwork and fostering a collaborative approach to care takes time, commitment and a willingness to work as a team. Constant change is an integral part of the National Health Service (NHS) and this creates an environment of uncertainty. Traditional roles and responsibilities are being re-examined in an attempt to reduce duplication throughout the service. Boundaries between nursing, medicine and social services are increasingly becoming blurred. One thing that remains constant however, is the centrality of the patient. Without this focus any care we deliver becomes meaningless.

Living with a chronic condition affects every aspect of a patient's life. Coming to terms with the diagnosis and the long-term implications of the disease takes time and the whole situation can become quite overwhelming for the patient. The skill of the team of professionals who are involved in the patient's care can have a fundamental impact on the patient's ability to learn to live with the condition. The patient should be seen as a partner who participates with the rest of the team in making decisions about how best to meet the identified needs. The patient should not be seen in isolation and any assessment of need has to take into consideration the needs of the family and informal carers.

Care and need

Before going on to explore the nature of the team and different approaches to teamwork in more detail, it is worth considering two words that are frequently used within health and social care, they are 'care' and 'need'. In considering their meaning it is important to recognize that they may mean different things to different people.

Care

Care has been defined as the most illusive concept within nursing (Kyle, 1995). It is frequently used as a blanket term for a variety of services. Care and caring can be used in different contexts, for example, you frequently hear professionals referring to the *care* that is being offered. An individual practitioner will refer to *caring* for a patient with a chronic condition. An informal carer will *care* for someone in a very *caring* way. The use of the word is very subjective and does not assist health care professionals to quantify their role. Sadler (1997) defined caring as: 'an individually and socially defined creative process, described by practising nurses as multidimensional work, where a holistic connection is made with a person to meet a recognised need.'

Despite the complexity of the nature of caring, it is vital that time is taken jointly to agree on what care means and take steps to ensure that the patient is not left with a vague idea of what 'care' is being offered.

Need

Defining need is a complex process and there has to be recognition that the patient may perceive their need differently to that of the health care professional. The distinction between the needs of a defined population and the needs of the individual patient may be different by the very fact that living with a chronic illness is a unique personal experience. Blackie (1998) refers to need as 'a condition to be fulfilled to maintain life or well-being'. However, Robinson and Elkan (1996) define it as 'the capacity to benefit from health care' and there is a clear distinction that health needs are not health problems. It is also important to note that needs vary and they may not be related to the nature and severity of the chronic condition.

Health and social needs are very much interlinked and cannot be seen in isolation from each other. Bradshaw (1972) outlined four different types of need and he referred to this as Bradshaw's taxonomy of need. This classification stems from the identification of social need but can be equally relevant to the health care.

Normative need

The need is defined by expert bodies, for example professional groups and government departments. A basic standard is set and if a population or an individual falls short of the agreed standard then normative need is identified.

Comparative need

This is when inequalities in the provision of care exist, either between two individuals or groups. An example would be access to specialist cancer services or the availability of continence products on the NHS.

Felt need

This is defined by what an individual patient wants. The felt need is personal to the individual and will be influenced by their perceptions of the situation. This can be a cause of conflict if the professional does not feel that the felt need is a priority in comparison with what they have identified. If this issue is not resolved to the patient's satisfaction then the patient–professional relationship could be compromised.

Expressed need

This is where the felt need is acted upon and the patient actively seeks resources from health and social care providers to meet these needs. A group of patients may collectively work to bring about change that will fulfil an unmet felt need. This could be the provision of day care for patients with Alzheimer's disease or complementary therapy provision for patients with cancer.

What is clear is that confusion can easily arise when different health and social care providers are not specific about which needs they have identified and what care they are providing. Health care professionals should pause and reflect on what they mean by 'care' and 'need' and go on to consider if the need identified by the health care professional corresponds with what the patient perceives as their need.

A successful team should have a shared vision, a common goal, therefore there are two fundamental questions that a health care team should ask: 'Are we truly working to meet the needs of the patient?' and 'What care are we providing?'.

Collaborative care

Collaboration is the central focus in the future delivery of health care (Department of Health, 1999, 2000). It should happen across all professional boundaries and especially between the providers of health and social care.

Collaborative care can enhance communication between different disciplines which will facilitate a clearer understanding of roles and responsibilities. Through effective collaboration duplication within social and health care provision can be reduced aiding the efficient utilization of resources. However, the most important outcome of successful collaboration between providers of care is that the patient feels valued.

Collaboration is not easy and it is fraught with problems associated with interdisciplinary and interagency working partnerships. The barriers to effective collaboration and teamwork are similar and they will be discussed later in the chapter.

If collaborative care is going to be successful and teamwork sustainable, then the degree of collaboration between different disciplines has to be at a level that will enhance these objectives. Armitage (1983) defined five stages of collaboration and identified that if teams are working at stage five then full integration of the service has been achieved. The five stages are outlined below:

Stage 1 – Isolation

This is when there is no verbal or written contact between different professionals and providers of care. They never meet on an informal or formal basis.

Stage 2 – Encounter

At this stage there is contact and information is shared but it stays at a level of passing on information or referring patients. There is no move to work jointly in identifying need.

Stage 3 – Communication

Information is readily shared and communication pathways between the different disciplines are open. There is a commitment to work together to agree jointly on the planned care for the patient.

Stage 4 – Partial collaboration

There is a clear commitment to work together and teams work effectively together with respect and understanding of each other's roles and responsibilities. However, within the working partnership professional boundaries and working patterns are debated. Joint working practices are embraced although the intricacies of the relationship still need to be defined from time to time.

Stage 5 – Full collaboration

A total integrated approach to care is implemented. The whole organization works collectively.

How easily teams manage to collaborate is dependent on numerous factors, which include a willingness to work together and the geographical location of the people involved. If all disciplines could be housed within the same building then informal networking will be easier and the ability to make contact on a day-to-day basis will enhance patient care. However, frequently professionals work in different locations and this limits the opportunities to discuss ongoing issues on an informal basis. Seamless care is the ultimate aim, where quality and consistency of care is continuous. The *focus* for the coordinated approach to care should be to meet the needs of the patient.

The team

The provision of health and social care varies around the country. Different working partnerships are being developed with social services, voluntary bodies and private agencies. Central to any partnership is the development of an effective team. Teams vary in composition and size depending on their defined function. In relation to patients with a chronic condition there tends to be a core team, utilizing the resources of an extended team as the need arises. Who is in the core team will be influenced by the needs of the patient, their family and informal carers. The core team composition will change over time, although it is likely that key members will remain constant, for example, the general practitioner.

The Queen's Nursing Institute, Scotland in 1997 hosted a conference entitled 'Multidisciplinary Care in the Community', which examined the patient's perception of the care offered by the various health and social care providers. At this conference a patient with a chronic condition gave his account of working in partnership with the various disciplines. From this patient's perspective the profession that outlined their service objectives the most clearly was the community pharmacist. The patient had a debilitating respiratory disease and it was vital that he felt confident that the supply of oxygen to his home would be maintained. He worked closely with the pharmacist who informed him about the drugs he was taking and the possible side effects. When things were not going well and the medication was not adequately controlling his condition he could rely on the pharmacist to liaise with the general practitioner and following assessment the medication would be altered accordingly. The patient's general practitioner remained constant and he knew that he would not have to repeat his whole life story every time he made an appointment, unlike when he visited the hospital and saw a different doctor every time.

Individual health and social care providers may perceive that their role is central to the care of the patient, however, when planning care it is important to ask the patient who they see as being important to enabling them to be as independent as possible.

Teamwork

Essentially if teamwork is going to be effective it comes down to working well together. Gilmore *et al.* (1994) recognized that for a team to be effective there had to be key characteristics present. These are:

- a shared common purpose
- a clear understanding of each other's role
- an identity within the team
- an awareness of each other's strengths
- the ability to pool resources
- shared responsibility.

The success of any team or collaborative partnership will be dependent on being able to meet regularly in an organized and structured way. The sharing of information is vital to facilitate seamless care. There has to be a recognition that protected time needs to be allocated to develop any new partnership and careful consideration has to be given to the communication pathways that will be adopted to enhance the delivery of care.

Time that is spent finding out about what another team member's role entails is never wasted. We live in an environment where it may not be possible to meet the people you refer patients to on a day-to-day basis. Sometimes, unintentionally we become cocooned in our own professional world and can become detached from the pressures felt by other disciplines. Consider when you last visited a social work department, an acute medical ward or spent a few hours with a community nurse. How can we expect to make effective referrals to each other if we have limited insight into the role each discipline undertakes? Collaboration can help the team to work together more effectively with the patient. This approach takes time and effort, however, the overall positive outcomes for all involved make this a worthwhile endeavour.

Teams within health care

Teams have been described as multidisciplinary, and more recently integrated or interdisciplinary.

Multidisciplinary team

The multidisciplinary team can be defined as a group of professionals who each have their own expertise, which is distinct from the skills used by other professionals in the team. Each professional in the multidisciplinary team will have their own professional code of ethics and standards of practice.

A patient with complex needs may require the services of several members of the multidisciplinary team. This model tends to compartmentalize the skills of each member of the team, promoting a task-orientated approach to care. A problem with this approach can occur when all members of the team are not fully consulted and work is allocated unevenly or inappropriately within the team. How effective multidisciplinary teamwork is will depend on the willingness of all team members actively to communicate with each other and be open to new ways of working together. Simply calling yourself a multidisciplinary team does not make you a multidisciplinary team.

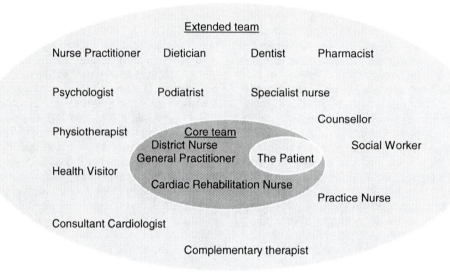

Figure 2.1 Example of a core team and extended team within primary care

The multidisciplinary team can be divided into the core team and the extended team and there will be movement between the two as the needs of the patient change. Some members of the team will come into direct contact with the patient and their family. However, some members will stay on the periphery and act in a consultative mode. Figure 2.1 is an example of a core team and extended team for a patient who has had a myocardial infarction, and has been discharged from hospital.

Integrated team

Ovretveit *et al.* (2000) refer to the 'patient's team', which is very apt for a patient with a chronic condition. The severity and progression of a chronic disease can vary tremendously and this means that the needs of the patient can change either dramatically or slowly over a period of time.

Integrated care means a multidisciplinary team extending their working partnership to meet the needs of a defined population. There should be common priorities, service objectives and a collective responsibility to the population they serve (Ovretveit *et al.*, 2000). Each member of the team will bring different skills, knowledge

and expertise to enable care to be prioritized (Young, 1997). The quality and comprehensiveness of the service will provide the measure of success of the integrated team.

The aims of integrated care include identifying health needs and deciding on the main priorities for the patient and the population served by the providers. The development of a range of skills and knowledge is integral to team development and duplication and gaps in the service should be identified (Vile, 1997). Integrated care is about endeavouring to improve teamwork among all disciplines involved in the care of the patient but particularly between health and social care providers.

Barriers to effective teamwork

Effective teamwork can be compromised by a number of factors. It is important that teams are conscious of the potential barriers to the team working effectively.

Professional rivalry

This can happen within one profession or between different professional groups and can be very destructive. As roles change it is important to recognize that the whole team may be affected by the change. There may be apprehension about the change in responsibility and concern among other team members that they may have to take on more responsibility themselves or that their post is being eroded. Therefore, it is vital that steps are taken to allay concerns among the rest of the team.

Different employers

Frequently within health and social care, team members are employed by different organizations. This can cause conflict if codes of practice and organizational processes and structures are different.

Personality differences between members of the team

It is only natural that if you like someone you will make more of an effort to work well together. Essential to any team is the ability to communicate openly with each other. If there are personal differences between team members these should be addressed before the whole team is compromised.

Power

Each team member should have an equal status within the team. However, traditionally the balance of power has been influenced by educational preparation, income, gender and perceived professional authority. Historically the nursing role was seen as submissive and non-professional and essentially there to provide care which was very much in the domain of the female role. The doctor traditionally assumed the more professional dominant role. Obviously society is changing but the legacy of patriarchal attitudes still exists. Vitally important is the patient's place within the team. The level of inclusion and influence can vary and formal meetings are often very intimidating to patients and their families and therefore they feel their voice is not heard.

Lack of understanding about each other's role and responsibility

Inappropriate referrals between professionals continue to happen because essentially health and social care providers lack a full understanding of each other's roles. Frequently patients are asked by health and social care providers how they can be supported. How do you know what you want if nobody tells you what you may need and what is on offer? A patient with a chronic condition should be empowered by health and social care providers to identify their needs and utilize the most appropriate resources.

Work place environment

The working environment of any professional is important. Comfortable and suitable accommodation can make a professional feel valued and thereby encourage 'harmony' within the workplace. However, poor amenities and the lack of suitable rooms for meetings can be a barrier to effective teamwork. Space is a valuable commodity and all too easily a team can disintegrate over the allocation of office and consulting rooms within a building. Territorial battles about who is entitled to use which rooms can be extremely detrimental to fostering collaborative approaches to care. Effective teamwork can also be hampered when team members work in different geographical locations.

An integrated approach to care sometimes evolves slowly over time and out of necessity. The following case history demonstrates how one team adapted to meet the changing needs of a patient with cancer. It provides a good example of a team who were employed by different organizations and came from a variety of different disciplines who were able to work together to achieve one common goal – to facilitate the patient being able to die at home.

Case history

The patient lived alone in an isolated village with minimal family support. Her ultimate wish was to die at home and sought guarantees from her general practitioner that if she lapsed into unconsciousness she would not be transferred to hospital. With no family or informal carers in the house, care had to be coordinated to ensure that someone visited every couple of hours to meet fundamental needs, for example getting a drink, helping her to the toilet or assisting her to change her position. It is important to note that each discipline represented in the core and extended team were not single individuals. For example, although the district nurse took on the coordinator role, there were a number of district nurses and community staff nurses who made up the district nursing input. The core team was defined according to whether they had access to the patient's house.

The core team

- District nurse
- General practitioner
- Home help
- Private home care staff
- Community pharmacist
- Marie Curie nurses

The extended team

- Macmillan nurse
- Social worker
- Occupational therapist
- GP out of hours service
- Dietician

As the patient's condition deteriorated and she became confined to bed the need to work together became more essential. Certain roles were retained by each discipline, for example the district nurse changed the syringe driver and managed wound care. However, assessment of pain involved feedback from all the team to obtain the necessary information about pain control over a 24-hour period. When the community pharmacist delivered morphine on a daily basis to avoid large quantities being left in the house she made a cup of tea or gave the patient a drink or washed her face. Who knows when you will fancy a lightly boiled egg or a bowl of ice cream? There had to be flexibility in the team and recognition that everyone had essential skills that had to be utilized if the patient was going to be maintained at home. No one service could afford to fund the care and therefore the cost of providing care over a 24-hour period had to be split between social services, the local NHS trust and local cancer charities.

Communicating with all members of the team and ensuring information was circulated to everyone involved in providing the care was challenging. The most valuable resource used by the team was the message book, which was left in the house. It became vital in communicating messages to each other, especially when the patient could no longer be as actively involved in her care. On reflection there was one piece of equipment, which would have been useful in the house and that was a fax machine. It sounds silly but when drug regimens are being changed and carers are being switched at the last minute having the ability to fax through valuable information could have prevented many journeys to the house. Sometimes care plans cannot be changed in the patient's home because different options need to be considered. However, the ability to fax through an altered care plan to a nurse who was due to be with the patient all night would have been invaluable, remembering that this patient lived a considerable distance from the health centre.

A small core team visited the patient but a larger extended team coordinated the resources. The patient felt confident with the team that had developed over time. As different problems emerged the team had to recognize their limitations and seek specialist advice. Early on the patient decided that she did not need the Macmillian nurse to visit, however, she recognized that the rest of the team needed to utilize this invaluable resource. Therefore the Macmillian nurse was used in a consultative mode.

The patient did die peacefully at home with two members of the team in the house. A month after the patient died the team came together to reflect on the case. The question was asked, why did it work and the group highlighted the following key points:

- respect for each other
- a clear understanding of each other's role and responsibilities
- flexibility
- willingness to blur professional boundaries
- common goal
- open communication between all members of the team
- a recognition of the team's limitations
- a recognition of when specialist advice was required.

One of the advantages of integrated care includes the abandonment of traditional hierarchical management structures. Care is assessed holistically rather than as a series of problems. Patient involvement is actively encouraged with the hope that that they will feel motivated and empowered to be involved in planning their care. Adopting an integrated approach will challenge different disciplines to review their traditional working patterns, recognize the potential to share skills and possibly extend roles. Moving from a multidisciplinary to an integrated team requires a high degree of motivation and commitment. Team building skills need to be fully utilized to ensure that any changes are sustainable in the long term.

Primary and secondary care interface

Patients now spend less time in hospital with the focus of health care shifting to the community. Advances in medical technology are enabling patients to reduce their stay in hospital with continuing care being provided in the community. As community health care services are strengthened, there are more opportunities to develop new and innovative ways of providing care. Recent developments include hospital at home schemes, whereby primary and secondary care providers work together to enable care to be provided at home (Coast *et al.*, 1998; Shepherd *et al.*, 1998).

Rapid response teams are also being developed throughout the country with the capability of accessing and mobilizing resources quickly to prevent a patient having to be admitted to hospital. This has the potential of being a tremendous step forward for patients who suffer from a chronic disease. The very nature of a chronic condition can mean that a patient's health and ability to cope independently can suddenly become compromised. In the past, if this happened the only alternative would be admission to hospital if existing services were unable to respond to the sudden need.

The key to an uneventful discharge from or the smooth admission to hospital is greatly influenced by the effectiveness of liaison

between primary and secondary care. This process is enhanced if liaison teams are in place to facilitate discharge planning and to mobilize the necessary resources. Liaison services vary but their ability to bridge the gap between primary and secondary care is invaluable.

There is a move for more specialist nurses, who are based within hospitals, to follow patients up in the community. This is called outreach and offers community-based staff the opportunity to enhance working relationships and use specialist nurses as an educational resource. Conversely inreach is when community-based staff undertake care within the hospital setting. Unfortunately, when traditional geographical working boundaries are challenged, professionals can become threatened and this can compromise effective health care delivery. There *must* be communication between primary and secondary care, with all care being coordinated to prevent duplication. A patient with a chronic condition should be able to feel confident that the relevant information is being transferred between the professionals involved in providing the care. As technology changes, for example, the introduction of video conferencing and electronic mail, so the opportunity to communicate with other providers of health and social care is enhanced.

Conclusion

The principles of teamwork apply at all levels of health service provision. It is essential that they are applied by teams who interface with the patient and their family and also by management teams who work with health care professionals to develop services for patients. At all levels it is important to be aware of potential barriers to teamwork and to strive constantly to redress these challenges. Integrated teamwork is effective in creating a collaborative and satisfying working environment for health care professionals and also in addressing the needs of the patient. Time spent in working towards integrated teamwork will result in rewards not only for health care professionals but, *most* importantly, for the patient.

References

Armitage P (1983) Joint working in primary health care. *Nursing Times* (occasional paper) **79** (28), 75–78

Blackie C (ed.) (1998) *Community Health Care Nursing.* Churchill Livingstone, Edinburgh

Bradshaw J (1972) The concept of need. *New Society* **30**, 640–643

Coast J, Richards S H, Peters T J *et al.* (1998) Hospital at home or acute hospital care? A cost minimisation analysis. *British Medical Journal* **316**, 1802–1806

Department of Health (1999) *The NHS Act.* HMSO, London

Department of Health (2000) *The NHS Plan.* HMSO, London

Gilmore M, Bruce N, Hunt M (1994) *The Work of the Nursing Team in General Practice.* Council for the Training of Health Visitors, London

Kyle T (1995) The concept of caring: a review of the literature. *Journal of Advanced Nursing* **21**, 505–514

Ovretveit J, Mathias P, Thompson T (eds) (2000) *Interprofessional Working for Health and Social Care.* Macmillan

Robinson J, Elkan R (1996) *Health Needs assessment: Theory and Practice.* Churchill Livingstone, Edinburgh

Sadler J (1997) Defining professional nurse caring: triangulation study. *International Journal of Human Caring* **13**, 12–21

Shepherd S, Harwood D, Gray A, Vessey M, Morgan P (1998) Randomised controlled trial comparing hospital at home care with inpatient hospital care. II: Cost minimisation analysis. *British Medical Journal* **316**, 1786–1791

Vile C (1997) Teamwork in the next millennium. *Practice Nurse* **14** (10), 623–624

Young L (1997) Improved primary health care through integrated nursing. *Primary Health Care* **7** (6), 8–10

3

Clinical governance

Linda Ward

It is a capital mistake to theorise before you have all the evidence. It biases the judgement.
(Arthur Conan Doyle, 1888)

Introduction

Clinical governance has been introduced into the UK health care system as a method of improving and assuring standards of care for the National Health Service (NHS Confederation, 2000). For people who live with chronic illness this should signal the end to inequity of service provision across the country and provide a means for enhancing the quality of the health service available to this group of people. In 1997 the Labour Government published its first strategy document for the NHS in a White Paper, *The New NHS Modern, Dependable* (DoH, 1997) which was soon followed by *NHS Wales: Putting Patients First* (Welsh Office, 1998a). Central to this strategy were six key principles, which would act as drivers for change in the NHS. These principles included the introduction of national standards for health care delivery, increased levels of working partnerships within the NHS, improving efficiency and service quality and restoring public confidence (DoH, 1997). The White Paper also included some very clear messages about the future of the health service's duties including some guidance on the roles and responsibilities of NHS staff members. One area singled out for specific mention was that of quality standards '*The new NHS will have quality at its heart. Without it there is unfairness. Every patient who is treated in the NHS wants to know that*

they can rely on receiving high quality care when they need it. Every part of the NHS, and everyone who works in it, should take responsibility for working to improve quality. This must be quality in its broadest sense: doing the right things, at the right time, for the right people, and doing them right – first time. And it must be the quality of the patient's experience as well as the clinical result – quality measured in terms of the prompt access, good relationships and efficient administration' (DoH, 1997; para 3.2).

This concept was further reinforced, following the publication of *The New NHS* White Paper (DoH, 1997), by the NHS Executive (NHSE) when they released an Executive Letter (EL) to senior NHS officials. It identified for them the main points of the White Paper and of the plans for the introduction of its proposals. In this EL (NHSE, 1997) Tom Langlands, the NHSE Chief Executive, makes a categorical statement regarding the responsibilities for the implementation of the White Paper requirements. He states '*The responsibility for implementing the White Paper proposals rests with everyone working in the NHS. I look to all concerned in Health Authorities, NHS Trusts and primary care to play their part. There is much work to be done locally, including:*

- *preparing for the first Health Improvement Programmes*
- *beginning the development of arrangements for the new Primary Care Groups*
- *developing the new clinical governance arrangements across the NHS*' (NHSE, 1997; para 4, p. 2).

The following year, in a speech given by Sam Galbraith, MP, Minister for Health for Scotland, emphasis was once again placed on the need to ensure that the public is confident regarding the standards of care and treatment provided by the NHS. However, he also includes a statement with regard to 'clinical judgement'. He says *'Clinical governance is the vital ingredient which will enable us to achieve a Health Service in which the quality of health care is paramount. The best definition that I have seen of clinical governance is simply that it means "corporate accountability for clinical performance". Clinical governance will not replace professional regulation and individual clinical judgement, concepts that lie at the heart of health care in this country. But it will add an extra dimension that will provide the public with guarantees about standards of clinical care'* (Galbraith, 1998).

It appears clear from these statements that responsibility for the implementation of the clinical governance agenda lies with all individuals working within the NHS, not just senior clinicians or managers, but everyone. We all, therefore, have a part to play, but how do we identify what that role is and how do we achieve it? The current situation in the NHS is that information and guidance documents in one form or another are appearing regularly and in reality most practitioners are finding it difficult to pinpoint accurately their individual or specific role in meeting the clinical governance objectives. This situation is further confused due to the differing stages of development and the approaches taken towards attainment of the required clinical governance outcomes within the UK. This national variability is currently affecting working practices throughout the four countries of the UK and practitioners in each country will need to consider different structures and processes within the clinical governance framework according to the regulations for that country. Each of the four countries has different policy documents which they must implement and these will reflect the national focus of the individual countries, while incorporating those elements of UK or Pan-European strategies or legislation which must be included.

In keeping with their pre-election pledge, the Labour Government pursued a process of devolution which was intended to allow more policy making at local level for Scotland, Wales and Northern Ireland. Although there have always been some differences in the ways in which the four countries have administered their health care services, much of the policy making has usually been considered with regard to the entire UK, not on an individual country basis. The effect devolution will have on health care planning and decision making in the future has been reviewed, the result of which is that the Department of Health and the devolved administrations have agreed to work in a coordinated manner with regard to future developments. Initially all parties committed to a 'Memorandum of Understanding' which was a general agreement of cooperative working and operated until December 1999 when it was replaced by a newly agreed 'Concordat on Health and Social Care' (DoH, 1999a). This 'Concordat' is to be supplemented by agreements made at a more local level, for example with health and social care departments. Areas of cooperation with regard to the 'Concordat' will include issues affecting the NHS, public health, social care and a range of wider health issues. The 'Concordat' appears to attempt to prevent the new administrations working in isolation and avoid the development of policies that may prove beneficial to one administration but detrimental to another. What the 'Concordat' does not do is impose any legal obligation or restriction upon the individual administrations, although the Department of Health will undertake the operational administration of the 'Concordat' 'wherever possible' (DoH, 1999a, p. 2). It will be interesting to see how equity in NHS service provision across the countries will be achieved in the future. It may be argued that the devolved administrations may choose to disregard any decisions that they felt may prove to be detrimental to the best interests of their individual population, especially if legal sanction is not a concern. Any such veto of service provision objectives may potentially result in a situation that would make it difficult to guarantee quality standards throughout the entire NHS system. The possibility, therefore, is that the Government may have to compromise on some of their proposed future plans in order to obtain a consensus agreement within the 'Concordat'.

Assuring service quality

In 1998 the Department of Health provided further guidance on how the NHS was to meet the required improvements in standards with the publication of the consultation document *A First Class Service: Quality in the New NHS* (DoH, 1998). This document built upon the concept of nationally required service standards being delivered and regulated locally through the clinical governance framework. Clinical governance was defined in *A First Class Service: Quality in the New NHS* as '. . . *a framework through which NHS organisations are accountable for continuously improving the quality of their services and safeguarding high standards of care by creating an environment in which excellence in clinical care will flourish'* (DoH, 1998, p. 33). It also highlighted the increased levels of public involvement and professional regulation as additional means of improving standards of care. In addition, it was also to incorporate a statutory duty for continuous improvement in the quality of care and service delivered by the NHS. This was to be overseen and guided by the newly formed bodies the Commission for Health Improvement (CHI) and the National Institute for Clinical Excellence (NICE) and by a series of National Service Frameworks (NSF). In Wales a comparative consultation document was also released in 1998, *Quality Care and Clinical Excellence* (Welsh Office, 1998b). The Health Act 1999 (DoH, 1999b) was introduced in order to amend the legislative framework under which the NHS was currently organized in England, Wales and Scotland and received Royal Assent on June 30th, 1999. The Health Act 1999 (DoH, 1999b) also allows for changes to the NHS and Community Care Act, 1990 allowing the Secretary of State for Health increased powers over the regulation of NHS Trusts' organizational functions.

The Commission for Health Improvement

The Commission for Health Improvement (CHI) is a 'non-departmental public body' which currently covers England and Wales. It is intended to be an inspectorate for the NHS which has statutory powers, but is independent of the Government (CHI, 2000). The role of the CHI was identified in the White Paper *The New NHS* as that of 'addressing shortcomings' within the NHS (DoH, 1997, para 3.4). The CHI organization was formally established as part of the 1999 Health Act (DoH, 1999b) on November 1st, 1999. It has been described as '*an independent body to provide external scrutiny of the quality of clinical care provided to NHS patients*' (Donaldson, 1999a, p. 7). It is anticipated that CHI, supported by the Audit Commission, will inspect each NHS organization a minimum of every 4 years (Secretary of State for Health, 2000a). If, as a result of this inspection process, however, any NHS organizations fail to meet the essential performance criteria, those organizations will be inspected at more regular intervals of at least every 2 years. These inspections will take the form of a clinical governance review and will consider aspects of the organizations' functional roles such as reviewing their implementation of NICE guidance and NSFs. Inspection reports will be published in summary form along with action plans produced by the individual organizations (Secretary of State for Health, 2000a). This routine review process will be undertaken in addition to the CHI's role in inspecting those organizations which, between inspection periods, are considered by the Government to be failing to provide adequate service provision (Secretary of State for Health, 2000a).

A system of assessing performance was introduced in 1999 and is currently in place for Health Authorities (NHSE, 1999a). It is intended that this Performance Assessment Framework (PAF) will be further developed in the future and encompass more of the NHS family. Currently the process focuses upon six areas of NHS performance, namely, health improvement; fair access to services; effective and appropriate delivery of health care; efficient use of resources, high quality experience of patients and carers and outcomes. The findings are then published in annual league tables allowing performance comparisons to be made. Following the publication of the NHS Plan (Secretary of State for Health, 2000a) changes and expansion of this system are intended with regard to the setting of performance standards and data collection and publication.

From April 2001, NHS organizational performance will be measured against a new complementary version of the Performance Assessment Framework and performance will be classified accordingly. The system will now incorporate all NHS Trusts and Primary Care Trusts and will utilize the relevant aspects of the current PAF, while also including some relevant Trust information regarding the views of patients, quality of care, levels of efficiency and the work-force. The performance classification based upon this framework will be illustrated by the use of a colour coding system of 'Red', 'Yellow' and 'Green'. Red will indicate those organizations that fail to meet some of the national core targets. Yellow will indicate those organizations that meet all or most of the core targets but are not in the top 25% of the performance ranking. Green classification will be used to indicate the organizations that meet all core targets but also achieve wider performance targets and attain the top 25% ranking. The colour classification will be initially awarded to all NHS organizations by the Regional Offices and will then be independently verified by the CHI (Secretary of State for Health, 2000a). In essence the Red, Yellow and Green classification will allow for national benchmarking of NHS performance, the results of which will form the basis of a reward or sanction scheme within the NHS. Annual publication of this information will now be the responsibility of the CHI in association with the Audit Commission, in an attempt to ensure public confidence in the independence of the reported data.

The outcomes of this scheme for NHS organizations will be in the form of financial incentive through the NHS Performance Fund and the potential for increased 'earned autonomy' for those performing well (Green) or satisfactorily (Yellow) (Secretary of State for Health, 2000a). Those organizations seen as underperforming (Red) will not be financially disadvantaged but their financial freedom and autonomy will be restricted. Those organizations which achieve Red classification will be subjected to financial restrictions as their share of the Performance Fund monies will be held by the Modernization Agency (DoH, 1997; Secretary of State for Health, 2000a), who will also supervise their spending activity. This will result in their share of the Performance Fund monies only being given, therefore, with restrictions to their operational freedom. They will also be under closer scrutiny by the CHI who will visit every 2 years. However, if the organization is deemed to be seriously failing they may also be subjected to direct intervention, increasing to the level of 'special measures', at which point external intervention, advice and support may be used in order to achieve change within the organization (Secretary of State for Health, 2000a). By contrast Green organizations will be allowed increasing freedom and autonomy. They will be given automatic access to their share of the NHS Performance Fund monies. They will also be visited by the CHI at the less frequent 4-yearly intervals and granted a more remote monitoring approach by the Regional Offices. Furthermore, they will be given greater autonomy regarding decision making and used as examples for NHS performance by the Modernization Agency (Secretary of State for Health, 2000a). In addition, Green organizations' clinicians and managers may be used to assist Red organizations in improving standards and performance.

The Government's intention as regard the Performance Fund is that it may be used to develop and improve services and facilities for NHS patients and staff. It is interesting to consider, therefore, the view expressed by the NHS Confederation who propose that the process of performance assessment will be damaging to the NHS (NHS Confederation, 2000). The Government suggestions on how this money is to be used are not binding but they do intend to pilot a system of 'team bonuses' in some NHS Trusts in 2000. The information gathered from this pilot scheme will be used as the basis for future decisions with regard to further developments in this area (Secretary of State for Health, 2000a).

The CHI will not, however, operate in either Scotland or Northern Ireland. In Scotland the function of external clinical governance monitoring is to be undertaken by the Clinical Standards Board for Scotland (Management Executive, 1998). Many of the functions undertaken by the Clinical Standards Board for Scotland will be similar to those of the CHI, namely, development and management of a national quality assurance and accreditation process based upon regular evaluation of clinical services (Health Department, 2000). In Northern Ireland there is no comparative organization to CHI and one possibility for the future is that CHI may be requested by the First Minister also to operate in Northern Ireland.

The National Institute of Clinical Excellence

The role of the NICE organization is to be that of a 'Special Health Authority' and this process was formally approved by Parliament on January 2nd, 1999 by the introduction of an 'Establishment Order' with the organization coming into official operation on April 1st, 1999. NICE has responsibility for the review of three areas of the NHS within England and Wales: appraisal of health technologies, development of clinical guidelines and clinical audit promotion. The intention is that NICE will appraise between 30 and 50 new and existing interventions per year and subsequently advise the NHS on their clinical and cost effectiveness (NICE, 1999a). The selection of guideline topics to be considered by NICE are the responsibility of the Secretary of State for Health and the National Assembly for Wales. In Scotland and Northern Ireland the situation is different, as there exists a different political process and structure which governs the NHS.

The production of specific policy documents was undertaken for Scotland and resulted in the White Paper *Designed to Care* (Scottish Office, 1999a) while Northern Ireland decided to undertake a consultation exercise following the publication of the NHS White Paper for England (DoH, 1997) before finalizing its approach (DHSS, 1998). Scotland received devolved power for health matters, following the Royal Assent of the Scotland Bill in November 1998, allowing devolution and the assumption of full powers by the Scottish Parliament on July 1st 1999. Despite the differences in such policy, and therefore guidance documents, the general principles applying to the quality improvements of NHS services remain broadly the same. However, the intention is that they will be tailored, with regard to their implementation, to suit the specific needs and structures of each country.

A further aspect of NICE's work will be the incorporation of functions previously undertaken by other groups and they will assume future responsibility for work of other organizations. These will include the National Prescribing Centre, the Prescriber's Journal, clinical guidance contained in PRODIGY, the National Centre for Clinical Audit, DoH funded National Guidelines Programme and Professional Audit Programme and the Effectiveness Bulletins. PRODIGY (Prescribing Rationally with Decision Support in General Practice Study) is a computer-aided decision support system for GPs which has been available on a national basis since November 1998, with the support

of the NHS Executive, to all general practices with compatible computer software systems. PRODIGY allows clinicians to enter a diagnosis, which triggers a decision-making support process that provides evidence-based management advice linked to the prescribing strategy. The system can be tailored to individual patient specification and will produce, for example, patient information leaflets, and advice on referral or investigation. In addition, the system allows for the editing of therapeutic recommendations in line with local prescribing policies and will also provide educational support information for professional updating. The most recent development phase of the PRODIGY programme is to focus upon the area of chronic disease management and is, therefore, of interest to all practitioners working with patients/clients with chronic care needs.

In August 1999 the first list of treatments for review by NICE was released (DoH, 1999c) and provided a wide ranging mixture of existing and new interventions from both the primary and secondary care arenas. In September that year there came an announcement from the DoH that NICE was to produce protocols for general practitioners (GPs) which would assist them in making specialist referrals more efficiently and effectively (NICE, 1999b). Shortly after this the Secretary of State for Health and the National Assembly for Wales published their first list of topic areas for guideline consideration by NICE (NICE, 1999c). These guidelines were to include various aspects of clinical involvement, including patient self-care and consider the whole experience of care delivery in both the primary and secondary settings. Some chronic conditions have been included for review in the first list of clinical guidelines, for example type 2 diabetes mellitus and hypertension, while others have been incorporated into the initial list of GP referral protocols, namely psoriasis, childhood eczema and acne.

The process of considering the patient perspective in the production of these protocols must be welcomed by practitioners, patients and carers alike as a means of improving both the process and outcome of any care intervention undertaken. Within the area of chronic illness, however, this development must be considered as even more significant due to the long-term nature of the condition and, as a consequence, the importance of the relationship between the individuals involved. Within health care there has for many years been an ongoing debate regarding the issue of patient 'non-compliance' with prescribed treatments and the best methods of dealing with this problem. In 1997 the Royal Pharmaceutical Society of Great Britain published the findings of their enquiry into the problem of patient non-adherence with prescribed medication. Their findings identified areas of concern that had previously been dismissed, ignored or undervalued by much of the research into this topic. They identified that the problem of patients' inability to comply with prescribed medication was multi-faceted and involved a range of issues including financial difficulties, psychological and social stigma of long-term medication requirements, professional and lay health beliefs, drug side effects, etc.

The Royal Pharmaceutical Society of Great Britain ultimately concluded that there needed to be a change in stance by the professions with regard to the way in which they approached the issue of non-compliance with prescribed treatments. They proposed that this could best be achieved initially with the substitution of the term 'compliance' by that of 'concordance' (see Chapter 1 for a full discussion focused on the issue of concordance). The Royal Pharmaceutical Society of Great Britain is currently undertaking further research into this area, which will hopefully be due for completion in 2002.

The structure of the NICE Board is also supportive of the inclusion of lay perspectives on care and service delivery standards. Board members will be appointed by the Secretaries of State for Health for England and Wales and will consist of both executive and non-executive roles with the Chief Executive accountable to the Board. In addition, there is a NICE Partners Council which will consist of key stakeholder groups, including patient and carer groups. At a local level NICE will liaise with a range of service providers, and patient and user groups in order to disseminate their recommendations and guidance at all levels of NHS involvement.

National Service Frameworks

The National Service Frameworks were first identified in the NHS White Paper (DoH, 1997) as a means of promoting improved quality and consistency of service delivery throughout the country. Previously, work undertaken in the area of cancer services and paediatric intensive care service provision provided a model for such development. The NSFs will be produced using an expert reference group of clinicians, social services, service managers, carers, users, partner agencies and other groups and individuals as necessary (Donaldson, 1999b). Donaldson sees the NSFs as delivering the aims of the recent governmental health policy, namely that of the NHS White Paper (DoH, 1997) and Public Health strategy *Saving Lives – Our Healthier Nation* (DoH, 1999d). A similar situation exists in Scotland through their legislative framework of the White Papers *Designed to Care: Renewing the National Health Service in Scotland* (Scottish Office, 1999a) and *Towards a Healthier Scotland* (Scottish Office, 1999b).

The intention of producing NSFs is to introduce national standards for service provision based upon specific, clinically focused conditions or more general areas of care which require greater levels of integrated service and inter-agency working. The NSF process, therefore, will identify specific role functions and objectives for the organizations involved. These will provide a measurable performance against agreed targets and a quality assessment and cost effectiveness capability. Progress monitoring of the NSFs will be achieved through the CHI inspection process, including the NHS Performance Framework, and information gathered from the NHS Patient Survey.

The NSFs will provide recommendations, in their identified area of care, on a series of service aspects. These will include research and development; information; clinical decision support systems; revenue and capital costs and human resources. The process will also include other programmes of intervention towards improving the nation's health and provision of quality services such as Health Improvement Programmes. Currently four NSFs have been announced with two already launched and the remaining two due for release in the near future. The first NSF launched was that for Mental Health (Secretary of State for Health, 1999), this was then followed by the NSF for Coronary Heart Disease (Secretary of State for Health, 2000b). Two further NSFs are next in line, namely the NSFs for Older People and for Diabetes, with future plans for additional NSFs still to be announced.

Beyond the initial four NSFs identified, no definitive information is available but it is clear that both clinicians and NHS users would benefit from improved care standards relating to areas of chronic illness. However, in order for this increase in standards to be universally achieved and maintained there is a clearly identified need for a commitment to continuing education and training from the entire NHS family. The process of Continuing Professional Development (CPD) has been proposed as a method of guaranteeing high quality care throughout the NHS by ensuring that clinicians keep up to date with the rapidly changing clinical environment they currently have to practise in. In addition CPD has been linked with future plans for professional regulation of clinicians.

Professional regulation

In *A First Class Service* (DoH, 1998) the linkages between clinical governance, CPD and professional regulation is clearly made. It further suggests that clinical governance should be based upon teamwork and partnerships, which includes practitioners, academics and managers (DoH, 1998, p. 35: 3.9). To some extent the identified requirements regarding the use of evidence-based practice, risk management and the introduction of standards monitoring, have influenced this emphasis upon partnership development. In addition, the NHS modernization programme has identified the need to introduce different working patterns and approaches to service provision. As a consequence of this process NHS services are being delivered in ever increasing numbers of ways by a widening range of health professionals, for example Walk-In Centres and NHS Direct. Although the manner in which new NHS services will be delivered to the public may differ greatly from that which the public currently experience, it is clear that the need to ensure service quality and the maintenance of the public's safety are still paramount. Therefore, there must be a rigorous process of professional regulation in place in order for this to be assured.

During the past decade there has been an increase in media focus upon failures within NHS care delivery. This has resulted in a change in public attitudes to health care professionals and their ability to provide consistent high quality care has ultimately been questioned. High profile failures, such as those of the Bristol Royal Infirmary paediatric cardiac unit and Alder Hey hospital retention of children's organs without informed parental consent, further undermined confidence in the health care professions. Other events, including the convictions of Beverly Allitt and Harold Shipman for the murder of patients in their care, has necessitated the need for a robust system of professional regulation for clinical practitioners and the introduction of a mechanism of risk management and risk reduction within the NHS.

In 1997 the United Kingdom Central Council for Nursing, Midwifery and Health Visiting (UKCC) introduced a method for revalidation of nurses on its professional register entitled Post Registration Education and Practice (PREP). This process works by the self-validation of nurses registered with the UKCC based upon their undertaking a programme of CPD as a requirement of their registration maintenance. The requirement equates to 5 days equivalent study over a period of 3 years. Details of the education undertaken are recorded in a Personal Professional Profile which ultimately forms the basis of a life-long learning programme and allows the nurse to demonstrate professional development and skills-based competence related to their professional practice. At the end of the UKCC mandatory 3-year re-registration period nurses will have to complete a self-validation declaration, failure to do so will result in a lapse in registration. The process of auditing PREP activity will commence nationally in 2001 as this year will mark the first 3-year cycle since the national introduction of PREP in June 1998 (UKCC, 1997). In 1999 the UKCC reviewed the audit system, as a result of information gathered from the pilot project, in order to ensure a quality outcome for the process.

In 1997 the four Health Departments for England, Scotland, Wales and Northern Ireland commissioned a review of the legislative framework which currently regulated the nursing profession. The review was undertake by J.M. Consulting Ltd. and their report, published in 1998, concluded that there was a need to reform the nursing professional regulation system. They proposed a new Nurses and Midwives Act which would allow legislative changes to be made to the regulation system which would include unification of the registration and education functions in one UK wide statutory body (J.M. Consulting Ltd, 1998). This would replace the current UKCC regulatory function and the education and training function of the four National Boards for England, Scotland, Wales and Northern Ireland. This resulted in the publication of the *Making a Difference – Strengthening the Nursing, Midwifery and Health Visiting Contribution to Health and Healthcare: Government Report on Strategic Interventions for Nursing, Midwifery and Health Visiting*, which introduced new structures and processes to the training and education of nurses (DoH, 1999f). These changes allowed for more flexible training and education opportunities and modernization of the professional regulation systems.

In August 2000 the DoH issued the discussion document *Modernising Regulation – The New Nursing and Midwifery Council* in order to gather opinion regarding the future requirements for nursing professional regulation and its proposals for the reorganization of the nursing regulatory bodies. It proposed the formation of a new Nursing and Midwifery Council which would be smaller than the UKCC and the National Boards but would include their role functions, in addition to the provision of a greater strategic role with strengthened lay involvement. The ratification of the changes required to create the new Nursing and Midwifery Council (NMC) formed part of the Health Act 1999 (DoH, 1999b). Under Section 60 of the Health Act 1999 (DoH, 1999b) the Nurses, Midwives and Health Visitors Act 1997 was repealed and the new NMC regulatory function ratified. The new Nurses and Midwives Council's jurisdiction will apply to the regulation of the nursing profession throughout the entire UK and, despite the absence of Health Visiting in the council's title, Heath Visitors will continue to hold separate registration and representation within the council structure.

Similar reviews of professional regulation systems are currently underway for other groups of clinicians and practitioners (Secretary of State for Health, 2000a). In August 2000 the DoH issued a further discussion document relating to the review of the Professions Supplementary to Medicines Act 1960 and its proposal for the development of a new Health Professions Council. The proposed changes to the regulatory functions to the current Council for Professions Supplementary to Medicine (CPSM) and its

12 Boards were based upon an independent review undertaken by J.M. Consulting Ltd, *Report of a Review of the Professions Supplementary to Medicines Act (1960) with Recommendations for New Legislation*. The repeal of the Professions Supplementary to Medicines Act 1960 and the ratification of the formation and proposed changes to the regulatory function of the new Health Professions Council were completed under Section 60 of the Health Act 1999 (DoH, 1999b) and will apply to the entire UK.

In addition, under Section 60 of the Health Act 1999 (DoH, 1999b), the Order also allows for modification of the professional regulation of pharmacists under the Pharmacy Act 1954, dentists under the Dentists Act 1984, opticians under the Opticians Act 1989, osteopaths under the Osteopaths Act 1993 and chiropractors under the Chiropractors Act 1994. These groups of health care professionals are not, however, subject to the same level of professional regulatory change as the nursing profession, Allied Health Professions (formally Professions Allied to Medicine (PAMs)) or the medical profession.

Following the consultation document *Supporting doctors, protecting patients* (DoH, 1999e), medical professional regulation will also incorporate a process of revalidation based upon doctors' participation in an annual appraisal and mandatory clinical audit (Secretary of State for Health, 2000a). All NHS contracted doctors, including general practitioners (GPs) and their locums, will have to participate in this annual performance assessment which will be undertaken at a local level through the postgraduate education system, supported by the individual medical Royal Colleges. The annual appraisal process will then be integrated with the mandatory 5-yearly revalidation system supervised by the General Medical Council (GMC) (GMC, 2000). This annual appraisal process is due to commence in 2001 with the GMC revalidation scheme beginning the following year in 2002 (Secretary of State for Health, 2000a). The legislation required for this change to medical professional regulation formed part of the Health Act 1999 (DoH, 1999b). Section 60 of the Act allowed for amendment to the Medical Act 1983 which was enacted through the Medical Act 1983 (Amendment) Order 2000 (DoH, 2000a).

From April 2001 locally identified failing or poorly performing medical practitioners may be referred to the National Clinical Assessment Authority (NCAA), a Special Health Authority within the NHS for expert assessment and advice through its Regional Assessment, Training and Development Centres (RATDCs) (DoH, 2000b). The NCAA can then recommend a programme of remedial action to deal with any identified problem. In addition, the NCAA will liaise with both the GMC and CHI in order to develop policies which will address any potential issues caused by the overlap in the activities of the three organizations in relation to the process of assessment of medical practice performance.

The mandatory requirement for medical practitioners to participate in clinical audit is seen as a means of improving the quality of medical interventions. While the process of clinical audit is now a common concept within the NHS, there may be a different emphasis placed upon its use in the future with the introduction of clinical governance and the use of clinical performance assessment. The NHS National Plan clearly states: *'For 50 years there has been no systematic way of independently assessing NHS performance. Independent inspection was, until the creation of the Commission for Health Improvement, completely lacking'* (Secretary of State for Health, 2000a: para 2.29) and goes on to add: *'A small minority of organisations and individuals within the NHS persistently fail to deliver high standards of care. The instruments for dealing with persistent failure are old fashioned and inadequate. The NHS needs a system which spots problems early, takes swift action and can act decisively. Persistent failure should be met with an escalating scale of sanctions'* (Secretary of State for Health, 2000a: para 2.30).

Previous clinical audit activity within the NHS was not set against a series of unified standards for the entire NHS and it is this aspect which will be the main change in the process. For example, the provision of evidence-based guidelines provided by NICE and the attainment of performance standards for the implementation of these guidelines as assessed by CHI, provides a universal assessment of NHS activity. The use of clinical audit set against these national criteria will provide NHS wide, measurable data collection for the first time. This will allow assessment of activity and attainment of pre-set targets for the service in the future and can provide a basis for agreed service standards improvements. Increasingly clinical audit is becoming

an important NHS organizational tool that supports and guides national and local initiatives. NHS leaders are providing information on ways in which the use of clinical audit may be strengthened (NHSE, 1999b).

While there is a requirement for mandatory participation in the clinical audit process for doctors as part of their professional regulation, the concept of team or multidisciplinary participation in clinical audit is still only a desirable outcome (NHSE, 1999b). However, experienced practitioners will recognize the capacity for individual performance assessment not to identify fully all aspects of the care intervention process or its quality. In order to consider fully the care provided to a patient or client there needs to be an appreciation of all elements of that care. It is possible for individual practitioners to perform well individually but still be part of a poorly performing or dysfunctional team. Likewise good team performance can mask practitioner failure or suboptimal functioning on an individual basis. In some of the initial CHI reviews team performance has been found to be variable even within the same NHS organization, with individual units performing as centres of excellence within a clinical speciality while others are barely meeting the required standards (Hine, 2000).

It is clear, therefore, that clinical audit in the future will be required to address a wide range of issues and elements of patient care and professional functioning. In order for the specified outcomes of the new NHS to be met, future clinical audit activity will need to operate at individual and team level and ultimately at interface areas. Such areas may include the interface between primary and secondary care; health and social care; formal and informal care; state and private care; state and charitable care etc. In addition, the undertaking of clinical audit is only one part of the process of improving the quality of service provision. Consideration will need to be given to the evidence-based identification of audit standards and criteria, the dissemination of audit findings, the identified changes to practice and lessons learned from the exercise.

In order to deliver this agenda the service will need to utilize all available expertise in the area of research and development in order for it to become integrated into the NHS culture. In time the initiation of research and the use of evidence-based practice must become a routine for all staff. In the past much of the research undertaken by individual clinicians and practitioners, often as a requirement for professional development, education and training, was rarely introduced into practice. It may be argued that the process of undertaking research which is never implemented or disseminated is counterproductive for the NHS, but it has produced a body of enquiring and questioning individuals who have begun the process of challenging practice and care delivery. Under the planned changes to the NHS not all practitioners will formally be involved in organizational research and development (R&D). However, if clinicians and practitioners are to implement the planned strategy they will need to develop the skills of critical analysis if they are actively to participate in the implementation of the NHS R&D initiative.

Conclusion

In conclusion it is clear that the process of clinical governance is complex and multifaceted. For it to work as the Government plans, the NHS will require the support of a wide range of individuals and groups. There will be a need for change in the future manner of service delivery which will only succeed if it is accepted by both health care users and providers. This will require a considerable change in cultural attitude regarding the NHS, at the heart of which needs to be openness and a desire to adapt. This may, however, be the hardest goal to achieve, as it will demand immense trust to be shown by all parties concerned. The fragile relationship between the public and the NHS has been identified and acknowledged (DoH, 1997) and the plan for rebuilding that relationship has been initiated (DoH, 1997; Secretary of State for Health, 2000a). Only time will tell if clinical governance proves to be the vehicle by which the NHS achieves its quality agenda.

Useful contact addresses/ e-mail/website addresses/ telephone numbers

Concordance web site – www.concordance.org/

NHS Clinical Governance Support Team
2nd Floor
6 Millstone Lane
Leicester LE1 5ZW
Tel. 0116 261 9068. Clinical Governance Helpline 0116 261 9062

Open Government web site, provides alphabetical links to all NHS and associated web sites – www.open.gov.uk

PRODIGY National Dissemination Office
Sowerby Centre for Health Informatics at Newcastle (SCHIN)
University of Newcastle Primary Care Development Centre
Newcastle General Hospital
Newcastle upon Tyne, NE4 6BE
Tel. 0191 256 3129
e-mail prodigy-ndo@schin.ncl.ac.uk
www.prodigy.nhs.uk

Royal Pharmaceutical Society of Great Britain web site – www.rpsgb.org.uk/

References

CHI (2000) *Frequently asked questions*. July. Commission for Health Improvement. http://www.doh.gov.uk/chi/faq.htm
DHSS (1998) *Fit For The Future – Executive Summary*. Department of Health and Social Services, Northern Ireland
DoH (1997) *The New NHS Modern, Dependable, Cm3087*. The Stationery Office, London
DoH (1998) *A First Class Service: Quality in the New NHS*. Department of Health, London
DoH (1999a) *Devolution: Concordat on Health and Social Care*. December. Department of Health, London
DoH (1999b) *Health Act, 1999*. Department of Health, London

DoH (1999c) *No place in the NHS for inequalities of care, Press Release I1999/0485* Friday August 6th. Department of Health, London

DoH (1999d) *Saving Lives – Our Healthier Nation, Cm. 4169.* The Stationery Office, London

DoH (1999e) *Supporting doctors, protecting patients: A consultation paper on preventing, recognising and dealing with poor performance of doctors in the NHS in England.* Department of Health, London

DoH (1999f) *Making a Difference – Strengthening the Nursing, Midwifery and Health Visiting Contribution to Health and Healthcare: Government Report on Strategic Interventions for Nursing, Midwifery and Health Visiting.* Department of Health, London

DoH (2000a) Medical Act 1983 (Amendment) Order 2000 (SI 20000 No. 1830). Department of Health, London

DoH (2000b) *The National Assessment Authority.* Department of Health, London

Donaldson L (1999a) *CMO's Update 24, Winter 1999/2000; December.* Department of Health, London

Donaldson L (1999b) *CMO's Update 23, August.* Department of Health, London

Doyle A C (1888) A Study in Scarlet, Chapter 3. Cited in (Knowles E, ed.) *The Oxford Dictionary of Quotations*, 5th edn. Oxford University Press, Oxford

Galbraith S (1998) Ministerial speech on Clinical Governance, June. http://www.show.scot.nhs.uk/sehd.cg.Sam%20Galbraith.html

GMC (2000) *Revalidating Doctors: Ensuring standards, securing the future.* General Medical Council, London

Health Department (2000) *Clinical Governance, NHS MEL (2000)29. June.* Directorate of Strategy and Performance Management, Health Department, Edinburgh

Hine D (2000) *CHI – Our Journey So Far, Dame Deirdre Hine, Chair, Commission for Health Improvement, Conference presentation, NICE Conference.* 29th November. Harrogate

J.M. Consulting Ltd (1998) *The Regulation of Nurse, Midwives and Health Visitors: Report on a review of the Nurses, Midwives and Health Visitors Act 1997.* J.M. Consulting Ltd, Bristol

Management Executive (1998) *Clinical Governance, MEL(1998)75.* Management Executive for Scotland

NHS Confederation (2000) NHS Management's Agenda for the National Plan. NHS Confederation

NHSE (1997) *The new NHS – Executive Letter, EL(97)81.* NHS Executive

NHSE (1999a) *The NHS Performance Assessment Framework, HSC 199/078.* NHS Executive, Leeds

NHSE (1999b) *Steps Towards Clinical Governance.* NHS Executive, Northwest Regional Office, Warrington

NICE (1999a) *NICE appraisals – Key Points.* National Institute of Clinical Excellence, London

NICE (1999b) *NICE to produce Primary Care Referral Guidelines. Press Release 1999/005, September 29th.* National Institute of Clinical Excellence, London

NICE (1999c) *Clinical Guidelines Programme, Press Release 1999/010, November 4th.* National Institute for Clinical Excellence, London

Royal Pharmaceutical Society of Great Britain (1997) *From Compliance to Concordance: Achieving Shared Goals in Medicine Taking.* The Royal Pharmaceutical Society of Great Britain and Merck Sharpe & Dohme, London

Scottish Office (1999a) *Designed to Care: Renewing the National Health Service in Scotland.* Department of Health, The Scottish Office

Scottish Office (1999b) *Towards a Healthier Scotland.* Department of Health, The Scottish Office

Secretary of State for Health (1999) *National Service Framework for Mental Health: Modern Standards & Service Models for Mental Health.* Department of Health, London

Secretary of State for Health (2000a) *The NHS Plan: A plan for investment. A plan for reform, Cm4818-I.* The Stationery Office Limited, London

Secretary of State for Health (2000b) *National Service Framework for Coronary Heart Disease: Modern Standards & Service Models.* Department of Health, London

UKCC (1997) UKCC agrees process for PREP self-validation and audit. *UKCC Council report, September; Issue 5.* United Kingdom Central Council for Nursing, Midwifery and Health Visiting, London

UKCC (1999) PREP evaluation update. *Register, Number 26; Winter.* United Kingdom Central Council for Nursing, Midwifery and Health Visiting, London

Welsh Office (1998a) *NHS Wales: Putting Patients First.* Welsh Office

Welsh Office (1998b) *Quality Care and Clinical Excellence.* Welsh Office

Chapter

4

Rehabilitation

Fiona Allan

Introduction

After World War I the issue of rehabilitation came to the fore. The hospitals seemed to be full of men who had returned from the Great War with chronic conditions caused by things such as wounds, gassing or shell shock. The rehabilitation services began with a very medical focus and were originally seen as a treatment to overcome, rather than live with, disability. For people who live with chronic conditions, however, rehabilitation cannot always mean a return to full independence, rather it has to involve an acceptance and adjustment to a new way of life which is likely to include limitations and difficulties. It is clear that the medical model is not adequate when we are dealing with patients who live with a chronic condition and we therefore need to seek alternative perspectives on rehabilitation to meet adequately the needs of this particular group of clients.

The World Health Organization (WHO) describes rehabilitation as 'The application of all measures aimed at reducing the impact of disability and handicapping conditions and enabling disabled and handicapped people to achieve social integration' (WHO, 1996). Willard and Spackman (1988) focus on the individual's functional restoration as the primary objective of rehabilitation as their definition of rehabilitation is, 'the combined and co-ordinated use of medical, social, educational and vocational measures for training or retraining the individual to the highest possible level of function'. In contrast to this, however, McLellan and Wilson (1997) state that rehabilitation can be seen as a set of influences, procedures and resources to be applied both to the disabled person and the environment and a process of active change by which a person who has become disabled, acquires the knowledge and skills needed for optimal physical, psychological and social function. McLellan and Wilson describe a 'social model of disability', which construes handicap as 'a mismatch between the functional ability of a disabled person and the environment' (McLellan and Wilson, 1997).

Rehabilitation is all these things, and can be summarized as the use of compensatory methods to achieve maximum independence for clients suffering from some temporary or permanent disability. Rehabilitation can and, in the ideal world, should involve every aspect of a person's life, from personal relationships to doing the shopping. To be truly effective it must treat the person as a whole being by considering the client's physical, emotional and spiritual needs.

Rehabilitation must take account of the fact that, in some cases, the individual has a condition which may get worse and which could cause a deterioration in the person's ability to adjust and adapt. Similarly, they may have a condition that is characterized by periods of illness alternating with periods of 'ability'. In each of these cases a broad definition of rehabilitation is necessary to help the health care professional and the client focus on realistic goals. In some cases it could be argued that rehabilitation should be called habilitation, because the skills being taught or acquired may be ones that the individual did not have before.

Rehabilitation may also be referred to as the *recapitulation of ontogenesis* (Hagedorn, 2000). Ontogenesis is the development of the individual's repertoire of occupational performance over time. The activities of daily living have been learned over time – and thus may need to be relearned over time.

Client-centred rehabilitation

When a client is fully involved in the rehabilitation process, and wherever possible given choices, he or she is likely to cooperate more fully and the outcome will be more satisfactory for all concerned. The imposition of the therapist's own wishes and values may result in outcomes which, while meeting the therapist's objectives, may not be the ones most important to the client. Being client centred means establishing a system where every individual is treated as just that – an individual. Each person is recognized as being a unique person and as having a life beyond what is evident to the professional. Implicit in the idea of personhood are the elements that make up the life experience of that person, their past, their present and their future, as well as their version of reality and their hopes and dreams. It also includes the notion of civil rights and societal responsibility. We must accept that everyone should have the 'freedom to make decisions regarding the way of life best suited to an individual disabled person's circumstances' (Prince of Wales Advisory Group on Disability, 1985).

A prime lesson in being client centred is recounted in the following true story. An occupational therapist was working with a lady, Mary, who had severe rheumatoid arthritis. The lady had lived with the disease for nearly 20 years and she had slowly come to terms with the constant pain and the encroachment of the disease on her functional abilities. She had bilateral hip and knee replacements, but her mobility was still extremely restricted. Her hands were gnarled and knotted and the simplest of activities such as washing her face, was almost impossible unaided.

The occupational therapist had assessed the lady in terms of her functional abilities, and had come up with a rehabilitation plan, which included the basic activities of daily living – washing, dressing and simple kitchen activities.

Mary, however, had another priority. When asked what she most wanted to do that she could not do currently, her answer was swift and sure, 'Take my dog for a walk!' Mary explained that she had a little Jack Russell terrier, called Topper, who was her boon companion and the delight of her life. As Mary's mobility had become more and more limited she had been unable to take him for a walk, and so had paid the young man from next door to exercise him. The young man was moving away and Mary was concerned that Topper would not get his regular walk. She felt that she had no right to keep a dog in her small terraced house, with only a small back yard for exercise. If she could not find a way to exercise the dog, then Topper would have to go to live with her sister.

Mary also explained to the occupational therapist that she had a very good group of home carers, and that they helped her with washing and dressing as well as food and drink preparation. This meant that Mary could concentrate on the things that she enjoyed doing, and not waste her precious and limited energy on things that she could let others do. The occupational therapist was able to help Mary find an electric buggy, which she could drive to the nearby park. They sorted out where it would be parked, stored and recharged. They found one, which had a luggage area and trained Topper to jump on it and sit there. They wrote to the local council and asked about having some kerbs lowered (although the buggy could climb kerbs). Mary got an extending lead and an extra big clip so that she could attach it. This phase of Mary's rehabilitation took quite a while, but had a successful outcome. Mary learned a new way of taking Topper for a walk and the occupational therapist learned a great deal about being truly client centred.

Being client centred of course, is not as simple as doing everything the client wants. There are instances where the client's desires and expectations may far exceed what is realistic or achievable. In this instance the therapist has to negotiate gently in order to make the rehabilitation plan workable. For example an individual, who has recently suffered a stroke, leading to a dense hemiplegia and fits, may wish to get back to driving their car. In the short term it is unrealistic and it would actually be illegal for them to do this. However, it could be put on the list of long-term rehabilitation goals and the immediate rehabilitation plan could be focused on short-term goals.

Care has to be taken, when negotiating the rehabilitation goals and aims, to balance reality with enthusiasm. It would be all too easy to say to the individual, 'You have just had bilateral below knee amputations and so you will never be able to climb Mount Everest'. The aim here has to be to focus the individual on the here and now, while retaining the optimism for the long term. Reality sometimes can be grim enough, without having it outlined bluntly by well-meaning professionals who 'don't want to raise peoples' hopes'. When setting client-centred goals and making rehabilitation plans, the professional has also to consider such factors as cost and availability, as well as the local policies and criteria for provision of help. It can be all too easy to raise the expectations of the client about the sort of equipment that will be available to them, only to have to back track when it is discovered that they do not actually meet the local criteria for provision of the equipment, or it will not fit into their home, or even that there is a better (and perhaps cheaper) alternative. It must be remembered that being client centred does not mean giving the client everything they want, but rather providing them with the things that they need – and there can be a big difference between the two! One such example of this is the client's expectation that a stairlift will be installed. The client may feel fobbed off or cheated if the reality is that, following assessment, they are provided with a second hand rail up the stairs.

While it is essential that rehabilitation is client centred, it must also be ethical. It can be argued that if it were not client centred it would be unethical and so the corollary of this is that if it is client centred then it is ethical. Here lie some hidden dangers. It can be difficult, for example, to be sure who the client is – is it always essentially the client? If the professional has been called in by the principal carer (for example when the patient is a child), who then is the client? Or is the client the person who pays for the service (for example when a health service professional is asked to do an assessment on behalf of another agency such as Social Services)? There are also times when clients want the professional to do something that the professional may not feel is in the client's best interests. A good example of this dilemma is that of George, a 21-year-old man

with a high spinal cord injury leaving him with little movement in his arms and none below the chest.

The occupational therapist made him some splints to enable him to hold cutlery and thus feed himself. George then asked her to make an adaptation to one of his splints, which would enable him to hold and smoke a cigarette. Medical evidence states that smoking is harmful to health, and so in acceding to his request she would be helping him to do something harmful. On the other hand smoking is not illegal, and as a consenting adult he has the right to make the same choices as the rest of us. This is a debate, which could run and run, but it demonstrates that often there is no clear-cut answer to some of the issues that have to be considered.

Rehabilitation should be focused, in that it is specific to the individual and targeted to achieve the best possible outcome for that person. This means that while the programme is specific to each individual, the activities contained therein may be carried out in a group. Some of the activities used are discussed later in this chapter.

Rehabilitation should involve the client's cognitive processes so that where they are able, they understand and agree with what is being done to them and with them.

It must include a behavioural component, in that it often involves changing, modifying or adapting the way the individual copes with and reacts to his or her environment and other people.

Rehabilitation should also be functional. It must work for the person. The planned activity must be something that the person can achieve. Goals must be set at a level that the person can reach. It is better constantly to reset the target than to set a target which the person feels is a long way off and therefore not achievable. The goals must be set and negotiated with the individual, taking into account their wishes and their personality. Some people like to set only a step at a time and would feel daunted by knowing how big the next hurdle is, whereas others like to see the whole picture, before setting out. Once the goals of rehabilitation have been achieved, new goals can be negotiated with the client and so progress continues.

The activities used to achieve the objectives should also be ones which the person enjoys and can relate to. Wherever possible they should be purposeful. For example if the aim is to get someone to compensate for hemianopia,

Table 4.1 Areas of rehabilitation

Physical dysfunction
Social or psychosocial dysfunction
Personal care
Mobility
Domestic work
Child care/parenting
Sexuality
Work and leisure

you may use reading as an activity. You may look for large print books, but it would be a mistake to use children's books or to use material which the individual perceives as too simple or insulting to their intelligence. For clients who are literate, newspaper headlines are much more appropriate.

Areas of rehabilitation

The following section outlines the many different areas in which a person with a chronic condition needs to experience rehabilitation. These areas are also summarized in Table 4.1.

Physical dysfunction

This relates to the situation where the person has to adapt to some temporary or permanent physical impairment. This may also include clients who face increasing physical dysfunction such as may occur in rheumatoid arthritis.

Social or psychosocial dysfunction

This may occur as a result of a mental illness, as well as physical problems. Rehabilitation may be aimed at helping the individual adjust psychologically to the presence of a chronic condition. The individual may experience many different emotions in regard to such a diagnosis. He or she will have to come to terms with the reality of living with the condition and dealing with its effects on a day-to-day basis. Each individual will react differently to their disease. Some will deal with it by ignoring it – by pretending that it is not happening, and thereby potentially putting themselves at risk (for example someone with diabetes being cavalier about what and when they eat). To others it may become the biggest factor in their lives – their lives will be completely dominated by it and they may feel they cannot do all the things they would like to do. It is difficult to say which way an individual should behave. Every situation is unique, but the role of rehabilitation should be to enable the person to achieve a way of living with their chronic condition which neither endangers their health, nor restricts their lives unnecessarily.

Personal care

This can be of paramount importance for a person's self-esteem and self-worth. For someone with a chronic condition they often feel the need to maintain this aspect of their independence for as long as possible. The loss of the ability to do this task is somehow equated with loss of independence generally and a submission by the person to other 'stronger' or 'abler' persons.

Mobility

The ability to be mobile impinges on all aspects of rehabilitation. It is the factor which gives the individual freedom to explore, control and interact with their environment. The person is able to expand their horizons and go out, rather than having to wait for the world to come to them. A person can be empowered by increasing their mobility, however, the means for achieving mobility, can in itself be problematic. Adapting to the use of a wheelchair makes a statement to the outside world that the user is in some way disabled and brings with it all the problems that this entails. Wheelchair users complain that they are treated as if they are stupid, just because they cannot walk. Similarly, the freedom that the wheelchair gives can be severely curtailed by the lack of access to places. Using other aids to mobility can also be problematic, as can driving adapted vehicles. This is not to say that any of these things should be shunned, rather that they should be adopted and used with caution, and with the user's eyes wide open to the limitations as well as the freedoms.

Domestic work

This can be an area where the 'trade off' takes place, in that some people decide that these tasks can be done satisfactorily by others, in order that they themselves can concentrate on activities, which for them are more meaningful or more important. However, to some, the ability to look after oneself and to control and maintain their immediate environment is very important. This sense of control can be linked to the person's self-esteem and their affirmation of who they are in relation to their home, their family and their world. It can be symbolic of their equality with the able bodied and they see it as making positive statements about themselves as capable and independent human beings.

Child care/parenting

This is an activity that few parents would wish to pass over to paid carers. They may accept that some adaptation may be necessary in terms of how things are done, but generally the disabled parent wants to continue for as long as possible to fulfil the role of parent to the very best of their ability. It can also be an area of fear. The disabled person fears, as all parents do, that they may not get it right. They fear that they may harm the child. They also fear that if they are unable to care properly for the child, then the child may be taken away from them. Society generally resists the idea of disabled people being parents. There are few, if any, images portrayed of families where one or both parents are disabled. This breeds a subliminal belief that disabled people do not have children, and worse, that disabled people should not have children. People who become disabled, or who develop chronic conditions have the same subliminal beliefs quite often, and so their fear that their children are going to be disadvantaged at best, or at worst, taken away, are heightened. Research shows that, while some of the children of cancer patients experienced problems related to their parents' cancers (Nelson *et al.*, 1994), anecdotal evidence tends towards the idea that, in the main, the children of a parent with a non-life-threatening condition can be mature and better adjusted to life than their contemporaries.

Sexuality

This is an area that is sometimes ignored. Disabled people complain that they are pigeon-holed by society as neither heterosexual nor homosexual, but rather as asexual. They sometimes feel that society discriminates against them as sexual beings. A client's sexuality is an important issue which should not be avoided, however, health care professionals sometimes do avoid any discussion of sexual health because of their own embarrassment. In instances where the topic has been raised the client is often relieved and grateful that it was discussed and that the door has been opened to finding solutions to the difficulties. The effects of this aspect of a person's rehabilitation on their relationship with their partner should not be underestimated.

Work and leisure

Because of the effects of a chronic condition, leisure may assume more importance in an individual's life, particularly if the effects of the condition mean that they will have to give up their job, or can no longer do the day-to-day activities they did prior to their illness. If the reality is that the person will be at home more, or will have more leisure time to fill, then they can be helped to do so, perhaps by linking them to groups or agencies that would interest them. Despite legislation such as the Disability Discrimination Act (1998), it is still a sad fact of life that it is more difficult for people with a chronic condition, especially one which involves disability, to obtain employment. This does not mean that it is impossible and people can be retrained for jobs which fall within their capabilities, particularly those involving the use of information technology, where even working from home is a possibility.

Aims of rehabilitation

Table 4.2 lists a number of common aims in rehabilitation, some of which may be very specific to the individual.

Table 4.2 Aims of rehabilitation

Restoration of function
Achieving maximum independence
Enhancement of life satisfaction
Improving competence in occupational tasks and developing and restoring normal roles and lifestyles
Enabling the individual to reach his/her maximum level of independence psychologically, economically and socially
Compensating for residual disability

Restoration of function

Functional restoration is achieved as far as is possible and within the constraints of an ongoing disability. Sometimes there has to be a trade off as was described earlier in the given example of Mary. She had decided that because of pain and tiring very quickly, she would not strive to achieve independence in many of the activities of daily living, such as dressing or cooking, but would conserve her energy for things she really wanted to do. Others may choose to make the same sort of trade off in order to pursue a hobby or spend quality time with their family.

Achieving maximum independence

This is usually a very important aim, particularly with regard to the activities of daily living. Paramount among these, usually, is the ability to go to the toilet and clean oneself. Most people can tolerate the idea of someone cooking and cleaning for them. They can even bear to be transported around. But the idea of having to rely on another person to help with going to the toilet and washing oneself can be abhorrent. It is even difficult for some people to discuss their difficulties, but their relief can be enormous when a solution is found to any of these very specific problems. Independence can relate to all other spheres of life and clients usually list it as one of their most important aims. It is important to define with each individual, what exactly they mean by independence. To some people it can mean being able to do everything

unaided, and to others it can be the ability to control what is done, when, where, how and by whom.

Enhancement of life satisfaction

Everyone needs some form of life satisfaction and it has been said that a life without satisfaction is no life at all. Sometimes it is necessary to help the person realize that they may have to change their horizons and gain satisfaction from other things. The paralysed mountaineer whose principal source of satisfaction was standing on the pinnacles, may have to learn to derive satisfaction from other activities. This may mean that the individual has to come to an acceptance of the fact that their life has changed in ways beyond their control, and may continue to change as their chronic condition changes. There may have to be a long period of adjustment to the new way of life. The rehabilitation process may have to incorporate a period of mourning for the life the person had and which they may see as gone, or at best changed, forever.

Improving competence in occupational tasks and developing and restoring normal roles and lifestyles

These two issues are linked together. The client needs to be able to do things around the house or in the wider environment because, by doing so, they establish their role and position in a family or in society. For example the housewife and mother who is disabled by a chronic condition needs to be able to continue to exercise some control over some, if not all, of the tasks which she formerly did around the house. By engaging in some familiar activities the client can assert who she is – wife, mother and homemaker. Through her actions she can affirm that she has not abdicated her role in the family merely by being disabled. There will inevitably be a period of readjustment and redefining, but the essence of the person's role has to be worked out, both by the client and by his/her family and friends. Even a client who lives alone, with no family, may need to re-establish their lifestyle and role. It is important to the individual's self-esteem and psychological well-being that this is done. Quite often this is an area which can be overlooked by health care professionals, particularly during a period of hospitalization. In hospital, the person takes on the role of 'patient' and often this is the only role that the professional sees them playing. It can be hard to see them as anything else. The focus can tend to be on physical preparation for discharge and the client's readiness to resume their formal roles in life can be overlooked.

Enable the individual to reach his/her maximum level of independence psychologically, economically and socially

The person can be helped to decide what that maximum is and this will be translated into aims. A variety of experts may be needed here to assist the individual in achieving these aims, ranging from the expert in welfare rights to a counsellor. It is important that they are able to retain their independence and be seen as a person in their own right, with their own thoughts and feelings. Their feelings of personhood are immensely important. They do not want to be seen or identified as 'the diabetic' or 'the paraplegic'. A person who lives with a chronic condition should be seen as a person first and the condition simply happens to form a part of that individual.

Compensating for residual disability

It should be remembered that sometimes like for like compensation is not possible and, in this case, an adjustment or adaptation has to be made. A good example of this is the man with paraplegia who had always enjoyed distance running. He took up a wheelchair marathon challenge. He compensated for the loss of one sport by adapting to another. Adaptation can be individual – which tends to focus on what the environment demands and what the person does to meet those demands. It may also involve an adaptation to the person's occupation, for example if a person's job requires particular physical abilities or aptitudes, or adaptation to

their social or physical environment, for example where the individual may have to move to a flat that is wheelchair accessible.

Methods of rehabilitation

The methods used for rehabilitation can be as diverse as the clients being rehabilitated. A client-centred programme will use methods that the individual feels comfortable with and understands. It is important to consider the aims of rehabilitation and to agree these with the client at the outset.

Rehabilitation can be very much about *education*. Education about the disease and the disease process; education about how to recognize signs and symptoms and what to do about them; and education about new methods of doing things.

It may be necessary to *modify the environment* in which the person lives. This can be their domestic environment or their work environment. The client may need to have adaptive and adapted equipment provided to help them deal with the environment.

Financial support is another important aspect of rehabilitation. The individual may need a review of the various benefits, which they may or may not be claiming. Money can be a great source of worry, particularly as the individual may not be in employment.

It may be necessary to provide the person with some *manual assistance*. This can take the form of someone coming into the house to carry out the tasks that the individual cannot physically do for themselves, or which they have chosen not to do, in favour of reserving their energies for activities which they value more. The tasks can be personal care tasks or domestic tasks. It can also take the form of someone coming to carry out tasks which the individual cannot do because of lack of skill or inclination, such as giving an injection.

One of the big obstacles to overcome can be fear. The person who is coming to terms with living with a chronic condition may be scared of doing even the simplest of tasks because the effort of doing the task could exacerbate their condition. They live with the fear that they will have another fit, another asthma or angina attack, or a flare up of their disease. Rehabilitation can be about helping people to *take control* of their disease or condition so that, wherever possible, they control it.

Rehabilitation techniques

When planning any intervention a full assessment should be carried out. This should incorporate all aspects of a person's life and would include aspects such as self-care skills and social skills. It may be easier and quicker to concentrate on a specific problem, but this can become reductionist and is not entirely suitable for some problems. Consideration should always be given to other aspects of a person's life and those around them. Any technique used should maximize function, build on strengths and should be aimed at problem solving with the client.

A rehabilitation assessment can be formal in that it follows a set format and is done within predetermined parameters. These tests would have their own particular type of documentation and would be analysed according to set criteria. The results of such a test would be able to be used both in treatment planning and in assessing outcomes of interventions. There is a very wide range of structured tests which can be used, such as the Model of Human Occupation (MOHO) (Kielhofner, 1995) or the Assessment of Motor and Process Skills (AMPS) (Fisher, 1999). There are also less formal ways of carrying out assessments which can be tailored to the needs of the individual and to the environment. These rely on the expertise of the professional to set the assessment and usefully interpret and apply the results. An example of this is the 'kitchen assessment', where the individual is asked to make a cup of tea and a slice of toast. This demonstrates that the individual is able to organize himself, to perform a task in the right sequence, is safely mobile, has some standing tolerance, is able to remember what he is doing, is safe pouring boiling water, can carry items in safety etc. This sort of test relies on the interpretation of the results by the professional. The professional has to decide what is 'safe' and how the results of one assessment can be transferred on to other things, for example if the person can make a cup of tea safely, how probable is it that they could cook for themselves and would they do so?

Following assessment a rehabilitation programme can be devised. Some of the specific

Table 4.3 Rehabilitation techniques

Graded enabling programmes
Specific programmes of remedial activities
Retraining or resettlement
Provision of aids and equipment
Environmental change
Orthoses and prostheses
Social skills training
Behaviour modification
Specific activities to redevelop cognitive, social, self-care or creative skills
Industrial therapy focused on work retraining and resettlement
Preparation for community living

---

techniques that can be utilized in such a programme are listed in the following section and summarized in Table 4.3.

Graded enabling programmes

These are designed to increase the person's ability and tolerance in a gradual way.

Specific programmes of remedial activities

These would be specific both to the individual and the task in hand. The programme would be designed around what the individual needed or wanted to do, and an analysis of the task. Sometimes the task may have to be broken down into component parts. The programme may be designed to start with simple tasks, getting progressively more complicated, until the individual can carry out a task from start to finish. It is rather like learning a new dance. You practise each of the steps on their own, then you practise stringing a few steps together, then you practise with the music and in the end you do the whole thing. Driving a car is learned in a very similar way.

Retraining or resettlement

This may be necessary. Learning new ways to do things, or perhaps something simple like learning to work within new timetables. For example carrying out tasks at a time when the individual is able to perform optimally, for example later in the day for a person experiencing morning stiffness, but not too late so they are not too tired. Practice in prioritizing and sequencing can be helpful too, as well as the importance of regular rest periods.

Provision of aids and equipment

This may be necessary, although it is a general rule that these should be as simple and as few as possible. It is far better to look at easier ways of doing something than to get in to the realms of complicated equipment. For example, learning to put just one cupful of water into a kettle and brewing the tea in the cup rather than filling it and using a heavy teapot, can keep the weight down and help a client deal with a lack of strength. The alternative would be cumbersome kettle tippers and teapot tippers. (This is not to say these items should never be used. Indeed, they are extremely useful at the right time and in the right situation. It is just that the simplest method of doing the task should always be the first option.)

Environmental change

Again this can range from simple alterations such as removing a loose rug which the individual can trip on, through to alterations to the house to provide an accessible bathroom and bedroom. If the environmental change is at the more complicated end of this continuum, it can be very time consuming and costly and mean the involvement of a number of professionals.

Orthoses and prostheses

These may be made and supplied to enable the person to perform a task, for example a writing splint for someone unable to grip a pen. Orthoses and prostheses may also be supplied to hold a joint in a good functional position when the person is resting, for example night resting splints for an individual with rheumatoid arthritis.

Social skills training

This can be given when the individual or the professional has identified that they have needs in that particular area. This can be something very basic like learning how to ask for help (as well as learning to ask for the right sort of help and how to refuse graciously) through to how to cope in new situations and how to be assertive without being aggressive. This can be very important for people who have lost confidence in their abilities.

Behaviour modification

This might be necessary when the individual needs to adapt their behaviour or responses to a particular situation. This can be allied to social skills training, but would go much deeper in that it seeks to enable people to understand themselves and the way they deal with situations.

Specific activities to redevelop cognitive, social, self-care or creative skills

This may involve individual or group work. This is not about learning new skills, rather it is giving people the opportunity to practise skills that they already have, but in which they may have lost confidence.

Industrial therapy focused on work retraining and resettlement

This can be done in collaboration with the employment services and can involve working with employers. It goes without saying that the most realistic work rehabilitation is that carried out in a real workplace. Disability discrimination legislation has strengthened the individual's right to obtain or continue in employment and a great deal of help is now available to ensure that this can happen.

Preparation for community living

This may involve habilitation in that the professional may be helping the individual to acquire skills that he or she has not had before, as well as learning to adapt old skills to a new situation. For example, the individual may be moving into single accommodation and have to learn to cook for themselves or they may be moving into a group home and have to learn to work with others.

Summary

Rehabilitation for people suffering from chronic conditions can involve a wide range of activities carried out in a wide range of environments. It usually occurs through medical or therapeutic interventions which are firmly focused on the individual, but may include several members of the multidisciplinary team. It can also occur through political change and cultural enlightenment. The person can only be rehabilitated in so far as society will let them. If society continues to discriminate against people who live with disabilities then the rehabilitation process will always remain incomplete. It is possible to reduce handicap by changing attitudes. The professional can strive to alter attitudes, both in the person's domestic circle and also in the wider society. In this way the rehabilitation process has more chance of success.

References

Disability Discrimination Act (1995) HMSO, London

Fisher A G (1999) *Assessment of Motor and Process Skills*, 3rd edn. Three Star Press, Fort Collins, Colorado

Hagedorn R (2000) *Tools for Practice in Occupational Therapy.* Churchill Livingstone, London

Kielhofner G (1995) *A Model of Human Occupation, Theory and Application*, 2nd edn. Williams and Wilkins, Baltimore

McLellan D L, Wilson B A (1997) *Rehabilitation Studies Handbook.* Cambridge University Press, Cambridge

Nelson E, Sloper P, Charlton A, While D (1994) Children who have a parent with cancer: a pilot study. *Journal of Cancer Education* **9** (1), 30–36

Prince of Wales Advisory Group (1985) *Living Options,* Prince of Wales Advisory Group on Disability, London (now called Disability Partnership)

Willard H S, Spackman W F (1988) *Occupational Therapy,* 7th edn. Lippincott, London

World Health Organization (1996) *Fighting Disease, Fostering Development* WHO, Geneva

5

Depression and its relation to chronic physical conditions

David Morning

Introduction

This chapter aims to equip the practitioner with information which will facilitate and enhance the process of understanding in relation to the assessment, treatment and care for an individual with depression and chronic physical illness. Accepting that depression, from a medical perspective, can be described and defined as a chronic disease in itself, features of clinical depression from this viewpoint will be identified and explored. A holistic perspective, where a psychosocial view will be taken, will complement this medical viewpoint. This in turn will be reflected in the therapeutic intervention section, equally recognizing the use of medication when appropriate.

For an individual with a chronic physical condition, depression can only exacerbate and complicate their personal suffering. Rodin and Voshart (1986) pertinently recognize that depression could be coincidental to a physical condition. Alternatively, it may well be caused by the physical condition itself or iatrogenically through the medication used to treat that condition. Equally, it could be an outcome of the pain or sense of loss experienced by the individual. Finally, it may be a reflection of the poor prognosis associated with the disease process.

Depression as a separate condition is recognized as one of the most common disorders in primary care. In the 1980s it was shown to affect between 15 and 20% of the adult population at any one time (Kiloh et al., 1988). More recent figures show that there has been little change in the prevalence of this disease, with

it affecting between 6 and 26% of those attending for health care (Rihmer, 1997). These figures focus on the occurrence of depression among the general population. Katon and Sullivan (1990) found that those suffering from chronic physical illness were even more likely to be affected by depression. McDaniel et al. (1995) comment that there is an increased chance of depression the more severe the illness. There have also been reports that those suffering from cardiovascular disease, diabetes mellitus, stroke, dementia and Parkinson's disease have a prevalence of depression between 20 and 50%, demonstrating that the incidence of depression is far higher for those suffering a chronic physical illness than the general population (Cunningham, 1994).

Depression has been referred to as the 'common cold of psychiatry' (Garland, 1996), however, only a small number of cases are actually seen by psychiatric services, usually the more severe end of the depressive scale. The majority of individuals are cared for within the primary health care team. Surprisingly for such a common illness, it remains unrecognized, misdiagnosed or inadequately treated in a number of cases (Roberts and Priest, 1995). The diagnosis of depression in those who are physically ill is further complicated by somatic symptoms, which can be misinterpreted as components of physical illness instead of depressive symptoms. Rihmer (1997) refers to this as 'masking' of the depression, which can often remain, unrecognized and untreated. Creed (1997, p. 6) outlines a contrary perspective associated with the presence of 'somatic symptoms such as fatigue, sleep loss, anorexia and weight loss', as these are often present in those who are physically ill, arising from the physical illness itself and not the presence of depression. In effect, the symptoms of the physical illness are similar to those that might be found in a person suffering from depression. This potential anomaly leads on to the need for an effective assessment of the individual.

Assessment

Once diagnosed, depression clearly responds to appropriate treatment. The variety of treatments will be discussed later. The main distinction to be made is between depression as a disease or as a state of 'normal' unhappiness. Rihmer (1997) states that depression is more than 'feeling blue' and recognized that it is a medical illness and not a personal weakness. This perception of not 'giving in to depression', can be a delaying factor in an individual seeking help. Once a person approaches for help and support, each individual will articulate and share their respective experiences in ways that are unique to them. This obviously is dependent upon the experience of the individual suffering from the disorder and the others who come into contact with them. Undoubtedly the practitioner has to be empathetic and endeavour to understand these experiences from the individual patient's perspective (Dexter and Wash, 1986).

Jenaway and Paykel (1997) reinforce the importance of being familiar with the condition of depression itself when considering its diagnosis in the presence of physical illness. In differentiating depression from physical illness it is helpful to be able to utilize diagnostic criteria. The Diagnostic and Statistical Manual IV (DSM, 1994) provides the most accepted diagnostic criteria for major depression. It offers a medical perspective for the practitioner with taxonomy of signs and symptoms indicative of clinical depression, viewing it as a disease process. Prior to the production of DSM-IIIR (DSM, 1988) there was no suggestion that these diagnostic criteria should differ in relation to those people who are also suffering from a physical illness. Since the updating of the DSM-IIIR there is now included a directive 'not to include symptoms which are clearly due to a physical disorder'. This provides clearer guidance in the assessment of those who are physically ill.

Table 5.1 Symptoms of a major depressive episode

1. Depressed mood, being present most of the day and nearly every day
2. Loss of interest and enjoyment (anhedonia)
3. Change in weight and lack or increase in appetite
4. Disturbed sleep, either difficulties getting to sleep or early morning wakening
5. Psychomotor retardation or agitation
6. Fatigue, diminished activity
7. Feelings of unworthiness, excessive and inappropriate guilt
8. Poor concentration, attention and indecisiveness
9. Recurrent thoughts of death and/or suicide, suicide attempts or plans for committing suicide

Adapted from the DSM-IV diagnostic criteria

A major depressive episode is defined by the DSM-IV as the presence of five or more of the symptoms found in Table 5.1. These should have been present during the previous 2 weeks and represent a change from the former functioning of the patient/client. At least one of the five symptoms would be either 1 or 2 in the diagnostic list, i.e. depressed mood and/or loss of interest.

As highlighted previously the diagnosis of depression is complex, as the origins of some symptoms are difficult to isolate to either a physical illness or depressive disorder. These are referred to as somatic symptoms and are included in the DSM-IV criteria. They include weight loss, fatigue and poor sleep pattern. Creed (1997) talks about the use of criteria specified by Endicott (1984), who substitutes the four somatic symptoms of sleep disturbance, weight gain, fatigue and diminished concentration for four psychological symptoms. These are social withdrawal, not talking, tearful, depressed appearance and non-reactive mood and brooding/pessimism.

To replace the somatic symptoms of depression with those of the 'Endicott' criteria would effect the validity of the DSM-IV diagnostic criteria, therefore the 'Endicott' criteria are useful only in offering another view point on the presentation of depressive symptoms in the physically ill. The criteria recognize that the somatic symptoms, although criteria for diagnosing depression, could be aspects of the physical illness. The four psychological symptoms acknowledge the cognitive/behavioural aspect of depression in the physically ill. This issue will be explored further within the therapeutic intervention section.

The signs and symptoms for depression have, so far, been presented in a list; however, Clarkson (1998) reminds the practitioner that depression is 'a complex entity', and not merely a 'collection of symptoms'. This, he comments, can cause difficulty in the assessment process, especially when presented or masked by disabling physical conditions and/or diseases. When assessing the individual it is necessary to take a wider view, exploring other deeper issues, than purely presenting symptoms. It is important to take a holistic view and include demographic and social factors as these may be influencing the prevalence of depression more than the severity of the physical illness (Creed, 1997). Lazarus and Folkman (1984) reinforce this perspective by reminding practitioners that cognitive appraisals are influenced by variables such as age and family. Specifically they refer to younger cancer patients experiencing significantly more emotional distress than older patients. However, as in physically healthy patients, issues such as having a past history of depression, including family history and previous response to treatment, should also be accounted for (Jenaway and Paykel, 1997). As has already been recognized, some of the potential somatic symptoms may be manifestations of a physical illness and not necessarily symptoms of depression. The somatic symptoms should only be used as diagnostic criteria when they are extreme and out of proportion with the physical condition. Dexter and Wash (1986) identify that, when assessing an individual suffering from depression, one of the most important skills is that of observation. Obviously it is important to listen to the content of what is being said, but equally important is the delivery, intonation and the non-verbal communication associated with the same.

Chernomas (1997) reminds the practitioner that while lists can be useful as a diagnostic tool, these lists represent the professional's view of depression. Kleinman (1986, p. 225) states that 'the disease experience is reinterpreted by practitioners in the terms of their theoretical models'. Chernomas refers to terminology that might be alien to the patient

and therefore the practitioner must be aware, when asking pertinent questions, to ask within a framework and style that will be understood and allow the individual to express their personal experiences and associated meanings. Accepting this, it is still useful for the practitioner to have a theoretical and conceptual framework to facilitate the assessment process.

There are a number of specific assessment tools that can assist in identifying the severity of experienced depression. Beck *et al.*'s (1961) inventory for measuring depression was a relatively early assessment tool which has since been updated (Beck and Steer, 1993). Others include The Hamilton Depression Rating Scale (HDRS) (Hamilton, 1960), The Montgomery–Asberg Depression Rating Scale (MADRS) (Montgomery and Asberg, 1979) and the Geriatric Depression Scale (GDS) (Sheikh and Yesavage, 1986). Specifically for postnatal depression is Cox *et al.*'s (1987) Edinburgh Postnatal Depression Scale. This is not an exhaustive list, but a representation of the screening tools available. While these tools can provide individuals with indicative questions and areas for exploration, like many assessment tools, practitioners require supervision and training in their application and interpretation.

Having identified some very specific assessment tools, Katona and Katona (1997) state that, in the cases of older people, four questions could be used to enable the practitioner in identifying depression in this group. These are listed in Table 5.2.

A low score of zero suggests that the person is not likely to be depressed, while a score of two or more indicates that they are suffering from depression. Katona and Katona (1997) are confident in the short questionnaire's sensitivity in detecting depression. It is important for the

Table 5.2 Four questions for identifying depression in the elderly

- Are you basically satisfied with your life? (Score 1 for no)
- Do you feel that your life is empty? (Score 1 for yes)
- Are you afraid that something bad is going to happen to you? (Score 1 for yes)
- Do you feel happy most of the time? (Score 1 for no)

practitioner to note that these four questions are taken from a more detailed 15-question questionnaire. However, they can be useful in providing practitioners with a foundation and baseline for assessment.

Assessment of risk

Depression, when treated appropriately, responds well and it is recognized that early detection and treatment is one of the most important factors in the prevention of suicide (Rihmer, 1997). There are about 5000 suicides each year in England and Wales, of which 400–500 involve overdoses of antidepressants and deliberate self-harm is 20–30 times more common (Hale, 1997). Not all people who commit suicide have a psychiatric disease but, among those who do, depression is the commonest disease and 15% of depressed patients eventually kill themselves (Kiloh *et al.*, 1988; Hale, 1997). Suicide rates in the physically ill are generally higher than in the general population. Specific conditions that indicate an increased risk include multiple sclerosis, spinal cord injury and renal disease (Harris and Barraclough, 1995; Mayou, 1997).

Gotlib and Hammen (1992) recognize that the psychological construct of hopelessness which is often found in depression can be added to the list of high-risk indicators, (see Table 5.3). Beck *et al.*'s (1974) Hopelessness Scale attempts to measure an individual's levels of pessimism. Dyer and Kreitman (1984) also report that hopelessness has been shown to be a contributor to possible suicide and is highly related to suicidal intent. Equally, demographic, social factors and denial all should be taken into account.

From Hale's (1997) criteria, in particular the variables of motive, precipitating and maintaining problems and hopelessness, could be extremely pertinent when associated with an individual with a chronic physical condition. Foote *et al.* (1990) recognize the importance of the construct of hope for individuals with chronic illnesses. In a study, which focused upon individuals with multiple sclerosis, they examined three psychosocial concepts – hope, self-esteem and social support. They reported that 'the possibility exists that individuals with a higher level of hope have a more positive attitude about themselves' (Foote *et al.*, 1990, p. 158). This potential link is important when

Table 5.3 Suicide or deliberate self-harm (adapted from Hale, 1997)

(a) Features to be assessed
- Motive
- Circumstances of attempt
- Psychiatric disorder
- Precipitating and maintaining problems
- Coping skills and support
- Risk

(b) High risk indicators for suicide
- Male
- Age >40 years
- Family history of suicide
- Unemployed
- Socially isolated
- Suicide note
- Continued desire to die
- Hopelessness sees no future
- Misuse of drugs or alcohol
- Psychiatric illness (especially depression, but also schizophrenia, personality disorder)

the practitioner links the sense of hopelessness to the risk of suicide in the individual who is depressed and has a physical illness. They also purport that individuals who have a higher level of hope and self-esteem may be more likely to attract supportive relationships. These areas will be explored next within the therapeutic intervention section.

Therapeutic interventions

The practitioner is reminded of the care programme approach (CPA) (Department of Health, 1990), which can provide an effective framework and structure for the coordinated care of an individual suffering from depression. This approach will usually only apply to those who have been referred to the specialist psychiatric services, e.g. community mental health nurse and/or psychiatrist. In the main, within primary health care, the primary health care team will provide support. However, it is worth clarifying with the patient/client and within the relevant records, if indeed there is a programme of care, as this could save the practitioner much time and effort in carrying out assessments needlessly.

The National Service Framework for Mental Health (Department of Health, 1999) reflects the government's commitment to integrate the CPA with Care Management (a social services framework).

The national framework sets out seven specific standards, of which standard two specifically focuses upon access to primary care services. In effect, any individual contacting their primary health care team with a common mental health problem should *'have their mental health needs identified and assessed'* and *'be offered effective treatments, including specialist services for further assessment, treatment and care, if they require it'.*

This reinforces the need for all practitioners to be familiar and confident with the assessment process. Even if it involves the clear recognition of referring on for further care and treatment.

Psychological and emotional support

When deciding on a care and treatment approach for an individual who is suffering from depression, it is vital that the team involved in this process remember that depression can have a multifactorial aetiology. Accepting this, then care and treatment do not necessarily have to include a single approach but could be a managed combination. This may include an approach that reflects the biological (physical), social and emotional/psychological aspects of the condition.

Focusing initially on the emotional and psychological aspect of depression, there are a number of approaches that have been shown to be relatively effective and could go under the broad umbrella of 'psychotherapy'. It is important to note at this stage that 'psychotherapy' can involve a number of short, limited contacts between the practitioner and individual and does not have to involve a long and protracted process. However, this is not to negate a more in-depth approach if it is appropriate. This is obviously dependent on the assessment, which was covered earlier.

There are a number of therapeutic approaches that have been utilized by practitioners in supporting and caring for the depressed individual. These have included behavioral therapy (Bandura, 1977; Rehm, 1979), rational emotive therapy (Ellis and Grieger, 1977) and cognitive

behavioural therapy (CBT) (Beck, 1974, 1983). For the purpose of this chapter, reflecting the relatively straightforward approach associated with CBT, this form of therapeutic intervention will be explored in more detail. The CBT approach attempts to explore the relationship between the individual's cognitions (thought processes), self-concept and associated behaviour, relative to their experience and situation. Lazarus and Folkman (1984), Liese and Larson (1995) and Morley *et al.* (1999) report on the benefits of a CBT approach in the psychological support of individuals with physical conditions and associated chronic pain. Liese and Larson (1995, p. 32) state that 'cognitive therapy is a time-limited, structured psychotherapy, well suited to individuals with life-threatening illnesses'.

Cognitive behavioural therapy

Aaron Beck, the originator of this approach, viewed the effect on an individual's mood from a psychological and social perspective. He believed that negative cognitions, which are the individual's view of their world and the future, are sustained through faulty information processing and a vicious circle is set up in which low mood increases. The negative cognitions are seen to arise from the reactivation of dysfunctional underlying beliefs known as schema. He believed that the cognitive theme in depression is one of loss.

This loss is either perceived, for example loss of status and role that can accompany events such as children leaving home or retirement, or actual loss, such as bereavement, divorce or redundancy. Of course, this perception of loss could be strong in an individual with a long-term physical illness, e.g. loss of mobility, independence and role.

Instead of involving the individual in a deeper exploration of identifying the cause of their depression, the challenge is related to the 'here and now' of the therapeutic intervention by empowering the person to challenge negative thinking and focusing upon a more positive way of appraising the situation. This then, arguably, has a reciprocal positive effect on lifting the individual's mood and associated emotions.

An awareness and understanding of depression is vital to the effectiveness of the CBT approach. In the initial stages of contact the individual is 'educated' and informed about the depressive process (Peden, 1996). This includes what Beck (1983) termed as 'faulty cognitions'. This faulty thinking, which may have become habitual, may have exacerbated the situation and been a compounding factor in the development of the depression. For example an individual can overgeneralize their experiences and situation, e.g. 'because my concentration is poor, my performance at work is not good, and therefore everything is bad'. Beck *et al.* (1979) believe these negative cognitions and faulty information processing can cause low mood. The aim of CBT is to identify the vicious circle between events, symptoms, negative thinking, behaviour and low mood.

The individual is facilitated to develop an awareness of this type of thinking and is encouraged to keep a diary in which they are asked to record thoughts, feelings, behaviour and level of mood in relation to an activity that they may be undertaking. The diary can provide the basis for sessions in which negative thoughts are challenged and where patients/clients are encouraged to suggest alternative positive thoughts, keeping a written note of when they challenge this type of negativity during an average day. In doing this the individual can use the diary to challenge thoughts and set small goals/objectives to work towards, on an ongoing basis (Beck *et al.*, 1979).

The emotional aspect is of course important within a CBT framework/approach. Basically, the premise rests upon the perception that attempting to change and develop the behaviour and associated thoughts of the individual leads to an overall positive change, rather than a deeper analytical approach where the goal is to discover why the person is feeling the way that they do. Peden (1996) in a study on women receiving help and support for depression identified the continued use of cognitive techniques to be essential in the management of their condition. Kramlinger *et al.* (1983) focusing specifically upon chronic pain patients did indicate that cognitive behavioural approaches could be effective in the alleviation of depressive symptoms in this patient group.

A note of caution, however, when caring for individuals with a chronic disease; the individual's outlook may be a very factual and insightful recognition that the future could be bleak, e.g. someone with a terminal illness. Noble (1996, p. 143) refers to the 'horror and dread which accompanies the prospect of the diagnosis of cancer'. To attempt to challenge this perception as a faulty cognitive process could be erroneous, as this negates the right of the individual to feel a sense of forbidding or hopelessness, which of course could be a symptom of depression or a realistic expectation of the future.

Pain and CBT

The severity of an individual's physical illness can of course have a bearing on their personal outlook. Bernard and Krupat (1993) recognized that the severity levels of arthritis sufferers were related to depression, helplessness and stress. The severity of a condition can also be linked to the associated pain experienced by the patient. Van Houdenhove and Onghena (1997, p. 465) comment that 'pain and depression can both be considered as perhaps the most serious forms of human suffering'. They also state that the treatment of depression in chronic pain patients, with an associated long-term physical illness, has the potential of improving their overall general well-being and quality of life.

Morley *et al.* (1999) conducting a 'systematic review and meta-analysis of randomized control trials of cognitive behaviour therapy and behaviour therapy for chronic pain in adults', concluded that psychological treatments, including CBT are effective for managing pain and enhancing positive coping skills. Thomas (2000) supports this perspective, seeing CBT as a positive intervention in the treatment of chronic pain, by reducing psychological distress and improving levels of self-confidence. Romano and Good (1994) identify that studies generally support CBT approaches for the treatment of chronic pain, but they remind practitioners that additional controlled research is required to evaluate both immediate and long-term outcomes.

Returning to the specific condition of depression and its link to physical illness and associated pain, Van Houdenhove and Onghena (1997, p. 428) report that 'treatment of a concomitant depressive disorder is likely to increase a patient's responsiveness to pain management techniques and diminish the risk of withdrawal from treatment'. The CBT approach would appear to complement this statement as it has the potential of a 'twofold' effect in improving an individual's depressive state and/ or any associated experienced pain.

Of course not every practitioner will need to be trained to become a CBT therapist, however, some of the principles associated with this approach can be taken to assist in the development of a therapeutic relationship, which could lead to positive change. Obviously, in some cases, patients/clients will have to be referred on to specialist services, e.g. community mental health nurse, psychologist or psychiatrist where a more intensive approach may be taken, still involving the referring practitioner in the care process. While recognizing the role of the statutory services, the role of the family and carers should not be forgotten in the support of the individual patient/client. Social support has been recognized to be important in the recovery of individuals suffering from depression.

Social support

The importance of receiving effective social support and its link to an associated lift in individual well-being, has been well recognized (Stevens, 1992; Scott, 1995; Ogden, 1996; Langford *et al.*, 1997). In developing their social comparison theory, Langford *et al.* (1997) state that individuals develop their self-concept by comparing themselves to others in their chosen reference groups. This process in the development of self-concept can enhance self-esteem and psychological well-being, thus leading to improved emotional adjustment and coping abilities. This issue of social comparison may not be successful in the development of self-concept without the process of social exchange. When assessing the individual patient, consideration should be given to the social support network of the person. Ogden (1996) refers to the potential benefits of joining social support groups. This could include specific groups supporting the individual with their management and coping abilities pertaining to their physical needs and associated condition.

Stevens (1992) identified a positive relationship between life satisfaction and the receiving of social support, as well as the giving of social support. Being socially competent is essential in the formation and maintenance of relationships which, in turn, is an essential aspect of social health. Some of the consequences of effective social support cited by Langford *et al.* (1997) are:

- Healthy coping abilities
- Increased personal competence in times of stress
- Sense of stability
- Recognition of self-worth
- Life satisfaction
- Decreased depression

They hypothesize that psychological well-being may 'be the ultimate outcome of social support' (Langford *et al.*, 1997, p. 97). When relating this variable to the treatment of depression it is an obvious beneficial state to attain and facilitate for the patient.

Interpersonal therapy (Klerman *et al.*, 1984) is a short-term approach, which concentrates on improving the individual's social relationships. This links with and complements Langford *et al.*'s (1997) social support construct, which has just been outlined. As previously identified, worthwhile and stable relationships are perceived as being vital for the development of well-being and self-esteem in a person. If, for whatever reason, a relationship comes under undue strain, for example marital difficulties, the individual suffers from this negativity and accordingly it can exacerbate an already low mood. Attempting to improve the communication and relationship skills, using assertiveness training and appropriately expressing emotions, attempts to build self-confidence and thus a more healthy self-image/perception which, in turn, could lead to a lift in mood for the individual (Scott, 1995). For the practitioner the objectives of this approach have the potential to integrate well with the principles of CBT, especially when time is limited.

Any improvement in relationships is of course dependent on the application of therapeutic strategies within the relationship itself. Occasionally it might be useful to meet respective partners, if both parties are willing to become involved in the change process. In particular, when a person is involved in caring for a partner suffering from a disabling condition, for example multiple sclerosis, diabetes mellitus or chronic obstructive airways disease, the need actively to involve them should be paramount, reflecting the physical closeness of the relationship as well as any emotional and psychological attachment. However, if the issues are complicated, referral on to an appropriate agency could be the way forward.

The above approaches (interpersonal and cognitive behavioural therapies) actively depend upon the patient/client's involvement in the therapeutic process. This application, in the main, takes place away from the one-to-one professional relationship and is utilized by the individual patient and/or relative within the context and associated environment of their day-to-day relationship. Reflecting this, the practitioner has to rely on the patient/client's commitment to the approach. Of course it has to be remembered that depression can affect an individual's volition and motivation. This has to be recognized as a factor, which could undermine the interventions. With this in mind, medication can play an active role in complementing an overall therapeutic strategy.

Medication

Psychological and emotional approaches are inherent aspects in supporting individuals suffering from depression which might be complicated by a physical, chronic condition. As previously noted the practitioner has to be aware not to negate and undermine an individual's right to see their future in a negative way. Alternatively, a person's mood might be so low as to warrant the use of medication and, in particular, antidepressants. As part of a unified approach antidepressants can play a positive role in elevating mood to the point where the patient can then begin to act upon their own volition, which might have been lost in the despair of depression itself. This is why the initial assessment process is so important in detecting the level and profundity of the depression.

Gill and Hatcher (1998, p. 1) conducted a systematic review 'to determine whether antidepressants are clinically effective and acceptable for the treatment of depression in people who have a physical illness'. The outcome of this review pointed towards a positive correlation between the prescription of antidepressants and an improvement in the associated mood of an individual with a physical illness. This reinforces the role that antidepressants have to play in an overall approach to treating and caring for the patient/client. They conclude the review by reiterating the importance of a detailed assessment in identifying a persistent low mood. They remind the reader that depres-sion is more frequent in those with a physical illness than individuals without. The outcomes are often poorer with increased morbidity and mortality (Lustman *et al.*, 1988; Katon and Sullivan, 1990; Frasure-Smith *et al.*, 1995).

The correct prescription of the required therapeutic dose is of course important. The efficacies of antidepressant treatments have been shown through many studies as described by Paykel and Priest (1992). A negative aspect of this form of treatment is that it can take 2–3 weeks to work and the individual patient/client may experience side effects from the first dose (British Medical Association and Royal Pharmaceutical Society, 2000). Due to these issues and clients' preference not to take medication there can also be problems with adherence (Hale, 1997). Practitioners should inform patients/clients that there is likely to be a delay in the therapeutic effects of the antidepressant and patience and adherence should be encouraged until the required improvements have been achieved. Hale (1997) is positive in his view that all antidepressants are equally effective, if prescribed at the recommended dosage. He goes on to identify, for mild and moderate depression, the efficacy of cognitive behaviour therapy and antidepressants.

The most commonly prescribed antidepressants today are those which come under the label of selective serotonin reuptake inhibitors (SSRIs). Of these, Prozac (fluoxetine) and Seroxat (paroxetine) are probably the best known and most prescribed to the general public (Donoghue, 1995, 1996). Other types from the same group include: Faverin (fluvoxamine), and Lustral (sertraline).

Other antidepressants which are still prescribed originate from the tricyclic group and include Triptafen (amitriptyline), Asendis (amoxapine), Prothiaden (dothiepin), Tofranil (imipramine) and Anafranil (clomipramine).

Monoamine oxidase inhibitors (MAOIs) include Nardil (phenelzine), isocarboxazid and Parnate (tranylcypromine).

The MAOIs generally are only prescribed when patients/clients do not respond to other types of antidepressants. This is mainly due to the complications associated with dietary intake and the associated metabolic interactions of the MAOI drugs. Certain foodstuffs can interact with the medication and may cause a dangerous rise in blood pressure. When patients/clients are prescribed MAOIs they are given a treatment

Table 5.4 Common side effects from some antidepressants

Name	Dose	Side effects
Prozac (SSRI) (fluoxetine)	20 mg daily	Nausea, vomiting, diarrhoea constipation, rash, tremor, dizziness, dry mouth, headache, drowsiness, nervousness, anxiety, sexual dysfunction
Lentizol (Tricyclics) (amitriptyline)	75–150 mg daily	Dry mouth, sedation, blurred vision, constipation, difficulty with micturition postural hypotension, tremor, sweating, rashes, increased appetite and weight gain
Nardil (MAOI) (phenelzine)	15 mg × 3 daily increased if necessary to 15 mg × 4 daily	Adverse effects commonly associated with MAOIs include postural hypotension and dizziness. Other side effects include drowsiness, headache, fatigue, dry mouth, constipation and other gastrointestinal disturbances, agitation and tremors, blurred vision, difficulty with micturition, sweating, convulsions, rashes and sexual disturbances

(Please note that the medication chosen and the highlighted side effects are only indicative and the BNF should be consulted at all times. This also includes any contraindications)

card which provides instructions outlining which particular food stuffs they have to avoid, e.g. cheese, yeast extracts and alcoholic beverages. They are also directed to show the card to any practitioner who may be treating them.

There are of course potential side effects, which can occur when taking antidepressants. Some of the common side effects can be found in Table 5.4 (please note the dosage outlined is for depression only and no other condition). For more side effects and other information, including contraindications, the reader is directed to the British National Formulary (BNF, 2000).

Fifteen to 20% of those who have been treated with medication alone experience a relapse (Garland, 1996). This figure can be reduced if the individual is treated with a combination of cognitive therapy and antidepressants (Blackburn *et al.*, 1986). The selective serotonin re-uptake inhibitors (SSRIs) have been shown to have the same efficacy and speed of onset as tricyclics but offer benefits in other areas. They have increased safety in overdose. The side effects are mainly gastrointestinal, which may be better tolerated and they are not as sedating, which can be less restricting for those who need to drive. These factors may lead to increased adherence (Blenkiron, 1998). Jenaway and Paykel (1997, p. 86) commenting on the subject of adherence and the efficacy of antidepressants report that 'the apparent reduced efficacy in medical treatments may be due to poor compliance and inadequate doses caused by difficulties of tolerability and drug interactions rather than

intrinsic differences in response'. Keshavan (1997) refers to adverse mood disturbances, which can occur when patients are administered or withdrawn from medication prescribed for both mental health and physical problems. Keshavan also refers to depression and manic depression being associated with the use of anabolic steroids.

The practitioner has to be aware of the possible side effects of antidepressants. This primarily recognizes the fact that if an individual is already suffering due to their physical illness, then potentially to exacerbate their situation and experience, as a result of taking antidepressants, can only complicate an already difficult situation.

Conclusion

This chapter has attempted to provide an overview of depression and physical illness using the application of different models of care and their associated influencing factors on the practitioner's approach. The medical model provides a diagnosis (DSM, 1988), which is not patient/client centred. It looks for presenting signs and symptoms to fit the diagnostic criteria and then treats with the appropriate medication. Assessment tools have been briefly reviewed, providing the practitioner with an aid to enhance the specific care approach. The cognitive behavioural model (CBT) (Beck *et al.*, 1979; Scott, 1995) acknowledges the client/patient as an individual and examines/explores their personal thoughts and behaviour. Interpersonal therapy (Klerman *et al.*, 1984) accepts that the individual exists within other relationships and improving these can be beneficial. This is supported by Langford *et al.*'s (1997) social comparison theory, where stable relationships are perceived as vital to an individual's sense of well-being. The application and use of medication is described, recognizing the potential side effects.

So referring once again to depression, it can be a stand-alone condition, but it can also be an added complication of a physical illness. The practitioner has to adopt a holistic approach, balancing the different models of care. All approaches are appropriate, depending upon the specific and presenting situation and an accurate assessment of the individual.

Information on support Depression Alliance is a UK charity offering help to people with depression, run by sufferers themselves. Their web site contains information about the symptoms of depression, treatments for depression, as well as Depression Alliance campaigns and local groups.

Depression Alliance
35 Westminster Bridge Road,
London SE1 7JB
Tel. 0207 6330557; www.depressionalliance.org.uk

References

Bandura A (1977) Self-efficacy: toward a unifying theory of behavioural change. *Psychological Review* **84**, 191–215

Beck A T (1983) *Cognitive Therapy of Depression: New perspectives in Treatment of Depression: Old controversies and New Approaches* (P J Clayton, J E Barrat, eds). Ravens Press, New York

Beck A T, Steer R A (1993) *Beck Depression Inventory Manual.* The Psychological Corporation, San Antonio

Beck A T, Ward C H, Mendleson M, Mock J, Erbaugh J (1961) An inventory for measuring depression. *Archives of General Psychiatry* **4**, 561–571

Beck A T, Weissrnan A, Lester D, Trexler L (1974) The measurement of pessimism: the hopelessness scale. *Journal of Consultant Clinical Psychology* **41**, 861–865

Beck A T, Rush A J, Shaw B F, Emery G (1979) *Cognitive Therapy of Depression: A Treatment Manual.* Guilford Press, New York

Bernard L C, Krupat E (1993) *Health Psychology: Biopsychosocial Factors in Health and Illness.* Harcourt Brace College Publishers, Florida

Blackburn I, Euson K, Bishop S (1986) A two-year naturalist follow-up of depressed patients treated with cognitive therapy. *Journal of Affective Disorders* **10**, 67–75

Blenkiron P (1998) The management of depression in primary care: a summary of evidence based guidelines. *Psychiatric Care* **5**, 172–177

BNF (2000) *British National Formulary.* British Medical Association and the Royal Pharmaceutical Society of Great Britain, London

British Medical Association and Royal Pharmaceutical Society of Great Britain (2000) *British National Formulary.* British Medical Association and the Royal Pharmaceutical Society of Great Britain, London

Chernomas W M (1997) Experiencing depression: women's perspectives in recovery. *Journal of Psychiatric and Mental Health Nursing* **4**, 393–400

Clarkson P (1998) Using screening instruments to detect depression in primary care. *Community Mental Health*, **1**, (4)

Cox J L, Holden J M, Sagovsky R (1987) Detection of postnatal depression: development of the 10 item Edinburgh Postnatal Depression Scale. *British Journal of Psychiatry* **150**, 782–786

Creed F (1997) Assessing depression in the context of physical illness. In (Robertson M M, Katona C L E, eds) *Depression and Physical Illness; Perspectives in Psychiatry* Vol 6. Wiley, New York

Cunningham L A (1994) Depression in the medically ill: choosing an antidepressant. *Journal of Clinical Psychiatry* **5** (suppl. 9), 90–97

Department of Health (1990) *The Care Programme Approach for People with a Mental Illness Referred to the Specialist Psychiatric Services.* HC(90) 23/LASSL(90) 11. Department of Health, London

Department of Health (1999) *National Service Framework for Mental Health: Modern Standards and Service Models.* Department of Health, London

Dexter G, Wash M (1986) *Psychiatric Nursing Skills: a Client Centered Approach.* Croom Helm, London

Diagnostic and Statistical Manual III (1988) *DSM III.* The American Psychiatric Association, Cambridge

Diagnostic and Statistical Manual IV (1994) *DSM IV.* The American Psychiatric Association, Cambridge

Donoghue J M (1995) A comparison of prescribing patterns of selective serotonin reuptake inhibitors in the treatment of depression in primary care in the United Kingdom. *Journal of Serotonin Research* **1**, 47–51

Donoghue J M (1996) Prescribing patterns of selective serotonin reuptake inhibitors in primary care: a naturalistic follow up study. *Journal of Serotonin Research* **4**, 267–270

Dyer J A T, Kreitman N (1984) Hopelessness, depression and suicidal intent in para-suicide. *British Journal of Psychiatry* **144**, 127–133

Ellis A, Grieger R (1977) *Handbook of Rational Emotive Therapy.* Springer Verlag, New York

Endicott J (1984) Measurement of depression in patients with cancer. *Cancer* **53**, 2243–2249. Cited in: Creed F (1997) Assessing depression in the context of physical illness. In (Robertson M M, Katona C L E, eds) *Depression and Physical Illness; Perspectives in Psychiatry* Vol 6. Wiley, New York

Foote A W, Piazza D, Holcombe J, Paul P, Daffin P (1990) Hope, self-esteem and social support in persons with multiple sclerosis. *Journal of Neuroscience Nursing* **22** (3), 155–159

Frasure-Smith N, Lesperance F, Taljic M (1995) Depression and 18-month prognosis after myocardial infarction. *Circulation* **91**(4), 999–1005

Garland A (1996) Cognitive therapy in the treatment of depression. *Mental Health Nursing* **16** (3), 28–31

Gill D, Hatcher S (1998) *Antidepressants for the Depressed Physically Ill*. The Cochrane Library, Issue 4, www.cochrane.org.uk

Gotlib I, Hammen C (1992) *Psychological Aspects of Depression*. NY Wiley, New York

Hale A S (1997) ABC of clinical depression. *British Medical Journal* **315**, 43–46

Hamilton M (1960) A rating scale for depression. *Journal of Neurology, Neurosurgery and Psychiatry* **23**, 65–61

Harris E C, Barraclough B M (1995) Suicide as an outcome for medical disorders. *Medicine* **73**, 255–260

Jenaway A, Paykel E S (1997) Managing depression in the physically ill patient. In (Robertson M M, Katona C L E, eds) *Depression and Physical Illness; Perspectives in Psychiatry* Vol. 6. Wiley, New York

Katon W, Sullivan M (1990) Depression and chronic medical illness. *Journal of Clinical Psychiatry* **56**, 3–11

Katona C L E, Katona P M (1997) Geriatric depression scale can be used in older people in primary care. *British Medical Journal* **315**, 1236

Keshavan, M S (1997) Iatrogenic depression. In (Robertson M M, Katona C L E, eds) *Depression and Physical Illness; Perspectives in Psychiatry* Vol. 6. Wiley, New York

Kiloh L G, Andrews G, Neilson M (1988) The long term outcome of depressive illness. *British Journal of Psychiatry* **53**, 752–757

Kleinman (1986) *Social Origins of Distress and Disease*. Yale University Press, New Haven. Cited in: Chernomas W M (1997) Experiencing depression; women's perspectives in recovery. *Journal of Psychiatric and Mental Health Nursing* **4**, 393–400

Klerman G, Weissman M, Rounsaville B (1984) *Interpersonal Psychotherapy*. Basic Books, New York

Kramlinger K G, Swanson D W, Maruta T (1983) Are patients with chronic pain depressed? *American Journal of Psychiatry* **140**, 747–749

Langford C P H, Bowsher J, Maloney J P, Lillis B (1997) Social support: a conceptual analysis. *Journal of Advanced Nursing* **25**, 95–100

Lazarus R S, Folkman S (1984) *Stress, Appraisal and Coping*. Springer Publishing Company, New York

Liese B S, Larson M W (1995) Coping with life-threatening illness: a cognitive therapy perspective. *Journal of Cognitive Psychotherapy* **9**, 19–34

Lustman P J, Griffith L S, Clouse R E (1988) Depression in adults with diabetes. *Diabetes Care*, **11**, 605–612

McDaniel J S, Musselman D L, Porter M R, Deed D A, Nemeroff, C B (1995) Depression with patients with cancer. Diagnosis, biology and treatment. *Archive of General Psychiatry* **52**, 89–99

Mayou R A (1997) Depression and type of physical disorder and treatment. In (Robertson M M, Katona C L E, eds) *Depression and Physical Illness; Perspectives in Psychiatry* Vol. 6. Wiley, New York

Montgomery S A, Asberg M (1979) A new depression scale designed to be more sensitive to change. *British Journal of Psychiatry* **134**, 382–389

Morley S, Eccleston C, Williams A (1999) Systematic review and meta-analysis of randomized control trials of cognitive behaviour therapy and behaviour therapy for chronic pain in adults, excluding headaches. *Pain* **80**, 1–13

Noble T W (1996) Psychosocial aspects of cancer and its treatment. In (Hancock B, ed.) *Cancer Care in the Community*. Radcliffe Medical Press, Oxford

Ogden J (1996) *Health Psychology: a textbook*. Open University Press, London

Paykel E S, Priest R G (1992) Recognition and management of depression in general practice: consensus statement. *British Medical Journal* **305**, 198–202

Peden A R (1996) Recovering from depression a one year follow up. *Journal of Psychiatric and Mental Health Nursing* **3**, 289–295

Rehm L (1979) *Behaviour Therapy for Depression*. Academic Press, New York

Rihmer Z (1997) Recognition of depression and prevention of suicide. *International Journal of Psychiatry in Clinical Practice* **1** (2), 131–134

Roberts A, Priest R G (1995) Depression in the community. *Primary Care Psychiatry* **1**, 5–13

Rodin G, Voshart K (1986) Depression in the medically ill: An overview. *American Journal of Psychiatry* **143**, 696–705

Romano J M, Good A B (1994) Recent advances in chronic pain. *Current Opinion in Psychiatry* **7**, 494–497

Scott J S (1995) Psychological treatments for depression: an update. *British Journal of Psychiatry* **167**, 289–292

Sheikh J A, Yesavage J A (1986) Geriatric Depression Scale (GDS): recent findings and development of a shorter version. In (Brink T L, ed.) *Clinical Gerontology: A Guide to Assessment and Intervention*. Howarth Press, New York

Stevens E S (1992) Reciprocity in social support: An advantage for the ageing family. *The Journal of Contemporary Human Services* 533–541. Cited in: Langford C P H, Bowsher J, Maloney J P, Lillis B (1997) Social support: a conceptual analysis. *Journal of Advanced Nursing* **25**, 95–100

Thomas V J N (2000) Cognitive behavioural therapy in pain management for sickle cell disease (SCD). *International Journal of Palliative Nursing*, **9**, 434–442

Van Houdenhove B, Onghena P (1997) Pain and depression. In (Robertson M M, Katona C L E, eds) *Depression and Physical Illness; Perspectives in Psychiatry* Vol. 6. Wiley, New York

art Two

ease management

Chapter

6

Diabetes

Alison Crumbie

Introduction and patient's perspective

The following is an extract from an interview with a patient who has lived with Type 1 diabetes mellitus for 20 years.

At the beginning

I thought I was getting the flu just before we went on holiday so I wasn't very excited about going. We were going with friends and their little girl for 2 weeks. The first week it was OK except I felt thirsty, it was unbelievable. We were in Devon and it was warm and my mouth got so dry and my lips stuck to my teeth. I was thinking 'ooo what's wrong with me?' And I couldn't get up, I was supposed to be sharing the housework but I couldn't force myself to get up. Then in the second week I thought I would need to get new glasses. My eyes had gone all fuzzy and out of focus. We managed to get to the seaside but I couldn't see the signposts or anything and I wasn't at all well.

Living with the condition

The day-to-day business is that you have to be quite in control. You have to think what you're going to do during the day and then compensate or add extra food. It's all concentration it seems to me and dedication. It gets ever so tiring sometimes you just get fed up and you want to forget it – perhaps most people feel like that. I must admit to feeling depressed now and again and thinking

'it's too much and I can't cope'. I don't think my routine changes, it's just how I feel at that particular time.

Sometimes you just feel like you're ploughing a lonely furrow. Nobody says 'oh you're doing really well, you've got good control' it's just one of those things you've got to face up to and you've got to do. It is becoming marginally better because you can chat to other people about it. In the last two years of my working life I worked with a chap who had diabetes, but everyone's an individual aren't they? You can't say 'oh wow I do so and so' it's just a bit of moral support that you two are in the same boat.

The problem with food

In the early days I didn't communicate well with the dietician. She kept talking about carbohydrates and I didn't know what a carbohydrate was in those days. It was very iffy this passing of knowledge. Anyway I did get some help from someone who was checking me and by doing some reading.

Lots of times I would just love more potatoes or a big piece of pudding and I don't have it so you feel (pause) and this is the thing, I felt in the beginning. You can feel quite deprived if you don't get these things but having said that I can eat certain amounts of ice cream and other bits and pieces.

When the TV adverts are on it's always in the middle of the evening and they're advertising chocolate bars or whatever and you think 'ooh I could just eat one of those'. You see when you've been free and easy and you've been able to eat whatever you want and then all of a sudden there's this restriction and you can't eat what you want, well you can but it's all measured and you certainly can't go around tucking into bars of chocolate and sweeties and things like that so you do feel, well I felt, quite deprived at first but I've got over that now.

I feel lighter about it these days, perhaps I concentrated on it too much before.

Prevalence of diabetes

In the UK 1.4 million people have diabetes (Diabetes UK, 2000a). The number has been estimated to reach 3 million by 2010 (Melville *et al.*, 2000). The cost to the UK National Health Service is estimated to be £4.9 billion a year (Diabetes UK, 2000b). The prevalence of diabetes in people of different ethnic groups, genders and people of different ages varies enormously. The Pima Indians have been found to have a 34% rate of Type 2 diabetes mellitus, while the general prevalence in the UK is 3%. High rates of diabetes have been found in the South Asian population living in the UK with rates as high as 16% in the 40–65 age group (Mackinnon, 1998). Afro-Caribbean people also have a slightly higher prevalence. It was thought that diabetes was more common in men than women (Diabetes UK, 2000a). However, more recently Diabetes UK (2001) have indicated that diagnosis is equally common in both genders. The prevalence of Type 2 diabetes increases with increasing age. Prevalence in the 40–49 year age group can be as low as 1% with the rate increasing to over 4% in the 70–79 year age group (Mackinnon, 1998).

Classification and terminology

In June 2000 the British Diabetic Association (BDA) adopted the recommendations of the World Health Organization (World Health Organization, 2000) to change the diagnostic criteria for diabetes mellitus. The classification and definitions of diabetes mellitus were also clarified at the time and the following section provides a summary of those recommendations.

Type 1 and Type 2 diabetes mellitus: the terms 'insulin-dependent diabetes mellitus' (IDDM) and 'non-insulin-dependent diabetes mellitus' (NIDDM) do not accurately reflect the type of diabetes a person has. A person with 'non-

insulin-dependent diabetes mellitus' could well be treated with insulin and therefore the terminology becomes problematic. It is for this reason that the use of the terms Type 1 and Type 2 diabetes mellitus are recommended. Type 1 diabetes mellitus was formally known as IDDM and Type 2 was formally known as NIDDM. Type 1 and Type 2 are terms that describe the cause of the diabetes rather than the method of treatment.

Impaired glucose tolerance: impaired glucose tolerance (IGT) is a stage of impaired glucose regulation (fasting plasma glucose <7.0 mmol/l and oral glucose tolerance test 2-hour value $>= 7.8$ mmol/l but <11.1 mmol/l).

Impaired fasting glycaemia: impaired fasting glycaemia (IFG) is the term used to classify those individuals who have fasting glucose values above the normal range but below those diagnostic of diabetes (fasting plasma glucose $>= 6.1$ mmol/l but <7.0 mmol/l). It is recommended that a person who has IFG should have an oral glucose tolerance test to exclude the diagnosis of diabetes.

IGT and IFG are not clinical entities in their own right; they are risk categories for cardiovascular disease (IGT) and/or future diabetes (IFG).

Gestational diabetes: gestational diabetes encompasses the group of people who have gestational impaired glucose tolerance and/or gestational diabetes mellitus. It is recommended that the stage of gestation at which the diagnosis is made should be recorded. As glucose tolerance changes with the duration of pregnancy, a diagnosis of impaired glucose tolerance in the third trimester should be treated with caution. The BDA recommend that clinicians should be aware of the clinical implications of impaired glucose tolerance in the third trimester and should use their own clinical judgement when diagnosing gestational diabetes in practice.

Control of glucose metabolism

Diabetes is the most common endocrine disorder with one of the defining characteristics being hyperglycaemia. In order to understand the pathophysiology of diabetes mellitus, it is helpful to begin with normal glucose metabolism. In this way we can more readily under-

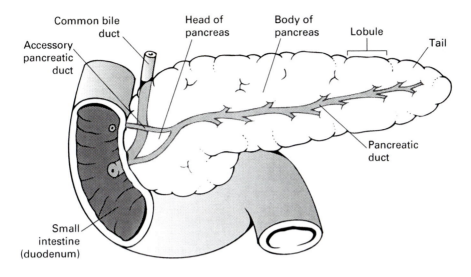

Figure 6.1 Gross anatomy of the pancreas

stand what is going wrong in diabetes and how the treatments work.

Insulin and glucagon are responsible for the regulation of glucose metabolism and these two hormones are produced by the pancreas. The pancreas is a slender organ which lies in the epigastric and left hypochondriac regions of the abdominal cavity (see Figure 6.1). The head of the pancreas lies in the curve of the duodenum and the body lies behind the stomach. The pancreas is both an exocrine and an endocrine gland. The *exocrine* pancreas represents approximately 99% of the overall volume of the gland and is responsible for producing an enzyme-rich fluid which reaches the lumen of the digestive tract and breaks down carbohydrates, proteins and fats. The *endocrine* pancreas is made up of a small group of cells scattered among the exocrine pancreas. These clusters of cells are surrounded by a capillary network and, therefore, the hormones produced by the endocrine pancreas are passed directly into the blood stream. The endocrine clusters of cells are known as islets of Langerhans and each islet contains four different cell types, alpha, beta, delta and F-cells.

The alpha cells produce a hormone called glucagon. Glucagon is responsible for raising blood glucose levels by increasing the rate of glycogen breakdown and glucose release from the liver. The beta cells produce insulin, which has the opposite effect to glucagon as it lowers blood glucose levels by increasing the rate of glucose uptake and utilization by most of the body cells. Insulin also stimulates glycogen synthesis in skeletal muscles and the liver and therefore is responsible for the storage of glucose in the body. The delta cells produce a peptide hormone called somatostatin and the F-cells produce a hormone called pancreatic polypeptide (Martini, 1995). We will focus on insulin and glucagon as these two hormones are responsible for the regulation of blood glucose.

Insulin is released when blood glucose levels rise above normal levels. The insulin molecule binds to receptor sites on the cell membrane producing a series of effects which cause the blood glucose levels to fall. This has resulted in the insulin hormone being described as 'the hormone of nutrient storage' (Hinchcliffe *et al.*, 1999, p. 218). There is an increase in glucose uptake by the cell, there is an acceleration in glucose utilization by the cell, glycogen formation is stimulated in the skeletal muscles and liver cells, triglycerides are formed in adipose tissues, amino acids are absorbed and protein molecules are synthesized. Not all cell types have insulin receptors and these are known as insulin-independent cells. Insulin-independent cells can absorb and utilize glucose without insulin stimulation and examples of these include cells in the brain, kidneys, lining of the digestive tract and the red blood cells. The neural tissue has a high demand for energy but the cells do not maintain reserves of carbohydrate, lipids or proteins. Neurons must be supplied with a reliable source of glucose because they are usually unable to metabolize other molecules. Therefore, if glucose levels drop, the central nervous system cannot continue to function and the person loses consciousness.

Glucagon is released from the alpha cells when blood glucose levels fall below normal. This results in energy reserves being mobilized. Glucagon binds to the receptor in the cell membrane and this results in stimulation of the breakdown of glycogen in the skeletal muscle and liver cells and the breakdown of triglycerides. In adipose tissue, glucagon is responsible for the stimulation of glucose production in the liver by absorbing amino acids from the blood stream and converting them to glucose. The result is that the blood glucose levels rise. The action of insulin and glucagon in maintaining glucose homeostasis is summarized in Figure 6.2.

Pathophysiology of diabetes mellitus

Diabetes is a condition where there is an absolute lack or relative lack of insulin. Without insulin the body cannot utilize the available glucose and the blood glucose levels rise. There are similarities between Type 1 and Type 2 diabetes mellitus as the effects of the raised blood glucose are similar. The pathogenesis of the 2 types is, however, different and so we will consider each one in turn.

Type 1

Type 1 diabetes mellitus is thought to develop as a result of autoimmune destruction of beta cells in the islets of Langerhans. The precise reason for this destruction is unknown, although it has been suggested that a beta-cell viral infection can be a factor. The damaged beta cells elicit an inflammatory response resulting in the cells being recognized as non-self. The signs and symptoms of diabetes emerge when 90% of the beta cells are destroyed and insulin secretion falls to a critically low level. It may be several

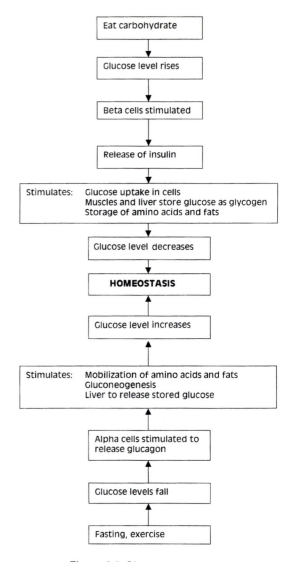

Figure 6.2 Glucose homeostasis

years before the lack of insulin secretion becomes critical but eventually the beta cell activity is unable to meet the demands of blood glucose regulation and the symptoms of diabetes become apparent. Familial patterns of Type 1 diabetes mellitus have been noted and this suggests that there may be a genetic predisposition to development of the condition.

Type 2

Like Type 1, Type 2 diabetes mellitus is thought to have a genetic component, however, the beta cells do not have the same sort of damage. Insulin levels in Type 2 diabetes may be insufficient to prevent high blood sugar or the insulin level can be normal or may even be elevated. One of the key features of Type 2 is a loss of target tissue insulin receptors and a flawed response to the binding of the receptors that are present. The patient becomes insulin resistant and the result is hyperglycaemia. Sometimes both the processes of insulin resistance and lack of insulin production occur together, however, either of these will produce the symptoms of diabetes mellitus. Both lifestyle risk factors and genetic disposition are linked to the development of Type 2 diabetes mellitus.

Risk factors for developing diabetes mellitus

The risk factors for developing Type 2 diabetes are being aged over 40 years, people of Asian and African Caribbean culture, being overweight, having a family history of diabetes, having a history of gestational diabetes in the past or any woman who has had a large baby (over 4 kilos in weight). It has been noted that the incidence of Type 2 diabetes decreases in food shortages. One theory has linked the intake of large quantities of sugar in childhood to the development of diabetes in later life (Mera, 1997). The increase in sugar intake results in large amounts of insulin being produced to deal with the sugar and ultimately this causes a decline in the capacity of the pancreatic cells to respond to the elevated glucose levels. Obesity is a risk factor for diabetes, however, not all people with Type 2 diabetes mellitus are obese and not all people who are obese have diabetes. Some studies have suggested that exercise can delay the onset of Type 2 diabetes (Mera, 1997).

The physiological effects of diabetes mellitus

The hyperglycaemia of Types 1 and 2 diabetes results in a wide range of consequences across several body systems. As the blood sugar rises it eventually exceeds the capacity of the renal tubules to reabsorb glucose and this results in the excess being lost in the urine. The loss of glucose in the urine also causes an osmotic diuresis as water molecules are prevented from being reabsorbed. The patient experiences polydipsia and polyuria and these are typical presenting symptoms of diabetes mellitus.

Reduced insulin secretion stimulates the liver to produce glucose from its stores of glycogen. This further increases the hyperglycaemia and the amount of glucose lost in the urine. As the production of glucose by the liver becomes chronic, proteins are broken down to supply the subunits for glucose synthesis, this results in weakness, fatigue and weight loss (Nowak and Handford, 1994). The reduced insulin levels also stimulate lipid metabolism resulting in hyperlipidaemia and the excessive production of ketone bodies. When there is an excess of ketones they will be excreted in the urine and through the lungs resulting in the sickly sweet smell of acetone. Ketone bodies are acidic and as they lower the pH they are toxic to the brain and the patient experiences nausea, vomiting and is at risk of acidotic coma. The physiological effects of diabetes mellitus are summarized in Figure 6.3.

The physiological effects outlined above can result in the presenting symptoms of polydipsia, polyuria, weakness, fatigue and weight loss. In addition to these symptoms, the patient may complain of blurred vision. There is always a concern in Type 2 diabetes that blurred vision may be a sign of one of the irreversible long-term complications, however, changes in the eye may be due to fluctuations in blood glucose. The lens of the eye is made up of cells and connective tissue. The cells obtain their nutrients from tissue fluid and the composition of this fluid alters according to the blood glucose concentrations. Large variations in blood glucose concentrations cause the lens to take up or expel water and this in turn alters the curvature of the lens (Mera, 1997). Once the blood glucose levels are under control the blurred vision can be corrected and the patient's sight returns to normal.

Chronic complications

The long-term complications of diabetes are due to damage to large and small blood vessels and to the peripheral nerves. The results of the Diabetes Control and Complications Trial (DCCT) (Diabetes Control and Complications Trial Research Group, 1993) proved that there

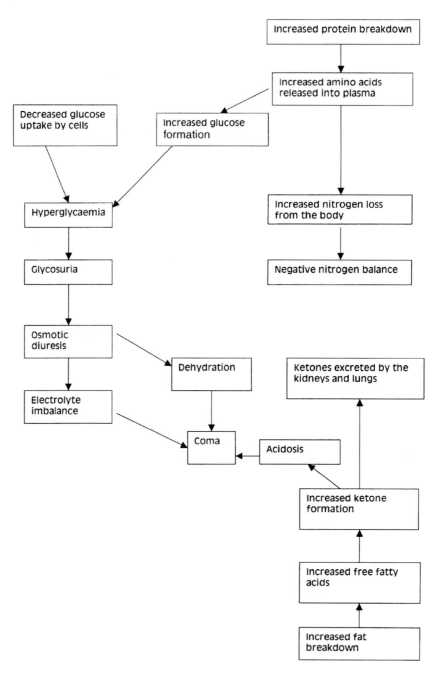

Figure 6.3 The physiological effects of diabetes mellitus. Reprinted from Hinchcliffe *et al.*, 1999, by permission of the publisher Baillière Tindall

is a link between the control of blood sugar and the development of the complications in Type 1 diabetes mellitus. The United Kingdom Prospective Diabetes Study (UKPDS) (United Kingdom Prospective Diabetes Study Group, 1998)

demonstrated not only the importance of glucose control in people with Type 2 diabetes mellitus but also the value of careful blood pressure control. Much of our work with people who have diabetes mellitus is aimed at the control of blood glucose and hypertension and hopefully the result of this is the prevention of long-term complications.

Macrovascular complications

People who live with diabetes are two to five times more likely to develop coronary heart disease, cerebrovascular disease and peripheral vascular disease (Mera, 1997). Mackinnon (1998) states that in younger patients the increased risk of dying from a heart attack is even greater at five times more likely in men and 11.5 times more likely in women. The increased risk of macrovascular complications is due to the long-term metabolic effects of hyperglycaemia. Mera (1997) states that there is evidence that excess glucose activates a protein kinase in vascular tissue. The activity of this enzyme alters the contractility of the vascular smooth muscles and alters the endothelial cell permeability. These changes result in the blood vessels being more susceptible to damage from lipoproteins and therefore the development of atherosclerosis is accelerated.

There is an increased risk of macrovascular complications in people with diabetes who also have nephropathy. Renal damage has been found to increase the prevalence of hypertension and hyperlipidaemia and accelerate the development of atheroma (Gatling *et al.*, 1997). Other risk factors for the development of coronary heart disease, cerebrovascular disease and peripheral vascular disease include hyperlipidaemia, hypertension, hyperinsulinaemia, smoking, obesity or a family history of ischaemic heart disease. The National Service Framework (NSF) for coronary heart disease (Department of Health, 2000) identifies people with diabetes as being at a high risk for the development of heart disease. The NSF recommends that people with diabetes should be targeted for assessment of their risk factors because there is no doubt that they would benefit from meticulous attention to their modifiable risk factors and stringent blood pressure control.

Hypertension is common in the diabetic population. In Type 1 diabetes, in the absence of nephropathy, the prevalence of hypertension is similar to that found in the non-diabetic population. In Type 2 diabetes, hypertension (defined as being >140/90 mmHg) is found in over 70% of patients (Ramsay *et al.*, 1999).

Hypertension has an important role in the development of the microvascular and macrovascular complications (Rottiers, 1999). In the United Kingdom Prospective Diabetes Study (UKPDS, 1998) tight blood pressure control in people with Type 2 diabetes mellitus was associated with a significant reduction in macrovascular and microvascular complications. (See Chapter 11 for a further discussion of hypertension.) Ramsey *et al.* (1999) state that optimal blood pressure targets in hypertensive diabetic people are systolic <140 mmHg and diastolic <80 mmHg.

Microvascular complications

The microvascular complications of diabetes mellitus include retinopathy neuropathy and nephropathy. Diabetic eye disease is the single most common cause of blindness in the 20–60 year age group (Gatling *et al.*, 1997) and diabetic nephropathy is the single most common cause of end-stage renal failure among adult patients starting on renal replacement therapy in the UK (NHS Centre for Reviews and Dissemination, 2000). The mechanism of the damage to the small blood vessels is unclear although a thickening of the basement membrane has been noted with increased permeability between endothelial cells.

Retinopathy

It has been estimated that 26–35% of the diabetic population will have retinopathy at any one time (Gatling *et al.*, 1997). Patients who present with Type 2 diabetes are often found to have retinal changes at the time of diagnosis. The pathological changes in the eyes develop in two main stages, the first stage being background retinopathy where the patient may not notice any change in vision and the second stage is maculopathy or proliferative retinopathy. In background retinopathy the small blood vessels have abnormally fragile walls and tend to leak. The leaked fluid can accumulate in the layers of the retina and in some areas capillaries become occluded causing ischaemia. The accumulation of fluid around the macula of the eye results in maculopathy and the patient will notice a decrease in visual acuity. The walls of the blood vessels in the fluid-filled area become fragile and dilated.

This results in microaneurysms, which are susceptible to haemorrhage (Mera, 1997). These haemorrhages can severely impair vision and, if they are present on the macula, they lead to blindness.

Ischaemia and retinal damage cause proliferation of abnormal new blood vessels. The new blood vessels have very thin walls and grow on the surface of the retina; they have a tendency to bleed and form scars on the retina. The formation of the scar tissue results in retraction of the tissues leading to retinal detachment, which again can cause irreversible blindness. In addition to retinopathy, people with diabetes are also susceptible to glaucoma, ocular motor palsies and cataracts. An efficient screening programme is essential to detect changes in the eyes at an early stage and to reduce the incidence of this disabling complication of diabetes.

Nephropathy

The pathological changes in diabetic nephropathy include renal hypertrophy, glomerulosclerosis and capillary basement membrane thickening. The damage to the kidneys becomes detectable when protein is excreted in the urine in higher concentrations than normal. As the condition progresses this eventually leads to renal failure. At an early stage in the progression of the damage, very low levels of protein can be detected in the form of microalbuminuria. Microalbuminuria has been defined as 20–200 µg/min in urine collected in patients at rest or 30–300 mg/24 h in a 24-hour urine sample (NHS Centre for Reviews and Dissemination, 2000). Fewer than 5% of deaths among people with Type 2 diabetes are directly attributed to renal disease. It has been found, however, that the death rate among people with Type 2 diabetes who also have microalbuminuria is more than double that found in people with normal urinary albumin levels (Dinneen and Gerstein, 1997).

Neuropathy

Neuropathy in the person with diabetes causes a great deal of discomfort and distress. There are three types of neuropathy: sensory, motor and autonomic dysfunction. The mechanism for the development of neuropathy in diabetes is poorly understood, however, accumulation of sorbitol and fructose within the nerve from the excess glucose is thought to cause the nerves to swell and this interferes with nerve conduction. Damage to small blood vessels supplying nutrients to the nerves also contributes. Demyelination and degeneration of the axons occurs resulting in neuropathy, which may be in a single nerve, for example the third cranial nerve leading to a palsy of the eyelid or it may occur in several nerves, for example in the generalized sensory loss in peripheral neuropathy.

Sensory neuropathy is common in people with diabetes. People complain of numbness or tingling in their toes and feet and eventually sensation in the feet is lost. This increases the risk of ulceration and damage to the feet. Neuropathy can also occur as autonomic dysfunction. Problems associated with autonomic neuropathy include poor heart rate control, loss of control over pupilomotor function, a change in gastrointestinal motility and changes in genitourinary function. Autonomic neuropathy associated with the heart can lead to postural hypotension, tachycardia and painless ischaemia or myocardial infarction. This can result in the patient with diabetes mellitus having a 'silent myocardial infarction' which may not be noticed until an electrocardiogram is recorded for other reasons. One of the more common neuropathies is associated with gastrointestinal function. This can result in the patient experiencing constipation or diarrhoea and has been found to be present in up to 25% of people with diabetes (Mera, 1997). It is important to distinguish between the gastrointestinal side effects of the antidiabetic medications and the potential for autonomic neuropathy because symptoms related to the side effects of medications will be treated differently to the symptoms of neuropathy.

Other symptoms associated with autonomic neuropathy include bladder disturbances and impotence. Bladder disturbances include a poor stream, overflow incontinence or urinary retention due to a neurogenic bladder. The neurogenic bladder is due to paralysis of the bladder and an inability to respond to the pressure as the bladder fills. Erectile dysfunction is another disturbance of the genitourinary system associated with neuropathy in people with diabetes. The prevalence is thought to be up to 30% of men with diabetes. The most common cause of erectile dysfunction in this group of patients is autonomic neuropathy, but it may also be due to vascular insufficiency, hormonal abnormalities, medications such as thiazides or beta-blockers, alcohol or psychological factors. The Erectile Dysfunction Alliance has issued guidelines on the management of erectile dysfunction (Alexander, 2000). (A full copy of the guidelines can be obtained by writing to Taylor Patten Communications Ltd, Communications House, 63 Woodfield Lane, Ashstead, Surrey KT21 2BT, UK.) As with all areas of assessment it is important therefore to consider the variety of differential diagnoses for the presenting symptoms.

Other complications of diabetes mellitus

Diabetic comas

People with diabetes may suffer from a loss of consciousness, either because their blood glucose is too high or because it is too low. The hyperglycaemia or hypoglycaemia effects the central nervous system resulting in coma.

Hypoglycaemia

Many patients are concerned about hypoglycaemia. They have heard that people with diabetes tend to lose consciousness and are frightened that the same will happen to them. This can often lead to patients aiming to keep their blood sugars high, which in itself is a problem because of the complications. Hypoglycaemia arises when blood sugars fall below normal physiological levels. The normal response to a fall in blood glucose levels is the release of adrenaline, glucagon and cortisol which produces gluconeogensis and production of glucose from glycogen stores and hence homeostasis is maintained. In a healthy human this system, which is driven by the nervous system, begins at blood glucose concentrations of 4 mmol/l, a continued fall below 3 mmol/l leads to cerebral dysfunction and the person is then unable to think properly. Confusion and drowsiness are evident below 2 mmol/l and coma below 1 mmol/l. If glucose is not replenished this will lead to fitting, cerebral hypoxia and death.

The symptoms of acute hypoglycaemia can be divided into autonomic and neurological. The autonomic symptoms include tremor, feeling hot, sweating, anxiety, nausea and palpitations. The neurological symptoms include dizziness, confusion, tiredness, difficulty in speaking, inability to concentrate, headache and visual disturbance. Other general symptoms include hunger, weakness, blurred vision, drowsiness and shivering. Individuals tend to have a certain pattern of symptoms, but sometimes the pattern changes and the patient is taken unawares. This can happen with ageing or in patients who have had diabetes for more than 15 years. Some patients experience hypoglycaemic symptoms with blood glucose levels which would usually be considered to be in the normal range. These patients have adapted to high levels of glucose and over time their receptors respond to a fall at a higher level than would normally be expected.

Friends or relatives comment that they notice a change in the patient's personality, mood, behaviour, disturbed sleep patterns or nocturnal sweating. These are the early signs which may then be followed by fitting or a loss of consciousness.

All diabetic people treated with insulin or sulphonylureas should be educated about hypoglycaemia and should be encouraged to educate their work colleagues and relatives. Patients need to know how to avoid hypoglycaemia and how to manage a hypoglycaemic episode should one begin to occur. Patients and family members can be advised that the blood glucose level should be raised as quickly as possible by eating quick-acting carbohydrate, such as three glucose tablets, a sweet drink such as 50 ml Lucozade or 100 ml Coca Cola. This represents 20 g of carbohydrate and should be sufficient to treat an attack. The blood glucose level should then be prevented from falling by eating a slowly absorbed carbohydrate in addition to usual snacks and meals. Examples of slow acting carbohydrates include a sandwich, two plain biscuits or one apple. It may take 10–15 minutes for symptoms to subside. If the patient is unconscious, 1 mg of glucagon can be administered subcutaneously. If consciousness does not return within 15 minutes, intravenous glucose is necessary. Family members can be advised on the use of subcutaneous glucagon as it is unsafe to force anything into the mouth of an unconscious patient.

When a patient experiences a hypoglycaemic attack there is a tendency to reduce the amount of insulin administered at the next scheduled dose or to omit or reduce the next sulphonylurea. The mechanism of hypoglycaemia should be discussed with the patient so that they can make an informed judgement about their treatment regimen. A hypoglycaemic attack can be followed by hyperglycaemia and this is known as the rebound effect. It is most likely that the regular insulin or sulphonylurea dose should be administered to avoid hyperglycaemia later in the day and with careful monitoring of blood glucose levels patients and their families can manage this quite safely. After the attack is over the patient should be encouraged to identify the reason for the hypoglycaemic attack to avoid the same thing happening in the future.

In order to avoid a recurrence of hypoglycaemia the causes of the event should be discussed with the patient. Check the patient's carbohydrate intake leading up to the episode and discuss dietary intake in general including alcohol consumption. In addition to causing hypoglycaemic episodes by inhibiting gluconeogenesis, alcohol also reduces awareness of the development of hypoglycaemia resulting in the patient's blood glucose level falling much lower than it might have otherwise done. Consider the role of exercise and whether adjustments to medication and/or dietary intake had been made in preparation for a period of exercise. Extra carbohydrate may be sufficient to cover the activity but you must also consider the period afterwards when the muscles are recharging their glycogen stores; this process can also cause hypoglycaemia. Review injection sites assessing for areas of lipohypertrophy or lipoatrophy and ask the patient where the injections are administered at each time of day. Review doses of insulin or sulphonylurea, which may need altering and consider the role of the menstrual cycle in women. Hot weather or a hot bath can accelerate insulin absorption and therefore result in hypoglycaemia. The issues to cover with a patient who experiences a hypoglycaemic episode are summarized in Table 6.1.

In the event of hypoglycaemia with a loss of warning signs, the patient is at an increased risk of suffering from a severe hypoglycaemic episode. The prevalence of asymptomatic hypoglycaemia tends to increase with increasing duration of diabetes (over 15 years). It is feasible

Table 6.1 The issues to cover with a patient who experiences a hypoglycaemic episode

Review what was happening prior to the hypoglycaemic episode:

- Carbohydrate intake
- Alcohol intake
- Level of exercise
- Consumption of food post exercise
- Adjustments to medication
- Was the patient having a hot bath

Consider the patient's usual management regimen:

- Review injection sites
- Review medications
- Consider menstrual cycle in women

to help patients regain their warning signs but these patients should be monitored very closely and usually need the expertise of the hospital diabetes team. The management involves avoiding hypoglycaemia completely to allow the warnings to return over a few weeks.

In all cases of hypoglycaemia, consider the patient's safety to drive or to operate machinery. The safety of others should be considered in addition to the safety of the patient.

Hyperglycaemia

Hyperglycaemia can occur for a variety of reasons such as the omission of medication, excessive consumption of food, or most often, during a period of intercurrent illness. Any type of infection generally causes the blood glucose levels to rise, this is due to the release of hormones such as cortisol and adrenaline. These hormones antagonize insulin and what insulin the patient has available becomes less effective. If a patient is suffering from vomiting or diarrhoea, the common mistake is to stop taking insulin (in the belief that this will cause hypoglycaemia in the absence of dietary intake). Another common error is to take syrupy cough linctuses when suffering from a cough. This further elevates the blood glucose level and puts the patient at risk of hyperglycaemia. There are two types of hyperglycaemic comas in people with diabetes, diabetic ketoacidosis (DKA) or hyperosmolar non-ketotic coma (HONK).

Diabetic ketoacidosis

The symptoms of DKA tend to develop over a period of 1–2 days, however, in obese people with Type 2 diabetes the onset can be insidious and the rising blood glucose level may only be found on routine blood testing or urinalysis. The symptoms may include polyuria, polydipsia, fever, nausea, vomiting, abdominal pain and fatigue followed by mental confusion, rapid deep breathing and a characteristic fruity odour on the breath. The end result of DKA can be death and therefore early detection of this condition is essential so that treatment and subsequent management can be initiated immediately. The health care professional can be aware of the major risk factors for DKA which include infection in young children with Type 1 diabetes and acute periods of stress such as myocardial infarction or infection in older people with Type 2. DKA may also occur in a patient who is undiagnosed as having diabetes mellitus, the lack of insulin causes hyperglycaemia and the patient subsequently develops ketoacidosis which becomes the presenting symptom for their condition. Other risk factors include anything that might cause a relative lack in the availability of insulin and these are summarized in Table 6.2.

The mechanism of physiological disruption for DKA commences with an inadequate production of insulin or an increased need for insulin. Due to the insulin deficiency the cells cannot utilize the available glucose and the blood glucose level rises. Glucose is lost in the urine causing an osmotic diuresis, weakness and fatigue. The low insulin level stimulates protein breakdown and lipid metabolism. Protein is broken down to provide the body with the subunits from which glucose can be synthesized in gluconeogenesis. The products of lipid metabolism are acetone and keto acids and as they accumulate they produce ketoacidosis. The body initiates compensation mechanisms to deal with the level of acidosis and therefore breathing becomes rapid in an attempt to remove carbon dioxide from the system and thereby increase the blood pH. Ketone bodies are volatile and produce the acetone breath found in DKA. Dehydration resulting from the osmotic diuresis causes a drop in blood pressure, tachycardia and shock. The marked dehydration also causes blood coagulation resulting in myocardial, brain and bowel infarction. The meta-

Table 6.2 Risk factors for diabetic ketoacidotic coma

Insufficient sulphonylurea or insulin dose

Poor injection technique with overuse of injection sites

Reduced activity

Infection or illness, such as myocardial infarction or stroke

Use of medication affecting glycaemic control (i.e. steroid therapy)

Life changes causing stress

Weight increase

Increase in food consumption

bolic acidosis resulting from the metabolism of lipids is toxic to the brain and causes confusion and coma. The combination of mechanisms occurring in DKA are life threatening and Mera (1997) estimates that 2% of people admitted to hospital with a primary diagnosis of DKA die. The mechanism of metabolic disturbances in diabetic ketoacidosis is summarized in Figure 6.4.

Due to the serious nature of DKA, patients and their significant others need to be educated about the causes of this condition and how to avoid it. An understanding of diabetes mellitus in general will help the patient to realize the significance of good injection techniques, the role of exercise, the importance of dietary management and the role of insulin or sulphonylureas. The patient should be introduced to sick day rules which will help them to cope in the event of intercurrent illness. A summary of the sick day rules can be found in Table 6.3.

In addition to a heightened awareness in patients and family members, health care professionals need to be acutely aware of this potential complication of diabetes. Immediate action includes a thorough assessment to confirm the diagnosis, determine precipitating causes and identify how severe the dehydration is. Gatling *et al.* (1997) suggest that the patient should be referred to secondary care if there is evidence of persistent vomiting for more than 4 h, there are signs of dehydration, any disturbances of consciousness, hyperventilation, inability to take oral fluids, significant ketonuria, acute illness in pregnancy, suspected myocardial infarction, stroke or trauma. If a patient is

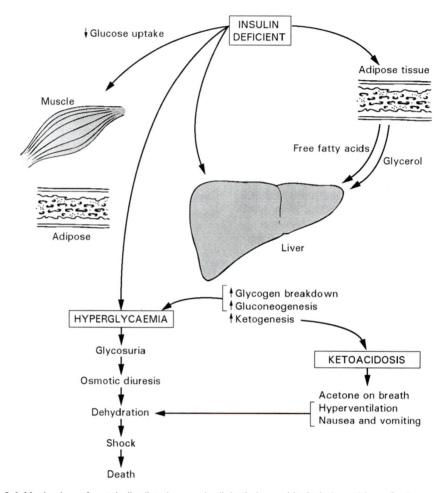

Figure 6.4 Mechanism of metabolic disturbances in diabetic ketoacidosis (adapted from Gatling *et al.*, 1997)

transferred to secondary care, the team will need to build upon the assessment made by the referring health care professional, initiate investigations and consider the need for fluid replacement, insulin, potassium and anticoagulation. Diabetic ketoacidosis is a complicated process involving dehydration, electrolyte imbalance, acidosis and possibly cerebral oedema at the same time. It takes a great deal of skill to manage such a situation and many units have strict guidelines to help staff cope should such a situation arise (Harrop *et al.*, 1999). It is essential to consider prevention of DKA as part of the holistic care of people with diabetes by providing the patient with information about the potential causes of hyperglycaemia and encouraging self-monitoring and self-care.

Hyperosmolar non-ketotic coma

In some cases of people with Type 2 diabetes a non-acidotic coma may arise. This condition is known as hyperglycaemic, hyperosmolar non-ketotic coma or HONK. The features of HONK are hyperglycaemia (can be as high as 60 mmol/l) with severe dehydration. There is a lack of ketoacidosis due to the small amount of circulating insulin which appears to inhibit ketogenesis. As the patient is not acidotic, they do not have the hyperventilation and acetone breath of DKA. HONK is, however, as serious as DKA, particularly in the elderly and therefore any patient suspected of having this condition should be referred to secondary care for immediate management. In secondary care the patient undergoes a thorough assessment and

Table 6.3 Sick day rules

Never stop or reduce your insulin dose

Measure blood glucose more frequently (four times a day)

If blood glucose remains below 11 mmol/l continue with your normal insulin dose

If blood glucose levels are above 11 mmol/l consider the need to increase your insulin and discuss this with your health care professional

If you are unable to eat, replace your normal carbohydrate with milk or a glucose drink and drink plenty of sugar-free fluids (at least 3 litres per day)

If you have a temperature take 2 paracetamol or 2 aspirin tablets up to four times a day

Test urine for ketones and if there is a moderate to large amount present contact your GP or diabetes team

If your blood glucose is above 17 mmol/l, if you are vomiting and cannot keep down liquids for 2 to 3 hours or if you are alone, contact your health care professional for support

(Gatling *et al.*, 1997)

investigations with management directed at correcting the hyperglycaemia and dehydration. Risk factors for developing HONK include undiagnosed diabetes, poorly controlled diabetes, infection, old age, consumption of large quantities of glucose and medications such as diuretics.

It is important to consider the potential differential diagnoses in the person with diabetes who lapses into a coma. Faced with the unconscious patient the clinician needs to consider the differences between hypoglycaemia and hyperglycaemia. A thorough assessment and history taken from relatives or friends can be helpful. A person with hypoglycaemia is likely to be drenched in sweat, whereas a person with hyperglycaemia is going to be dehydrated and is more likely to have vomited. The pupils are often dilated in hypoglycaemia and the person with hyperglycaemia is going to be hyperventilating with the sweet smell of acetone on the breath. A finger prick blood test will determine hypo- or hyperglycaemia and urinalysis (which should not be relied upon for glucose detection) will determine if there is an excess of ketones in the urine, strongly suggestive of DKA. With a careful assessment the patient can be treated

effectively and the likelihood of developing devastating consequences can be reduced.

The assessment of the patient with diabetes mellitus

Diagnostic criteria

It has been estimated that a quarter of patients who are diagnosed with Type 2 diabetes have long-term complications at the time of diagnosis and that the average time of onset of Type 2 diabetes to diagnosis is 10–12 years (Brashers, 1998). It is essential therefore to be alert to the signs of diabetes mellitus and to be aware of the risk factors for the development of this disorder. Early diagnosis will result in improved glucose control from an early stage in the disease process and this should therefore prevent the long-term complications of diabetes and improve quality of life for the patient.

The diagnosis of diabetes has important legal and medical implications and therefore it is essential to be accurate in this clinical decision. A diagnosis should never be made on the basis of glycosuria or a finger prick blood glucose alone and HbA1c is not recommended for diagnosis.

The following diagnostic criteria are based on the World Health Organization's publication *Definition, Diagnosis and Classification of Diabetes Mellitus and its Complications* (WHO, 2000). The British Diabetes Association (BDA) recommended that all health care professionals in the UK should adopt these criteria in June 2000 (British Diabetic Association, 2000).

Diabetes symptoms (polyuria, polydipsia and unexplained weight loss) plus:

- a random venous plasma glucose concentration $>= 11.1$ mmol/l or
- a fasting plasma glucose concentration $>= 7.0$ mmol/l or
- a 2 hour plasma glucose concentration $>= 11.1$ mmol/l 2 hours after 75 g anhydrous glucose in an oral glucose tolerance test.

With no symptoms diagnosis should not be based on a single glucose determination but requires confirmatory plasma venous determination. At least one additional glucose test result on another day with a value in the diabetic range is essential either fasting from a random sample or from the 2 hour post glucose load. If the fasting or random values are not diagnostic the 2 hour value should be used.

Children frequently present with severe symptoms and diagnosis should be made in this instance on a single raised blood glucose result and referral to the paediatric diabetic team should not be delayed.

Diabetes UK recommends that all those with impaired fasting glucose should have an oral glucose tolerance test to exclude the diagnosis of diabetes and, in addition, these people should be actively managed with lifestyle advice. In patients who continue to have an elevated blood glucose lifestyle advice still needs to be continued; however, treatment with antidiabetic medications will have to be considered.

Treatment

Once a person with diabetes has been diagnosed with the condition some form of treatment plan will have to be considered. No person with diabetes should be considered as having 'mild' diabetes, however, some patients may only require diet to manage their condition. Other patients may require a whole range of medications in addition to the diet, depending upon their blood glucose levels, blood pressure readings and urinalysis. Whatever level of intervention is required it is important to always remain aware that each patient is an individual. Each patient will need a varying amount of education and support and their families will have a varying amount of involvement in their care. We need to remain sensitive to the needs of the patient and be prepared to adapt the treatment plan to achieve a balance that is acceptable to them. The following covers some of the main areas of treatment for people with diabetes including, diet, antidiabetic medications, insulin and antihypertensive medications.

Diet

Diet has long been the cornerstone of diabetes management. In recent years, however, we have moved away from the idea of a 'diabetic diet' and the restriction of food exchanges that was generally involved in such a diet. Today the message is that a good diet for people with

diabetes mirrors the healthy eating that is recommended for the whole population. Even though this sounds more straightforward, each person who is diagnosed with diabetes should be referred to a dietician on diagnosis and should be reviewed annually thereafter. In between those times it is the role of the whole health care team to reinforce healthy eating messages and to evaluate clinical outcomes such as lipid levels, HBA1c and body weight. At least 80% of patients who are diagnosed with Type 2 diabetes are overweight (McGough, 2000) and therefore some of the dietary advice might include weight reduction. General recommendations for dietary intake for people who are newly diagnosed with diabetes mellitus include the items listed in Table 6.4.

The results of various studies are continually updating our knowledge of diet in diabetes and more recently studies have shown that sucrose intake (the sugar used to add to tea or coffee) need not be totally restricted as sucrose is not detrimental to blood glucose control (McGough, 2000). Artificial sweeteners have no benefit over sucrose and foods marketed as 'suitable for diabetics' tend to be as high in fat and calories as standard products and are often more expensive. In addition, the sorbitol content of these foods can have a laxative effect. There is now more flexibility in the proportion of energy a patient might get from carbohydrates versus the energy taken in from fat due to the promotion of the use of mono-unsaturated fat, which has been found to

Table 6.4 Broad dietary guidelines for people who are newly diagnosed with diabetes

- If you are thirsty drink low-calorie, sugar-free squashes and fizzy drinks. Water, tea or coffee without sugar are ideal. Do not add sugar to drinks
- Try to avoid very sweet foods such as sweets, chocolates, sweet biscuits and cakes
- Eat at least five portions of fruit and vegetables every day
- Fried and fatty foods should be eaten only occasionally
- Eat regular meals which include some starchy foods such as bread, potatoes or cereal. High fibre foods are particularly good, such as wholemeal bread, high fibre breakfast cereals, jacket potatoes etc.

reduce low density lipoprotein and therefore improve lipid profiles.

Oral antidiabetic medications

Biguanides

The only biguanide available is metformin. Metformin acts by increasing the use of glucose in the peripheries and by decreasing gluconeogenesis. It is only effective in Type 2 diabetes. Metformin is the drug of choice in patients who are obese. The gastrointestinal side effects of metformin are common when the patient first begins treatment; these include anorexia, nausea, diarrhoea and vomiting. The side effects can be minimized by starting treatment with a low dose and working up to a higher dose and by advising the patient to take their medication with food. The dose of metformin is 500 mg every 8 h or 850 mg every 12 h (BNF, 2000). Metformin may provoke lactic acidosis, a serious and life-threatening diabetic emergency. It is therefore particularly important to ensure that this drug is avoided in hepatic or renal impairment, severe infection, heart failure, trauma, pregnancy and breast feeding as these conditions predispose the patient to the development of lactic acidosis.

Sulphonylureas

Sulphonylureas stimulate the pancreas to release insulin and increase the sensitivity of the peripheral tissue to circulating insulin. They can lead to weight gain and therefore should be prescribed only if poor control persists in spite of dietary management. Sulphonylureas are absorbed rapidly from the gut, although the rate of absorption is reduced if they are taken with food.

As the sulphonylureas augment the action of insulin there is the potential to cause hypoglycaemia. Patients should therefore be advised to be alert to the symptoms of low blood sugars and they should be provided with information about how to manage should such a situation arise. The risk of hypoglycaemia is particularly problematic in the elderly and in people with hepatic and renal insufficiency. Other side effects include gastrointestinal disturbances and headache, but these are usually mild and transient.

There are several different sulphonylureas, the longer acting chlorpropramide and gliben-clamide and the shorter acting gliclazide and tolbutamide. The long duration of action of chlorpropramide and glibenclamide increases the risk of hypoglycaemia in elderly people significantly and therefore the use of these drugs in this group of patients should be avoided.

The dose of the sulphonylureas varies according to which one is being used. An example is gliclazide which is taken at a dose of 40–80 mg daily up to 160 mg as a single dose and 320 mg in divided doses. Glibenclamide is taken at 5 mg daily, adjusted according to response, up to a maximum of 15 mg daily.

Thiazolidinediones (glitazones)

Rosiglitazone and pioglitazone are examples of a new class of drugs known as the peroxisome proliferator-activated-receptor-gamma (PPAR-gamma) agonists. They work by reducing the body's resistance to insulin. The National Institute for Clinical Excellence issued guidance on the use of rosiglitazone in August 2000. They recommend that rosiglitazone should only be offered to patients who are unable to tolerate the combination therapy of metformin and a sulphonylurea. It should be taken in combination with metformin or with a sulphonylurea in those patients who are unable to take metformin (NICE, 2000). The dosage of rosiglitazone is 4 mg daily and may go up to 8 mg daily after 8 weeks if used with metformin. The side effects include increased risk of infections affecting the nose, sinuses and larynx. It may also cause headaches, weight gain, anaemia and oedema. The risk of oedema is particularly increased with the concomitant use of non-steroidal anti-inflammatory drugs. Rosiglitazone should not be taken by anyone who has a history of heart failure or liver problems and it should not be taken with insulin. Liver function tests should be carried out prior to commencing treatment and then should be checked regularly for the first year. Pioglitazone became available on prescription in the UK from November 2000 and it offers further choice of medical treatment for people who live with Type 2 diabetes.

Alpha glucosidase inhibitors

An example of an alpha glucosidase inhibitor is acarbose. This drug in an inhibitor of intestinal glucosidase and therefore delays the absorption and digestion of starch and sucrose from the gut. It can be effective in reducing the postprandial hyperglycaemia in Type 2 diabetes and it can be used either on its own or in combination with metformin or a sulphonylurea. The side effects can be difficult to tolerate and include flatulence, abdominal distension and diarrhoea. The dose is 50 mg daily and it can be increased to 50 mg three times daily.

All of the oral antidiabetic treatments are for people who have Type 2 diabetes. At times of intercurrent illness such as myocardial infarction, coma, infection, trauma or planned surgery, the patient may need temporarily to use insulin treatment. It is also possible that a person with Type 2 diabetes may need eventually to progress on to treatment with insulin in combination with their oral medication. The UKPDS trial (1998) proved that tight glycaemic control would prevent complications in people with Type 2 diabetes and therefore, if oral antidiabetic treatments are not having an adequate effect you may need to encourage the patient to move on to treatment with insulin.

Insulin

There are many different insulins available for the treatment of people with diabetes. The basic principle is to provide the patient with the insulin that is lacking due to the inability of the pancreatic beta cells to produce it. There are three main types: those that have a short duration such as soluble insulin and insulin lispro; those that have an intermediate action such as insulin zinc suspensions; and those that have longer durations such as crystalline insulin zinc suspensions. It is important to consider the onset, peak activity and duration of action of the insulin being used. A useful guide to this can be found in the Monthly Index of Medical Specialities (MIMS, 2000). The administration of insulin should be tailored to the needs of the individual. Blood glucose level is only one part of the picture when deciding which form of treatment to use. You also need to consider the patient's occupation, shift pattern, exercise pattern, visual acuity, motivation and ability to manage the delivery system. Some patients may choose to use a pen to inject their insulin, others may choose a needle

and syringe. Insulin pumps are also available, although not widely used at this time.

Insulin should be administered 20–30 minutes before a meal. Insulin lispro has a rapid onset of action and can be administered immediately before a meal or, if necessary, during a meal. The injection is delivered at a 90° angle or if the patient is thin the skin should be pinched and the angle may need to be 45°. Needles come in 12 mm, 8 mm and 6 mm sizes. It is important to choose the site of injection carefully. Insulin is absorbed most quickly from the abdomen and absorption will also be increased if the injection is delivered into a limb that is then used for exercise. It is helpful for the patient to develop a rotation regimen, where they might use the abdomen in the morning and at lunch time and the thigh later in the day. Injection sites should be checked for signs of lipoatrophy or lipohypertrophy and the patient instructed on rotating around each site to avoid this complication. Insulin that is not being used should be stored in the fridge at 2–8°C, however, pens or the vial that is currently being used can be left at room temperature for 28 days.

The major side effect of insulin treatment is hypoglycaemia. The patient should be provided with information on how to avoid this problem. You may want to refer to the notes on hypoglycaemia earlier in this chapter. Other side effects include local reaction at the injection site, lipohypertrophy and lipoatrophy.

Other medications

In addition to the reduction of blood glucose it is likely that the person with diabetes will need to be treated for their hypertension and hyperlipidaemia. Cardiovascular disease is the biggest cause of morbidity and mortality in Type 2 diabetes (Jones, 2000) and therefore the prevention of cardiac events needs to be taken seriously in this group of patients. (For a full discussion of the use of antihypertensive and lipid lowering treatments see Chapter 11.)

Self-monitoring

In most patients with diabetes self-monitoring of their condition will be necessary. Some patients may have been advised to test their urine to check for glucose and ketones. This is an unreliable test, however, as individual patient's renal thresholds for glucose vary and the test result is based on urine that may have been in the patient's bladder for some time. Blood glucose monitoring is more accurate, although it is more expensive and involves an invasive procedure. There are many blood glucose monitors available and the choice of machine will depend on individual preference and dexterity. The test results will rely upon the patient using a correct technique and this includes washing the hands before carrying out the technique and being able to produce an adequate amount of blood. Blood glucose monitoring provides essential information both to the patient and to the health care professional. It can hand control back to the patient as they learn to fine tune their medication and diet according to the results.

The annual review

In addition to the patient's own monitoring of their health status, the health care team should monitor annually every person with diabetes; this can occur in the hospital, the surgery or a combination of the two. Most areas in the UK now have a diabetes register which is maintained centrally. This is an attempt to ensure that all patients are monitored regularly and that no person with diabetes is slipping through the net. The annual review includes education, support, counselling, monitoring and review. Elements of the review should be checked at every possible opportunity. When a patient with diabetes interacts with the health care system for any reason, the health care team should be considering whether this patient has had any foot care advice recently, a blood pressure check or urinalysis. The rational for including all the elements of the annual review follows, however, a summary can be found in Table 6.5.

The annual review includes:

1 Ask about general health and well-being including symptoms of vascular diseases and symptoms of neuropathy. A review of the patient's general health will help you to determine if the patient is experiencing any new symptoms, if they are feeling generally tired and if they have noticed any change

Table 6.5 Summary of the elements in the annual review

The annual review includes:

Blood test for	HBA1c and blood glucose level
	U&E
	Serum creatinine
	Lipid profile (depending on age)

Early morning urine for microalbuminuria

Urinalysis for protein, ketones and glucose

Weight, height, BMI

Ask about general health and well-being including:
 symptoms of vascular diseases
 symptoms of neuropathy (include erectile
  dysfunction as appropriate)
 alcohol and smoking
 review self-monitoring results
 measure BP sitting and standing
 ensure that retina has been examined within
  the last 12 months
 examine feet including vibration, sensation,
  position sense, pulses, light touch and reflexes
 examine injection sites
 review medications
 review dietary management
 check travel plans
 young women: check plans for pregnancy
 check understanding of hypoglycaemia and
  hyperglycaemiaplan for further review

Check membership of Diabetes UK and other sources of support

in their health. This allows the patient to start with anything that might be troubling them and it also clues you into areas of the review that may require special consideration. For example, if the patient reports that they have noticed they have been more breathless recently you might consider an examination of the cardiovascular system.

2 Many patients will have been carrying out some form of self-monitoring. It is very important to take notice of these results, whether you feel they might give you some useful information or not. The patient will have spent a great deal of time compiling the information relating to blood glucose or urinalysis and this is part of their active role in the management of their diabetes. Taking the results seriously helps to emphasize the importance of their contribution to the process and therefore it is important to focus on these results in detail. If the patient

has been monitoring blood glucose regularly this will give you a great deal of valuable information upon which to make decisions about treatment.

3 At least once a year the patient will need to be investigated with blood tests for HbA1c, blood glucose level, urea and electrolytes, serum creatinine and lipid profile. Blood glucose level provides an immediate record of the patient's blood glucose control but this does not tell you anything about their average control over the preceding months. HbA1c is a record of glycosylated haemoglobin and it provides an invaluable tool in the management of diabetes as it represents the average plasma glucose concentrations over a period of 2 months. Glucose in the blood combines with proteins to form permanently glycated proteins. The percentage of glycated protein in the plasma depends upon the glucose concentration and the half-life of the particular protein. Haemoglobin is found in red blood cells and as they live for 120 days the half-life is 60 days or 2 months. In the non-diabetic person HbA1c would be in the range of 3–5%. This can rise as high as 20% in a person with poorly controlled diabetes, however we should be aiming for 7% or less in a person who is well controlled. A record of HBA1c on more than one occasioin each year can check for control in between annual reviews.

Urea, electrolytes and creatinine provide valuable information about the patient's renal function. Not only is nephropathy a complication of diabetes, it is also a potential side effect of many of the medications which may be used in the person with diabetes. Renal impairment is also a contraindication for the use of metformin in diabetes. It is therefore important to make an accurate assessment of the patient's renal profile.

It has been suggested that in patients with diabetes, lipid profiles can predict mortality more closely than glycaemic control (Florkowski *et al.*, 1998) and that diabetic patients without previous myocardial infarction may be at as high a risk of myocardial infarction as the non-diabetic patient who has had a previous myocardial infarction (Haffner *et al.*, 1998). Leese *et al.* (2000) found that even though hyperlipidaemia was identified in people with diabetes both in the hospital and primary care setting, it was not well treated or monitored. It is therefore important to screen all people with diabetes for lipid profiles. The person with diabetes should not be screened for lipid levels at the time of diagnosis as the hyperglycaemia present at this time may falsely elevate the result. Screening should take place approximately 3 months after diagnosis and then once a year. If lipids are found to be elevated a plan for management needs to be developed, however, it is also important to consider testing for secondary causes of the hyperlipidaemia such as thyroid disorder or liver dysfunction. For a more detailed discussion of hyperlipidaemia in relation to coronary heart disease see Chapter 11.

4 A sample of the patient's early morning urine should be tested for glucose, ketones, protein and microalbuminuria. A dipstick urinalysis can take place to determine if the patient has glycosuria to provide some information about the patient's general glycaemic control. Urinary glucose is, however, a very unreliable predictor of blood glucose levels as different people have different renal thresholds for glucose. A positive urinary glucose would, however, provide the clinician with information that might be valuable when this information is related to the patient's symptoms. It is worthwhile checking for ketones in the urine as the patient may be developing diabetic ketoacidosis without any symptoms. A dipstick should also be carried out for proteinuria. If protein is present there is no point in further testing the urine for microalbuminuria. The test for microalbuminuria is more expensive than the ordinary dipstick and therefore you should consider the quality of the urine sample before arranging to have this test done. There are several reasons why a microalbuminuria might be inaccurate and these are listed in Table 6.6. There is no doubt that microalbuminuria can be present for months or even years before renal damage progresses to overt proteinuria and it is therefore worthwhile screening for the presence of microalbumin so that progression to proteinuria and damage to the kidney can be reversed with appropriate treatment.

5 It is important to measure the patient's weight and height and to calculate body

Table 6.6 Factors which interfere with screening for microalbuminuria

---

Increases microalbuminurea:
  haematuria
  congestive heart failure
  exercise
  excessive protein intake
  fever
  uncontrolled diabetes
  uncontrolled hypertension
  urinary tract infection
  contamination of specimen

Decreases microalbuminurea:
  ACE inhibitors
  malnutrition
  NSAIDs

---

mass index (BMI – weight/height^2). The incidence of Type 2 diabetes mellitus has been found to be directly proportionate to the BMI and those with a large waist:hip ratio (i.e. central obesity) have an even higher risk (Gatling *et al.*, 1997). A patient's glucose tolerance can be improved through weight loss and conversely can decline with increasing weight. It is therefore important to monitor the patient's BMI on at least an annual basis. Targets for BMI can be found in Table 6.7.

6 Ask about smoking and alcohol consumption. The person with diabetes is at a high risk of cardiovascular complications due to the nature of the disease process, however, if they also smoke this increases the risk even further. All people who smoke should be provided with every opportunity to stop, however, this is vitally important in the person with diabetes. Smoking cessation assistance should be available for the person when they feel ready to access this service and therefore they need to be reminded of this whenever the opportunity arises. For a more detailed discussion on

Table 6.7 BMI targets

	Good	*Borderline*	*Poor*
Men	<25	<=27	>27
Women	<24	<=26	>26

smoking cessation see Chapter 8. The person with diabetes can safely consume alcohol so long as they remain within the recommended guidelines of 14 units per week for women and 21 units per week for men. This quantity of alcohol should be consumed over the period of the full week rather than in two binges at the weekend. People who take insulin or sulphonylureas should be reminded of the potentiating effects of alcohol and the potential for hypoglycaemia. If alcohol has been consumed the patient should be reminded to take a bedtime snack.

7 The measurement of blood pressure both sitting and standing is as important as the measurement of blood glucose levels, particularly in Type 2 diabetes. The blood pressure should be measured using the British Hypertension Society's guidelines as discussed in Chapter 11. The difference between sitting and standing blood pressure will help you to decide if the patient has postural hypotension and if so this would indicate the potential for autonomic nervous system dysfunction and the potential for cardiac complications. Measuring the blood pressure also provides the opportunity to listen to the rate and rhythm of the heartbeat. You should be alert to any arrhythmias or tachycardia and follow this up with a full cardiovascular examination if necessary.

8 Ensure that the patient has received an eye examination within the last 12 months. An appropriately qualified person should check the retina through dilated pupils at least annually. Due to the increased risk of eye disease in diabetes the patient needs to have a thorough examination of the eyes. The lens is checked for opacities, the pressure of the eye is checked for signs of glaucoma and the retina is examined for signs of retinopathy. On examination the clinician might observe dots, blots, hard exudates, cotton wool spots and/or new vessels. See Table 6.8 for an overview of these findings.

9 The patient's feet should be examined for signs of neuropathy or microvascular disease by carrying out a structured examination of the feet. The examination should include vibration, sensation, position sense, pulses, light touch and ankle reflexes. During the assessment of the feet the practitioner should use the opportunity to discuss with the patient methods of preventing damage

Table 6.8 Findings on examination of the retina

Feature	Type	Appearance
Dots	Microaneurysms or microhaemorrhages	Small round red lesions
Blots	Haemorrhages	Medium-sized round red lesions with an indistinct outline
Hard exudates	Oedema/lipid deposits	Irregular yellowish white deposits with a sharp outline
Cotton wool spots	Ischaemic areas	White or grey areas with indistinct outlines
New vessels	New vessels	Fine tangled mess of vessels

Gatling *et al.* (1997)

to the feet. The patient can be advised to check their feet daily for signs of broken skin, and areas of pressure and they should check between the toes for signs of fungal infection. They should wear shoes and socks that fit well and never walk around the house or garden with bare feet. If the patient has good vision, and has no unusual findings on foot examination they may be able and willing to cut their own toenails. If there is any sign of increased risk on the foot examination, however, the patient should be referred to a podiatrist or chiropodist for regular attention to their feet. It is also important to advise the patient to test the temperature of the water in their bath by using their hand before stepping into it and care for the skin of their feet by using moisturising creams to keep the skin supple and reduce the risk of cracking dry skin.

10 Repeated injection of insulin into the same sites leads to tissue damage. Injection sites should therefore be examined for signs of lipohypertrophy or atrophy as this will make the absorption of insulin erratic. An examination of the sites at the annual review provides an opportunity for the health care professional to emphasize the importance of site rotation and to point out the potential hazards if care is not taken with insulin administration.

11 It is always valuable to ask the patient what medications they are taking and to allow them to tell you in their own words. It is easy to ask the question 'you are taking the gliclazide twice a day aren't you?' and the patient simply answers 'yes', but you may not have discovered what the patient is really taking. If you allow them to tell you how they are managing their diabetes you

should also be prepared to be told that they occasionally miss a dose depending upon what they are doing or how they feel. An assessment of all the medications that the patient is taking will help you to determine if there are any interactions between the drugs or if other medications might be adversely effecting glycaemic control.

12 The patient's understanding of dietary management should be assessed. There tends to be an assumption that a patient who has lived with diabetes for many years will have an accurate working knowledge of the diet required to manage diabetes. In many cases this is accurate, however, it is always worthwhile discussing issues relating to diet with the patient as they may have some concerns over conflicting messages in the media or they may have picked up information from other sources which may need some clarification. Discussing the diet also emphasizes the fact that dietary management represents the cornerstone to the control of diabetes mellitus and this will serve to raise awareness of this issue with the patient.

13 Check travel plans with the patient. There are some destinations that require some extra planning to ensure that the person has access to the necessary equipment while away from home. Diabetes UK can help to advise on insurance policies for travel abroad and can also provide some specific advice for people who need to carry insulin equipment and other supplies overseas.

14 If the patient is a young woman, check her plans for pregnancy. A pregnancy in a woman who has diabetes is considered to be a high-risk event in obstetric terms. At one stage 50% of pregnancies in women who had diabetes ended in the death of

the fetus (Mera, 1997). The outlook now is much improved and the majority of women can expect to deliver a healthy baby. The key to this improvement is tight glycaemic control both before conception and during the pregnancy. If the woman is considering pregnancy she should be referred to secondary care for specialized management and advice prior to conception and this support should continue throughout the pregnancy.

15 Check the patient's understanding of hypoglycaemia and hyperglycaemia. If the patient is being treated with a sulphonylurea or insulin there is always a risk of hypoglycaemia. The patient needs to be aware of the risk and ways to be aware of what is happening, how to treat it and how to avoid it (see Management of hypoglycaemia on p. 67). It is also important to determine who else needs to know about hypoglycaemia and whether the patient has discussed this with them. This may include family members, friends or people at work. The person needs to be alerted to the fact that an infection, such as vomiting and diarrhoea, the 'flu or a cold for example, could potentially elevate the blood glucose level (see Development of hyperglycaemia on p. 68). The patient's understanding of the sick day rules should be checked (see Table 6.3).

16 Regardless of where the review of the patient takes place a plan for follow up is essential. It may be that you meet the patient in a walk-in centre and that you are simply covering a few of the annual review items listed here. However, it is important to determine that the patient is being reviewed fully either in the hospital outpatient clinic or at the surgery.

17 Check where the patient is getting support from and ensure that the contact details for local self-help groups are made available and that details relating to Diabetes UK and other relevant organizations are provided for the patient.

18 Provide an opportunity for the patient to discuss any other issues that might be worrying him or her. You may need sensitively to provide an opportunity to discuss erectile dysfunction for example or concerns about work issues. It is important to let the patient know that you have time for this and that you are interested in the patient's agenda and not just the collection of information to meet the targets of your clinic.

The aim of this extensive review is to work with the patient to promote the tightest possible glycaemic and blood pressure control in an attempt to avoid the onset of the complications of diabetes. We are also aiming to educate patients so that they might understand how to avoid the complications and recognize the importance of their condition. Every interaction with a person who has diabetes is an opportunity to address any one of these issues, to clarify misconceptions and to provide support.

Conclusion

The Department of Health is about to publish a National Service Framework (NSF) for Diabetes in England and Wales. At the time of writing this chapter the NSF was not available. However, they have announced that the scope will cover the prevention, identification and management of diabetes (type 1, Type 2 and gestational) and surveillance for and management of complications and include rehabilitation and continuing care (Department of Health, 2001). Diabetes UK has issued a position statement on their vision for the NSF and they have suggested that the following areas should provide a focus for the framework:

- All people with diabetes should be provided with up to date, consistent and ongoing information and education
- All people with diabetes should have access to integrated diabetes services which meet their individual needs
- All people with diabetes must have access to high quality care, assured through regular performance management
- Communication and coordination should be a priority across primary and secondary care
- Research should be focused on quality of life issues, models of good practice, evidence-based practice and efficacy of new treatments (Diabetes UK, 2000c).

We recognize in writing this chapter before the publication of the NSF that we have been unable to refer to specific targets which may be issued by the Department of Health later in 2001. However, we hope that this chapter, when studied alongside other chapters in this book, will assist health care professionals in meeting many of the priorities identified by Diabetes UK in its position statement which is underpinned by the vision that the Diabetes NSF should be patient centred and based on the principle of equality. As stated by the patient at the beginning of this chapter, each person with diabetes is an individual. We have to be attuned to the patient's individuality in order to have any chance of success in helping them to manage this challenging condition.

Contacts

Diabetes UK
10 Queen Anne Street
London W1G 9LH
Tel: 020 7323 1531
www.diabetes.org.uk

References

Alexander B (2000) Erectile Dysfunction Alliance Guidelines. *Practical Diabetes International* **17** (5), 139–140

Brashers V L (1998) *Clinical Applications of Pathophysiology. Assessment Diagnostic Reasoning and Management.* Mosby, New York

British Diabetic Association (2000) *New Diagnostic Criteria for Diabetes.* Circular BDA

British National Formulary 39 (2000) *British National Formulary.* British Medical Association, London

Department of Health (2000) *National Service Framework for Coronary Heart Disease.* HMSO, London

Department of Health (2001) *The Diabetes National Service Framework.* HMSO, London http://www.doh.gov.uk/nsf/diabetes.htm February 2001

Diabetes Control and Complications Trial Research Group (1993) The effect of intensive treatment of diabetes on the development and progression of long-term complications in insulin dependent diabetes mellitus. *New England Journal of Medicine* **329**, 977–986

Diabetes UK (2000a) Diabetes in Practice Fact Sheet 18. *Diabetes Update,* Autumn 2000

Diabetes UK (2000b) Missing million. *Balance,* July–August 2000, 27–30

Diabetes UK (2000c) Priorities for the NSF for England and Wales *Position Statement.* Diabetes UK, London

Diabetes UK (2001) Fact sheet No 2 – Diabetes: The figures. September 12th 2001. http://www.diabetes.org.uk/info/fact/fact2.htm

Dinneen S F, Gerstein H C (1997) The association of micro-albuminuria and mortality in non-insulin dependent diabetes. A systematic overview of the literature. *Archives of Internal Medicine* **157**, 1413–1418. Cited in: NHS Centre for Reviews and Dissemination (2000) Complications of

diabetes: Renal disease and promotion of self management. *Effective Health Care* **6** (1), 1–12

Florkowski C M, Scott R S, Moir C L, Graham P J (1998) Lipid but not glycaemic parameters predict total mortality from Type 2 diabetes mellitus in Canterbury, New Zealand. *Diabetes Medicine* **15**, 386–392

Gatling W, Hill R, Kirby M (1997) *Shared Care for Diabetes.* Isis Medical Media, Oxford

Haffner S M, Lehto S, Ronnemaa T, Pyorala K, Laakso M (1998) Mortality from coronary heart disease in subjects with Type 2 diabetes and in nondiabetic subjects with and without prior myocardial infarction. *New England Journal of Medicine* **339**, 229–234

Harrop M, Thornton H, Woodhall C, Ratcliff J (1999) Improving paediatric diabetes care. *Nursing Standard* **13** (51), 38–43

Hinchcliffe S, Montague S E, Watson R (1999) *Physiology for Nursing Practice* p. 221. Bailliere Tindall, London

Jones I (2000) Type 2 diabetes: a cardiovascular rather than an endocrine disease? *Practical Diabetes International* **17** (7) suppl., S2–S4

Leese G P, Andrews S, Wijenaike N, Lucas A, Leese R A, Gill G V (2000) Management of lipids: comparison between patient with diabetes and ischaemic heart disease. *Practical Diabetes International* **17** (3), 81–83

Mackinnon M (1998) *Providing Diabetes Care in General Practice,* 2nd edn. Class Publishing, London

Martini F (1995) *Fundamental of Anatomy and Physiology,* 3rd edn. Prentice Hall, New Jersey

McGough N (2000) Diet in diabetes care. *Diabetes Update,* Summer 2000, 16–18

Melville A, Richardson R, Lister-Sharp D (2000) Type 2 diabetes. *Health Service Journal* March 2000, 32–33

Mera S L (1997) *Pathology and Understanding Disease Prevention.* Stanley Thornes, Cheltenham

MIMS (2000) *Monthly Index of Medical Specialities.* Haymarket Publishing Ltd, London

NHS Centre for Reviews and Dissemination (2000) Complications of diabetes: renal disease and promotion of self management. *Effective Health Care* **6** (1), 1–12

NICE (2000) NICE issues guidance on rosiglitazone for Type 2 diabetes. http://www.nice.org.uk/nice-web/Article.asp?a=8080&c=476 August 2000

Nowak T J, Handford A G (1994) *Essentials of Pathophysiology.* Brown Publishers, Oxford

Ramsay L E, Williams B, Johnston G D *et al.* (1999) Guidelines for management of hypertension: report of the third working party of the British Hypertension Society. *Journal of Human Hypertension* **13**, 569–592

Rottiers R (1999) Cardiovascular disease in diabetes: the rennin angiotensin system and beyond. *Practical Diabetes International* **16** (8), suppl., S1–S8

United Kingdom Prospective Diabetes Study Group (1998) Tight blood pressure control and risk of macrovascular and microvascular complications in type 2 diabetes. UKPDS 38. *British Medical Journal* **317**, 1886–1892

World Health Organization (2000) *Definition, Diagnosis and Classification of Diabetes Mellitus and its Complications.* WHO, Geneva

7

Asthma

Gail South

A patient's perspective

I had a coughing problem when I was tiny. The doctor said it wasn't asthma because I had a high peak flow. They just kept saying it couldn't be asthma. But when I was 11 or 12 years old my breathing really started to deteriorate and I was up all night coughing so they said that it was asthma. They gave me some salbutamol and that helped. The trouble really started when I was 14 or so and it got really bad. I couldn't sleep because I was coughing so much and throwing up everything. They started me on becloforte and after that I went to see a paediatrician. I was put on serevent – so I have been around the block with drugs, but after a while you get used to it. I'm meant to take the drugs every day but I have to admit I don't.

It is really strange to talk about my asthma because, well, I don't think about it. You just have to learn to get on with it. It scares you at first, because you and everyone else take breathing for granted – well I can't anymore. It really used to scare me not being able to breathe. I would cough so much. It starts off with a cough and then you manage to get your breath back then it gets worse and the inhaler doesn't work. You just think here it goes again and you must try not to panic because then you don't concentrate on breathing and well, once that goes you really are in trouble. I wouldn't say that asthma rules my life, I am just aware of it. I can't go into a pub when I am ill and being on steroids is nasty at times. But all in all, it's OK. I don't tell too many people I have asthma because I don't want to be an invalid. However, you have to tell a few people in case you have an attack.

Epidemiology

Asthma is a common and chronic condition involving widespread narrowing of the airways which is variable and resolves spontaneously or as a result of treatment (O'Byrne and Thomson, 1995). It can affect all age groups and has a wide range of symptoms. The effects vary between individuals and can also vary in the same person at different times. It affects approximately one in 25 adults (over 16 years) and one in seven children (aged 2–15 years) in the UK (National Asthma Campaign, 1999).

Asthma begins most often in early childhood and is more common in boys than in girls. It is estimated that 23% of boys and 18% of girls (aged 2–15 years) have been diagnosed as having asthma at some point in their lives (Joint Health Surveys Unit, 1998). It can, however, begin at any age.

In 1997 there were 1584 deaths registered as caused by asthma which represents 0.25% of the total deaths (Office of National Statistics, 1997). It continues to cause people to die prematurely with 33% of deaths from asthma in England and Wales being in people below the age of 65 years. The figure for premature deaths is even higher in Scotland and Northern Ireland (Office of National Statistics, 1997).

Despite a fall in mortality rates, there is an increase in disease prevalence and severity. The morbidity associated with asthma remains extensive. In the *Impact of Asthma Study* (National Asthma Campaign, 1996), 27% of respondents said that asthma totally controlled or had a major effect on their lives. How someone experiences asthma as a whole is a complex interaction of several factors including disease severity, treatment and psychological reactions to chronic and acute illness (Hyland *et al.*, 1993).

Asthma morbidity describes the reduction in quality of life ensuing from such things as endless disturbed nights, inability to participate in sporting activities and the consequent knock on effect that this has on the general health and well-being of individuals and families. Like many chronic conditions, asthma affects not only the sufferer but the whole household.

Aetiology and pathophysiology

It is now widely accepted that airway inflammation is central to the pathogenesis of all the clinical manifestations of asthma (O'Byrne and Thomson, 1995). Airway inflammation can be defined as the presence of activated inflammatory cells. It is characterized by bronchial hyperresponsiveness (Kumar and Clarke, 1990), which is generally defined as an abnormal response of the airways to a provoking stimulus (Edgar, 1995; O'Byrne and Thomson, 1995) (see Figure 7.1).

In the person without asthma, antibodies are produced which attach themselves to antigens (allergens) and render them harmless. Hypersensitivities (allergies) are abnormally vigorous immune responses in which the immune system actually causes tissue damage as it fights off a perceived threat that would otherwise be harmless to the body. The process of sensitization in asthma involves the production of large quantities of the antibody immunoglobulin E (IgE). This antibody is secreted by plasma cells in the lining of the skin, the gastrointestinal tract and the respiratory tract, and is frequently specific to a certain allergen. In asthma the common allergen triggers are:

- House dust mite
- Pollens and spores
- Animals
- Specific industrial chemicals, for example isocyanates (spray painting), anhydrides (plastics/adhesives/glue), platinum salts (photographic industry)
- Food hypersensitivity

Under normal circumstances IgE attaches onto the allergen and prevents any reaction. However, in individuals who have become sensitive to an allergen, the IgE binds to mast cells in the tissues and eosinophils in the blood. When

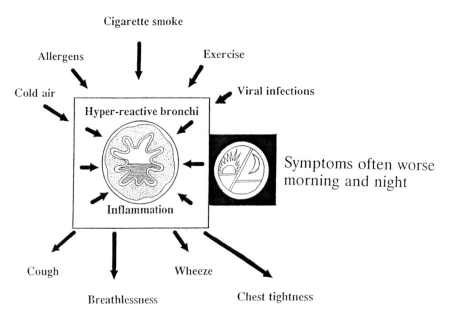

Figure 7.1 Abnormal responses to environmental stumuli (reproduced by permission from the National Asthma Training Group)

the body encounters more of the same allergen it reacts with the IgE attached to the mast cells causing a process known as degranulation, which allows the release of potent chemical mediators including histamine, prostaglandins and leukotrienes, from within the cell (Marieb, 1991). When the respiratory system is the site of allergen entry, as in asthma, the action of these mediators causes the pathological features of bronchoconstriction, namely:

- Contraction of bronchial and bronchiolar smooth muscle, this is known as broncho-spasm. If this is frequent and prolonged the muscle can become permanently thickened (hypertrophied). This results in long-term airway narrowing.
- Vascular permeability is increased causing the epithelium and submucosal layers of the bronchioles to become engorged leading to oedema.
- Hypersecretion of mucus is caused by a multiplication of the mucus secreting cells. This process starts within minutes, peaks within 15 minutes and disappears within about 3 h. It is known as the 'early asthmatic response'.

Approximately 50% of allergic adults and 70% of allergic children go on to develop a 'late asthmatic response', several hours after exposure to an allergen and lasting 18–24 h. This occurs as a result of more toxic and longer lasting

mediators which are released from other inflammatory cells and are 'recruited' to the area as a result of the early mediators (mentioned above). These include eosinophils, macrophages, neutrophils and lymphocytes. Studies have demonstrated the presence of activated eosinophils and mast cells in the airway wall and lumen of people with even mild asthma (Alderoth *et al.*, 1990). Figure 7.2 shows lung function in early and late asthmatic responses.

Predisposition of individuals

Although the precise sequence of events is as yet unclear in asthma, certain individuals are thought to be more at risk of developing hypersensitivity reactions due to the presence of a condition known as atopy. This is defined as 'increased levels of circulating IgE, specific to environmental allergens' (O'Byrne and Thomson, 1995). It can manifest itself as asthma, hayfever or eczema, with one or more conditions being present in the same individual. It is believed that 25–30% of the population is atopic (Hubbard, 1993), however, the possibility of developing asthma depends on both the genetic and environmental factors to which the individual is exposed (Meighan-Davies and Parnell, 1999). The risk for developing asthma in childhood where one parent has asthma is doubled. If both parents have asthma the risk

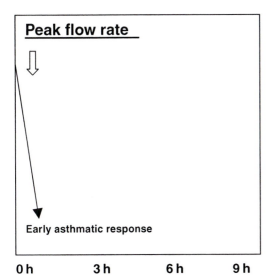

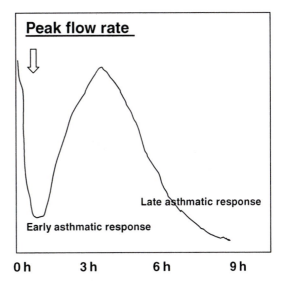

Figure 7.2 Lung function in early and late asthmatic responses

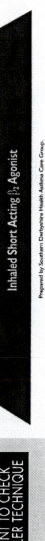

Figure 7.3 Management of chronic asthma (reproduced by permission from the Southern Derbyshire Health Asthma Care Group)

may be as high as 40% (Hall, 1996). 'Skin prick testing' can be used to diagnose individuals who are atopic to common inhalant allergens (as mentioned above). It should be noted, however, that atopy is not an essential prerequisite for asthma.

Other trigger factors

There are other non-specific triggers to asthma about which much less is known of the chain of events leading to bronchoconstriction. These include:

- Exercise
- Emotional stress
- Respiratory infections.

As well as other triggers such as:

- Smoking – it is known that maternal smoking increases the likelihood of a child developing asthma, and in children with established asthma parental smoking is associated with more severe disease (Lewis *et al.*, 1995; Strachan and Cook, 1998). Similarly, exposure to tobacco smoke worsens lung function and respiratory symptoms in adults with asthma and increases circulating IgE (Coultas, 1998).
- Certain drugs, including non-steroidal anti-inflammatory drugs (NSAIDS), betablockers and aspirin.

Assessment

The British Thoracic Society Guidelines for the Management of Asthma (BTS, 1997) have been widely accepted as the gold standard for the diagnosis, assessment and management of this condition. Figure 7.3 provides an excellent example of how these guidelines have been adapted to suit local circumstances.

Presenting symptoms

Asthma affects all the airways, including the trachea and the bronchioles. Clinically asthma is characterized by:

- Breathlessness. This can be intermittent or variable and often occurs during or after exertion or at night.

- Wheeze. Patients may describe this as 'noisy breathing'.
- Chest tightness. This often occurs after exercise.
- Cough, either dry or productive. As with breathlessness, it occurs during or after exertion and can also occur on breathing in cold air or after an upper respiratory tract infection. A particular symptom of asthma is a nocturnal cough. In children, cough may be the only or main presenting symptom.

The difficulty in asthma is that patients can present with one or all of these symptoms. As can be seen by its very definition, asthma is a variable condition and therefore symptoms are not constantly present. Specifically, the symptoms may not be present when the patient consults a doctor or nurse in general practice. The assessment process will therefore be different for the patient presenting in a non-acute state to, for example, the practice nurse, compared with a patient presenting to the Accident and Emergency Department with an acute attack.

History

As symptoms may or may not be present at the time of consultation, it is important to take a careful history from the patient in order to make an accurate assessment. This will include:

- Year of onset of symptoms
- Family history of asthma, hayfever or eczema
- Occupational history
- Drug allergies
- Current and past treatment of symptoms
- Other medical conditions and drug therapy
- Trigger factors
- Number of days off work/school in the last year
- Present symptoms can be analysed using a structure such as PQRST (Morton, 1993). Provocative/palliative, quality, radiation, severity and timing. What makes it better, what makes it worse? Ask the patient to describe how it feels in his own words. Are there any other parts of the body affected? How severe is the condition and when does it occur, time of day, time of week and/or seasonal.
- Smoking status.

Physical examination

Physical examination is important in the diagnosis and assessment of acute exacerbations of asthma. It may also be helpful in patients where the diagnosis is blurred between asthma and chronic obstructive pulmonary disease (COPD). (See Chapter 8 for a full description of the physical examination.)

Objective measurements

It is necessary to assess the following factors in order to make the following measurements of pulmonary lung function reproducible and meaningful. These, along with a careful history are used to confirm a diagnosis or to assess the progression of the condition:

- Age
- Sex
- Height
- Ethnic origin.

Peak expiratory flow rate (PEFR)

This is the maximum flow rate that can be generated during a forced expiration. It is a simple reproducible measure of airway obstruction (O'Byrne and Thomson, 1995). PEFR has also been found to correlate well with the FEV_1. (FEV_1 (forced expiratory volume in 1 second) is fully explained on p. 107 in relation to spirometry.) PEFR can be measured with inexpensive and portable meters, allowing patients to monitor their condition when symptoms occur.

Spirometry

This is also described in more detail in Chapter 8. Although less useful in the ongoing management of asthma, spirometry is recommended in the initial assessment and diagnosis as it will distinguish between restrictive and obstructive disease.

Establishing the diagnosis

If the patient's history and symptoms are suggestive of asthma, a baseline recording of PEFR or FEV_1 should be recorded. Further objective

---

1. Measure peak flow rate and record

2. Give inhaled Beta Agonist 400 mcgs via large volume spacer device

3. Wait 15 minutes

4. Record peak flow rate again

5. A rise in peak flow of >15% is diagnostic of asthma

Figure 7.4 Reversibility test

testing can then be undertaken to confirm or refute the diagnosis.

Reversibility test

If the PEFR is less than 80% of predicted then a reversibility test should be undertaken (Figure 7.4). A rise of 15% or more in peak flow rate after 15 minutes indicates asthma.

Serial peak flow monitoring

As previously discussed, symptoms may not be present at the time of the consultation as this is a variable condition. The reversibility test will be negative in such patients. The patient can then be asked to monitor their PEFR over a number of days (Figure 7.5). A variation of 15% or more between the lowest and highest reading indicates asthma. The normal diurnal variation is around 5%.

---

1. Lend patient a peak flow meter

2. Ask patient to record morning and evening peak flow (best of three) for one – two weeks

3. Variation of >15% (5% is normal) between the highest and lowest are diagnostic of asthma

Figure 7.5 Serial peak flow monitoring

1. Measure and record peak flow rate

2. Ask patient to run for 6 minutes (preferably outside)

3. Measure peak flow rate at 5 minute intervals for 15 minutes

4. A fall in peak flow rate of >15% is indicative of asthma

Figure 7.6 Exercise test

Exercise testing

This is a particularly useful test in children and younger adults as almost all people with asthma have exercise-induced bronchoconstriction (Figure 7.6). It is an unsuitable test for anyone who is unused to vigorous exercise. It is not always necessary to perform this test in the surgery or clinic. If the patient is willing, they can perform the test while undertaking their normal exercise routine. Again, a fall in PEFR of 15% or more from the baseline indicates asthma.

If none of the above tests prove positive, but the symptoms and history remain suggestive of asthma, then a further test can be undertaken.

Steroid trial

Prednisolone tablets, 30–40 mg, are taken daily after breakfast for 1–2 weeks. A 15% improvement in PEFR is indicative of asthma. (See page 91 for a discussion of the side effects of steroid treatment.)

Occupational asthma

This describes asthma that is caused by an agent that has been inhaled at work. Occupational asthma is now the most common occupational respiratory disease, representing 26% of all cases of occupational respiratory disease in 1989 (Meredith *et al.*, 1991). It is also estimated that only one-third of people with occupational asthma are identified.

If occupational asthma is diagnosed at an early stage and the patient is removed from the agent causing the symptoms, then there is more chance that permanent impairment/disability can be prevented (Chan Yeung *et al.*, 1982). Obviously the diagnosis can have serious social consequences if the patient has to leave their employment, with the ensuing financial and personal loss. Objective evidence and assessment by an appropriate professional is necessary.

Diagnostic tools

These include:

- Medical questionnaire. A detailed history should be taken. The symptoms may be caused by exposure to causal agents in a previous occupation, therefore an accurate assessment of the starting time of asthmatic symptoms should be made. Questioning as to whether symptoms improve at times when not at work, for example holidays or days off, can help identify occupational asthma.
- Serial peak flow monitoring. You may be able to identify a pattern by asking the patient to record serial peak flow measurements. A low and variable peak flow while at work which resolves to a stable pattern when not at work can provide a great deal of information about the patient's condition.
- Immunological testing. Although atopic individuals may be more susceptible, anyone may develop occupational asthma. Skin prick testing and subsequent sensitivity diagnosis do not automatically confirm occupational asthma. To do this the airways must be shown to be hyperresponsive to the particular substance in question.
- Assessment of airway responsiveness. This is usually done in a controlled environment by estimating the bronchoconstrictive response to a pharmacological agent, usually histamine. This should be done on a working day after a period of at least 2 weeks at work because the patient's lung function may be normal if he or she has not been exposed to the substance for some time. A negative response to such testing will virtually rule out occupational asthma.

It is important, once an occupational cause of asthma is suspected, to refer the patient to a specialist respiratory physician experienced in dealing with occupational asthma, as compensation may be paid if there is conclusive evidence that asthma has been triggered by an industrial substance.

Diagnosis in children

In children, the diagnosis of asthma will be made primarily on the history from the child and/or parent. In any child consulting for respiratory symptoms more than once a year, asthma should be considered.

Objective measurements of PEFR are unreliable in children under the age of 5 years. In the younger child, therefore, the only option is to monitor their response to treatment. Generally, if they show an improvement in symptoms using a trial of bronchodilators for one week, a diagnosis of asthma can be made.

Ongoing monitoring and management of asthma in primary care

The principal aim of management in working with people who have asthma is to provide individualized care in the form of both physical and psychological support. The successful management of asthma in adults involves an increasing awareness by the individual of factors in the environment, psychological influences and physiological reasons for their condition and their ability to adapt to and accept these influences. Most patients, with appropriate education and understanding of their condition, will be able to follow a self-management plan to an individualized level.

Frequency

New patients should be seen weekly until their symptoms are controlled and then less frequently. Patients with established asthma should be seen 3–6 monthly, depending on the individual, for example patients with severe disease will need to be reviewed more often. Some patients with clearly defined seasonal asthma may only need to be reviewed once a year prior to the anticipated commencement of symptoms.

Review process

It is usual for general practices to compile an asthma register for call and recall purposes. At each visit there should be a systematic review of identified criteria. This task has been simplified by the increased use of computerized records, allowing for easy identification of asthma patients.

- Record asthma symptoms including days off work/school since the last review
- Record medication and dosage
- Review treatment, making any necessary alterations
- Check inhaler technique
- Record bronchodilator usage
- Record PEFR and check technique
- Review self-management plan
- Assess asthma knowledge and provide education and information appropriate to the individual's needs
- Measure height, particularly in children, who can grow dramatically in only a few months.

Self-management

This involves teaching the patient with asthma to manage their own condition to a level which is appropriate to the individual. It is based on either symptoms or PEFR or both. These plans focus on the early recognition of unstable or deteriorating asthma and studies have shown that there is greater benefit when self-management is accompanied by written plans and regular medical or nursing review (Fishwick *et al.*, 1997). Figure 7.7 shows an example of a simple self-management card.

Self-management is more successful when individualized as the needs of all patients cannot be met through the use of one particular version. They should be developed in conjunction with the patient and reflect individual cultural needs.

Quality of life

In a chronic disease such as asthma, cure is not possible and the majority of sufferers lead lives that are characterized neither by good health nor by severe impairment (Jones, 1995). Health

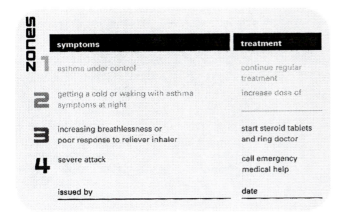

zones	symptoms	treatment
1	asthma under control	continue regular treatment
2	getting a cold or waking with asthma symptoms at night	increase dose of
3	increasing breathlessness or poor response to reliever inhaler	start steroid tablets and ring doctor
4	severe attack	call emergency medical help
	issued by	date

Figure 7.7 Example of an asthma self-management card (National Asthma Campaign)

care practitioners have a responsibility to ensure that we understand what is important to the individual and attempt to measure health accordingly. An assessment of symptoms, medication use, airway responsiveness and expiratory flow rates may provide valuable information about the effect of a medication on the airways but it does not tell us whether a patient feels better or functions better in every day life. Improving these measures does not necessarily improve quality of life in the patient with asthma. A study using the St George's Respiratory Questionnaire, showed a significant decrease in quality of life with PEFRs at 90–95% of predicted (Jones, 1992).

There is a fairly wide selection of tools, both disease specific and generic, which are, or could be, applicable to asthma sufferers, such as 'The Asthma Quality of Life Questionnaire' (Juniper *et al.*, 1992), or 'The Sickness Impact Profile' (Bergner *et al.*, 1981) (see Table 7.1 for examples).

These measures are certainly more comprehensive than most histories taken in general practice. It could be debated whether the additional cost and time to administer an instrument such as these to every patient with asthma seen in routine consultations would be justified. Jacobs and Barnes (1995), however, reported that the use of the Asthma Quality of Life Questionnaire by practice nurses (given to patients prior to the asthma clinic) maximized the information gained from consultations, reduced consultation time and made it more client focused and individual. We should consider whether the use of such tools allows us to tailor the interventions we make to what is actually important

to the patient as opposed to what we think is important.

Diagnosis and assessment in the acute setting

A major nationwide survey of the impact of asthma showed that more than 1 in 10 respondents had visited a hospital Accident and Emergency (A&E) department in the last 12 months due to a severe asthma attack (National Asthma Campaign, 1996). Other studies show that A&E attendees have good access to general practice and asthma clinics, yet choose to present habitually to the A&E department when their condition deteriorates (Hill and McEntegart, 1995). It is therefore important to consider the assessment of the patient presenting with an acute asthma attack. There are clear guidelines for the management of asthma in the A&E department which are included in the BTS guidelines for the management of asthma (see Figure 7.8).

Presenting symptoms

The main presenting symptoms of the acute attack are:

- Too wheezy or breathless to complete a sentence in one breath
- Respiratory rate
  - adults >25 breaths a minute
  - children >50 breaths a minute

Table 7.1 Selection of health assessment tools for use with asthma patients

Subject	Measuring tool	Mode of admin.	No. of items	Scale	Reference
Knowledge/ understanding	The knowledge attitude and self-efficacy questionnaire.	Q	29		Wigal *et al.*, 1993
Attitudes	1. The Living with Asthma Questionnaire	Q	68 32	4 point category point	Bowling 1995 Rutten van Molken *et al.*, 1995 Juniper *et al.*, 1992*
	2. The Asthma Quality of Life Questionnaire	Q or I	60 31	4 point Likert	Bowling 1995 Rutten van Molken *et al.*, 1995 As above
	3. The Knowledge, Attitude and Self-Efficacy Questionnaire	Q			Bowling 1995
	4. Attitudes to Asthma	Q or I			
Behaviour	The Asthma Quality of Life Questionnaire	Q or I	32	7 point	As above
Acute attacks	The Asthma Symptom Checklist	Q	50	5 point	Hyland *et al.*,1993 Bowling 1995
Psychological distress	The Asthma Bother Profile		22	7 point	Hyland *et al.*, 1995*
Generic	1. The Sickness Impact Profile	Q or I	136	Score 0–100	Bowling 1997 McDowell and Newell 1996*
	2. The Short Form 36	Q or I	36	Max. 6point	Bowling 1997 McDowell and Newell 1996*
	3. The Dartmouth Coop Charts	Q	6 charts	Visual analogue	Bowling 1997 Jenkinson 1994* McDowell and Newell 1996*

Notes: Q = Questionnaire, I = Interviewer, * = copy of full instrument included

- Heart rate
  - adults >110 beats a minute
  - children >140 beats a minute
- PEFR 50% or less of best or predicted value for age and height
- Relief medication ineffective or lasting for less than 4 h.

In adults the PEFR is used as the principal assessment tool in the acute situation. This should distinguish those patients who are hyperventilating from those with acute airways obstruction (who may also be hyperventilating). Figure 7.8 shows a local adaptation of the British Thoracic Society's guideline for the management of acute asthma in the A&E department.

Although the development of valid guidelines must often take place at a national level because insufficient resources are available locally (Ayres *et al.*, 1995), research has supported the adaptation of published guidelines for local use (Grimshaw and Russell, 1993).

Brittle asthma

Sudden fulminant attacks of asthma are sometimes referred to as 'brittle asthma'. In patients with brittle asthma, attacks develop very rapidly without the usual warning signs. Often general practices and hospitals develop 'fast track' arrangements for these identified patients. Patients at increased risk of this sort of attack are those with previous hospital admissions for acute asthma, those who need regular courses of inhaled steroids, and those with previous fulminant attacks.

Management of the acute attack

The immediate treatment of acute severe asthma consists of:

- High flow oxygen (6–8 l/minute) if available
- High dose inhaled $\beta2$ stimulant, for example nebulized salbutamol 5 mg (adults) or 2.5 mg (child) or an equivalent dose using a metered dose inhaler and large volume spacer. If using a nebulizer this should be oxygen driven where possible
- Oral steroids (IV hydrocortisone if vomiting)
- If life-threatening features are present (see Figure 7.8) then IV bronchodilators and/or

nebulized ipatropium bromide may be added
- Response to treatment should be monitored after 15 minutes. If there is no improvement or if life-threatening features are present then the patient should be admitted to hospital. Continue to treat until the ambulance arrives.

Ongoing management following the acute attack

Following an acute asthma attack it is important to ensure prompt follow up and review, usually within 24–48 h.

A full history of the patient's activities and condition in the days prior to the attack will help to identify any new factors that could be responsible. Have they moved house or started a new job? Adopted any new pets?

The treatment should be reviewed, including compliance. Are they taking sufficient preventative medication? Are they actually taking their inhaled medication as prescribed? It has been reported that only 50% of patients with chronic diseases take their medication in therapeutically effective doses (Marinker, 1998).

Does the patient have a good understanding of their inhaled medication and how it works?

The patient's inhaler technique should be reviewed. You may want to consider if the delivery system is appropriate.

Does the patient have a self-management plan? If so does it now need to be refined? As described above, the aim of asthma management should be to empower patients to manage their condition by themselves to a level appropriate to the individual patient. Part of the management should include what to do in the event of an acute attack. Written action plans for acute exacerbations of asthma have been shown to be effective (Woolcock *et al.*, 1988; Charlton *et al.*, 1990).

Differential diagnoses

The possible differential diagnoses include COPD, acute bronchitis, bronchial obstruction due to an inhaled foreign body, bronchiectasis, croup, cardiac causes of breathlessness or hyperventilation. Probably the most important differential diagnosis, particularly in the elderly, is

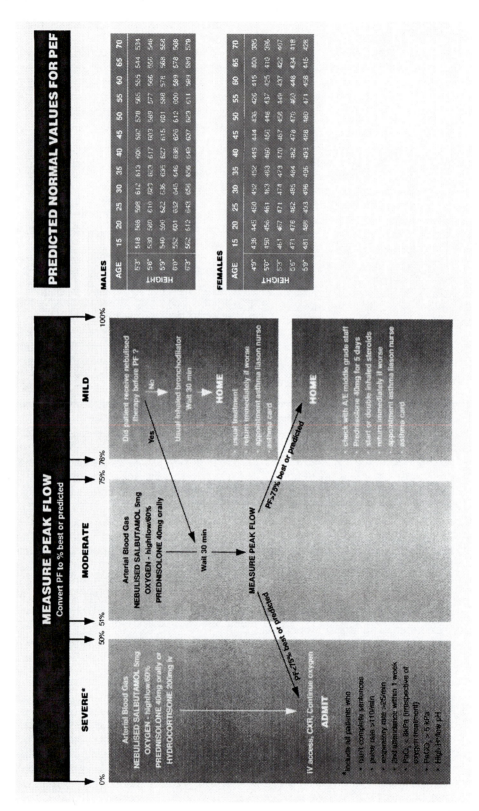

Figure 7.8 Local adaptation of the British Thoracic Society's guidelines for the management of acute asthma in the A&E department (reproduced with permission from the British Thoracic Society)

between asthma and COPD, as the approach to treatment and management is quite different. (See Chapter 8 for further description of differential diagnosis between asthma and COPD.)

Guidelines

The British Thoracic Society published guidelines on the management of asthma in 1993, which were revised in 1997 (BTS, 1997). The participants involved in producing these guidelines covered a broad spectrum of clinical practice with physicians ranging from academic professors to hospital and family doctors. They were posted to every general practitioner in Britain and are widely available from the National Asthma Campaign (address at end of chapter). They are based on research where it is available and accepted best practice where it is not. As with any guidelines, they are an attempt to improve all practice to an optimal level and to reduce variations in practice. A selection of these guidelines is reproduced in Figure 7.9.

Treatment of asthma

The pharmaceutical management of asthma is commonly divided into two main groups:

- Drugs which relieve symptoms as they occur, these are called 'relievers'
- Drugs which prevent worsening or progression of the disease, these are called 'preventers'.

The inhaled route is the route of choice in the administration of asthma medication. In 1969, salbutamol, the first inhaled beta agonist was licensed to reverse constriction of bronchial smooth muscle. This was followed in the early 1970s by the first inhaled steroid, beclamethasone diproprionate, in recognition of the role of inflammation in the pathogenesis of the disease. In 1977, the cholinergic receptor antagonist, ipatropium bromide was introduced. The ensuing years have seen the further development of these three classes of inhaled treatment. Over the last decade the development of leukotriene receptor antagonists and leukotriene synthesis inhibitors is of particular interest in the management of asthma, since they represent the first new therapeutic class to be intro-

duced for more than 20 years and they are administered orally.

The aim of the pharmaceutical treatment of asthma is to achieve the maximum control of symptoms and minimum disruption to normal activities of daily living with the minimum medication. The British Thoracic Society Guidelines for the Management of Asthma (BTS, 1997) recommend a step-wise approach to the pharmaceutical treatment of asthma (see Figure 7.9).

Relievers

This term is used to describe those drugs classed as bronchodilators. This class is further divided into short-acting and long-acting bronchodilators.

Bronchodilators work in different ways:

- On the sympathetic nervous system by stimulating $\beta2$ receptors causing bronchial smooth muscle to relax, for example short-acting $\beta2$ stimulants such as salbutamol or terbutaline. These are the most widely prescribed bronchodilators. They have an almost immediate effect, which peaks at 15 minutes and can last for up to 4 h. Although the inhaled route is the one of choice, these drugs are available orally as tablets or syrup and they are introduced at Step 1 of the BTS guidelines (1997).
- On the parasympathetic nervous system by blocking the cholinergic receptors and therefore preventing bronchoconstriction, for example the short-acting anticholinergic ipatropium bromide. This drug is prescribed exclusively by the inhaled route. It has a slower onset of action, taking 30–40 minutes to be effective. However, its effects can last up to 6 h. In general, asthmatic patients will respond better to $\beta2$ stimulants than to anticholinergics, however, a significant proportion will respond equally to both (Van Schayck *et al.*, 1991). These drugs are introduced at Step 4 of the BTS guidelines.
- By inhibiting the enzyme phosphodiesterase, which leads to an increase in cyclical AMP levels and thus bronchodilation, for example the methylxanthine, theophylline. These preparations are not available as inhaled preparations. They have a wide and toxic side-effect profile as well as a narrow therapeutic range (10–20 mg/l). They are

- Avoidance of provoking factors where possible
- Working towards a self-management plan
- Selection of best inhaler device

Starting out:
Patients should start treatment at the step most appropriate to the initial severity. A rescue course of prednisolone may be needed at any step (<1 year 1-2 mg/kg/day; 1-5 years 20 mg/day)

Step 1:

Occasional use of relief bronchodilators

Short acting β agonists "as required" for symptom relief but not more than once daily. Before altering a treatment step ensure that the patient is taking the treatment, the inhaler is appropriate, and inhaler technique is good. Address any concerns or fears. Mildest cases may response to oral β agonists.

Step 2:

Regular inhaled preventer therapy

Inhaled short acting β agonists as required plus (i) cromoglycate as powder (20 mg 3-4 times daily) or via metered dose inhaler and large volume spacer (10 mg thrice daily), or (ii) beclomethasone or budesonide up to 400 µg or fluticasone up to 200 µg daily. Consider a 5-day course of soluble prednisolone (dose given above) or temporary increase in inhaled steroids (double dose) to gain rapid control.

Step 3:

Increased dose inhaled steroids

Inhaled short acting β agonists as required plus beclomethasone or budesonide increased to 800 µg or fluticasone 500 µg daily via a large volume spacer. Consider short prednisolone course. Consider adding regular twice daily long acting β agonists or a slow release xanthine.

Step 4:

High dose inhaled steroids and bronchodilators

Inhaled steroids (up to 2 mg/day) and other treatment as in step 3. Slow release xanthines of nebulised β agonists.

Stepping down:

Regularly review the need to decrease treatment and step down as indicated. Monitor all changes in treatment by clinical review.

Avoidance of provoking factors where possible
- Patient's involvement and education
- Selection of best inhaler device
- Treatment stepped up as necessary to achieve good control
- Treatment stepped down if control of asthma good

Notes
- Patients should start treatment at the step most appropriate to the initial severity. A rescue course of prednisolone may be needed at any time and at any step. The aim is to achieve early control of the condition and then to reduce treatment.
- Until growth is complete any child requiring beclomethasone or budesonide >800 mg daily or fluticasone >500 mg daily should be referred to a paediatrician with an interest in asthma.

Prescribe a peak flow meter and monitor response to treatment

Stepping down:

Review treatment every three to six months. If control is achieved a stepwise reduction in treatment may be possible. In patients whose treatment was recently started at step 4 or 5 or included steroid tablets for gaining control of asthma this reduction may take place after a short interval. In other patients with chronic asthma a three to six month period of stability should be shown before slow stepwise reduction is undertaken.

Step 5:

Addition of regular steroid tablets

Inhaled short acting β agonists as required with inhaled beclomethasone or budesonide 800-2000 μg daily or fluticasone 400-1000 μg daily via a large volume spacer and one or more of the long acting bronchodilators plus regular prednisolone tablets in a single daily dose

Step 4:

High dose inhaled steroids and regular bronchodilators

Inhaled short acting β agonists as required with inhaled beclomethasone or budesonide 800-2000 μg daily or fluticasone 400-1000 μg daily via a large volume spacer plus a sequential therapeutic trial of one or more of
Inhaled long acting β agonists
Sustained release theophylline
Inhaled ipratropium or oxitropium
Long acting b agonist tablets
High dose inhaled bronchodilators
Cromoglycate or nedocromil

Step 3:

High dose inhaled steroids or low dose inhaled steroids plus long acting inhaled β agonist bronchodilator

Inhaled short acting β agonists as required plus either beclomethasone or budesonide increased to 800-2000 μg daily or fluticasone 400-1000 μg daily via a large volume spacer or beclomethasone or budesonide 100-400 μg twice daily or fluticasone 50-200 μg twice daily plus salmeterol 50 μg twice daily. In a very small number of patients who experience side effects with high dose inhaled steroids, either the long acting inhaled β agonist option is used or a sustained release theophylline may be added to step 2 medication. Cromoglycase or nedocromil may also be tried.

Outcome of steps 4-5: best possible results
- Least possible symptoms
- Lease possible need for relieving bronchodilators
- Least possible limitation of activity
- Least possible variation in PEF
- Best PEF
- Least adverse effects from medicine

Step 2:

Regular inhaled anti-inflammatory agents

Inhaled short acting β agonists as required plus beclomethasone or budesonide 100-400 μg twice daily or fluticasone 50-200 μg twice daily. Alternatively, use cromoglycate or nedocromil sodium, but if control is not achieved start inhaled steroids

Step 1:

Occasional use of relief bronchodilators

Inhaled short acting β agonists "as required" for symptom relief are acceptable. If they are needed more than once daily move to step 2. Before altering a treatment step ensure that the patient is having the treatment and has a good inhaler technique. Address any fears.

Outcome of steps 1-3: control of asthma
- Minimal (ideally no) chronic symptoms, including nocturnal symptoms
- Minimal (infrequent) exacerbations
- Minimal need for relieving bronchodilators
- No limitations on activities including exercise
- Circadian variation in peak expiratory flow (PEF) <20%
- PEF ≥80% of predicted or best
- Minimal (or no) adverse effects from medicine

NATIONAL ASTHMA CAMPAIGN

Working for Healthier Lungs

In association with the General Practitioner in Asthma Group, the British Association of Accident and Emergency Medicine, the British Paediatric Respiratory Society and the Royal College of Paediatrics and Child Health

Figure 7.9 Management of asthma in (a) pre-school children and (b) adults and schoolchildren. (The British Guidelines on Asthma Management, *Thorax*, **52** (suppl. 1), S1–34, 1997, with permission from the BMJ Publishing Group)

therefore used mainly when bronchospasm persists, despite full use of other agents. They are introduced at Step 4 of the BTS guidelines.

All of the above bronchodilators have a long-acting equivalent.

In 1990 the first long-acting $\beta2$ stimulant, salmeterol, became available, followed by eformoterol a few years later. These drugs are intended for regular twice-daily use as maintenance therapy, and should not be used for quick symptom relief. They have been found to be effective in controlling exercise-induced and nocturnal symptoms. Recently there has been debate as to their effectiveness in the management of patients whose asthma is uncontrolled on a low to moderate dose of inhaled steroid, as an alternative to increasing the inhaled steroid dose. A meta-analysis of studies designed to investigate the effects of adding salmeterol to a low-to-moderate dose of inhaled steroid, compared with at least doubling the inhaled steroid dose, showed that the addition of salmeterol produced greater benefits, using a variety of outcome measures (Shrewsbury *et al.*, 2000). Further evidence that the addition of an inhaled long-acting bronchodilator to an inhaled steroid has a beneficial rather than a negative effect on exacerbations, comes from the FACET study by Pauwels *et al.* (1997). These drugs are recommended at Step 3 of the BTS guidelines.

Oxitropium is an anticholinergic with a longer duration of action (10–12 h). It is used as a supplement to $\beta2$ stimulants, or an alternative in the elderly and those with COPD. The addition of an anticholinergic is recommended at Step 4 of the BTS guidelines.

Slow-release preparations of methylxanthines are available, which reduce the risk of toxic side effects. These have largely superseded the use of standard tablets. They can be given in twice or once daily doses and are mainly used at bedtime to control nocturnal symptoms as their duration of action is up to 12 h.

Preventers

This term is used to describe drugs that control airways inflammation in asthma. Corticosteroids are the main group of drugs described under this heading. Their precise mechanism of action is not fully understood, but they are thought to have direct inhibitory effects on many of the cells involved in asthmatic inflammation – T lymphocytes, eosiniphils, macrophages and epithelial cells. Although they may not have direct inhibitory effects on mast cell mediator release, they reduce the number of mast cells within the airways. Steroids may also directly inhibit plasma exudation in inflamed airways and airway mucous secretion.

By reducing airway inflammation, inhaled steroids are effective in reducing airway hyper-responsiveness in both adults and children. This reduction takes place over several weeks and may not be maximal until after several months of therapy.

Corticosteroids

These drugs, again used mainly in an inhaled form, are now widely considered to be the most effective therapy in the treatment of asthma (Barnes, 1995). The recognition that airways inflammation is present even in the mildest of asthmatic patients has led to the introduction of inhaled steroids at a much earlier stage. The most widely used inhaled steroids in the UK are beclamethasone diproprionate, budesonide and fluticasone dipropionate. These drugs must be taken regularly. They are equally effective in both children and adults. In the inhaled form, corticosteroids have few systemic side effects. There has been concern that the use of corticosteroids could cause stunting of growth in children, however, asthma itself has been shown to have an effect on growth patterns which becomes more pronounced with more severe disease (Russell, 1993). Many studies have now shown that there is no significant effect on growth in children of inhaled steroids in doses of up to 800 µg daily (Allen *et al.*, 1994). Their introduction is recommended at Step 2 of the BTS guidelines.

Oral or parenteral steroids are used in the treatment of acute exacerbations of asthma. The first choice is usually prednisolone orally or hydrocortisone hemisuccinate parenterally. Oral steroids are also used as a last resort in maintenance therapy for severe asthma. However, their toxic effects, which include hypertension, diabetes, osteoporosis and adrenal insufficiency, require that the costs and benefit to the patient are carefully considered on an individual basis. Their addition is recommended at Step 5 (the final step) of the BTS guidelines.

Mast cell stabilizers

Mast cell stabilizers were introduced in the late 1960s. They are thought to stabilize mast cell membranes, therefore inhibiting the release of inflammatory mediators, although their mode of action is not fully understood. These drugs have been found to be most effective in atopic children and in exercise-induced asthma. Sodium cromoglycate is the most frequently used mast cell stabilizer in the UK. It is recommended at Step 2 of the BTS Guidelines as a possible alternative to an inhaled steroid.

New drug therapies

The leukotriene receptor antagonists, montelukast and zafirlukast, as mentioned above, represent the first new therapeutic class to be introduced in the treatment of asthma in the last 20 years. Leukotrienes are divided into the cysteinyl leukotrienes LTC, LTD and LTE, and the non-cysteinyl leukotriene LTB. The cysteinyl leukotrienes were identified in 1979 as being the major bioactive constituents of SRS-A (slow-reacting substance of anaphylaxis) (Drazen, 1994). LTC and LTD are the most potent bronchoconstrictors studied in human subjects (O'Byrne and Thomson, 1995). LTE (the metabolite of LTC and LTD) is excreted in the urine and increased levels have been clearly demonstrated in patients presenting to hospital with acute severe asthma (Taylor *et al.*, 1989). By blocking the receptors for these potent chemical mediators, the contractile responses of the three cysteinyl leukotrienes are therefore antagonized, as well as preventing leukotriene-induced increases in vascular permeability leading to oedema and leukotriene-induced influx of eosinophils into the airway.

Both of these new drugs are administered orally representing a diversion from the inhaled therapy we have come to expect in the treatment of asthma. They are effective in reducing exercise-induced asthma and benefit aspirin-sensitive asthmatic patients. They do not as yet have a place in the BTS guidelines, but are recommended as an 'add-on' therapy in patients with mild to moderate asthma who are uncontrolled on oral steroids and bronchodilators.

The latest drug therapy which will impact on the management of some asthmatic patients is bupropion HCL, a new nicotine-free tablet treatment for smokers who are motivated to quit. It is purported to break the cycle of nicotine addiction by acting on the brain to modify the neurotransmitters involved in nicotine addiction and withdrawal. It has been shown to be almost twice as effective as a nicotine patch in achieving smoking abstinence at one year (Jorenby *et al.*, 1999).

Drug delivery systems

The majority of asthma medication is delivered in the inhaled form as it makes sense to apply the medication directly to the lungs as opposed to the entire body. Bronchodilator aerosols have been used in the treatment of asthma since the 1930s, with the pressurized metered dose inhaler being introduced in 1956 (Crompton, 1995). Spacer devices allow inhaled medication in a pressurized metered dose inhaler to be delivered to patients of almost any age. Dry powdered devices have provided an alternative delivery system (although their use is limited in children under the age of 4 years). Nebulizers, although less convenient can have a role in the long-term treatment of children with moderate to severe asthma, and in the management of acute severe asthma in both children and adults.

The metered dose inhaler

These are still the most widely used inhaler systems, but although the instructions appear simple, many adults find the technique difficult to master. The main problem experienced is difficulty in coordinating dose release during inspiration (Crompton, 1982). Later versions of this device have attempted to overcome this problem, for example the breath-activated devices. In addition to the difficulty in using the inhaler, some patients find that the high velocity of the aerosol jet (the 'cold freon' effect) makes it difficult to continue inhaling when the propellants are released into the oropharynx. This causes particular problems when corticosteroids are inhaled as their deposition can cause oral candidiasis and dysphonia (Pearson, 1990).

Spacer devices

These were initially devised to reduce the 'cold freon' effect and to help overcome coordination problems. However, they have been found to increase drug availability to the lung, while decreasing drug deposition in the oropharynx (Lindgren *et al.*, 1980). Their use in adults is therefore recommended when corticosteroids have to be given in large doses. In children, spacer devices are used regularly because of their ease of use. A mask attachment is available for most spacers, making them particularly suitable for infants.

Dry powder devices

These devices depend entirely on the patient's inspiratory effort and are usually easier to use. However, the dry powder can cause a para-doxical cough and mouth rinsing is important after inhaled steroids to prevent the local side effects mentioned above. Many of these devices need to be loaded either singly or in a day's supply. This requires a degree of manual dexterity in some cases, which may cause problems for certain groups of patients.

Nebulizers

There are two types of nebulizer: jet or ultra-sonic. Jet nebulizers work by compressed air or oxygen entering a chamber in the nebulizer through a narrow tube. The liquid is broken up into large droplets and then a fine aerosol which is inhaled through a mouthpiece or face mask. There are many different types of jet nebulizer with widely differing characteristics and performance. They are influenced by factors such as the flow rate of the driving gas (either air or oxygen), the nature of the solution being nebulized and the amount of liquid in the chamber.

Ultrasonic nebulizers use high frequency sound waves produced from a crystal. The vibra-tions are focused on the surface of the liquid to create a fountain which generates droplets. They are usually less efficient than jet nebulizers.

The chief advantage of nebulized therapy is that less inspiratory effort is required by the patient, therefore this method is used in the acute attack and often with children (although

there is debate as to whether a spacer device is equally effective). However, a much higher dose of the drug is required. There is a danger that some individuals have a tendency to self-treat for too long with a home nebulizer before seek-ing further help. Potentially this can be danger-ous and even fatal.

Choice of device

Different pharmaceutical companies have devel-oped different and varied devices. The choice of device can be as important as the drug itself. Several factors should be taken into account when choosing the delivery device. If the patient requires more than one inhaler it is less confus-ing if the same device can be used for all inhaled medication, although it is not always possible to achieve this.

It is important to consider the patient's ability to use the device. Some devices, although excel-lent for some patients, require a degree of manual dexterity which is not always achievable, particularly in elderly people who may have arthritic changes in their hands. Some manufac-turers however have produced aids, for example the Haleraid® to overcome this. Other devices, particularly the metered dose inhaler, require coordination in addition to dexterity.

Patient preference should be considered. Some devices appeal more than others depend-ing upon the patient's age for example, therefore, involving the patient in the choice of delivery system is important. This also empowers the patient and gives them a degree of control over the management of their condition.

The patient's lifestyle and the dosing regi-men of their medication will also influence the choice of device. Some devices are more bulky than others, for example the large volume spacer, which makes them less suitable for patients who need to take their medication away from the home on a regular basis.

The age of the patient is another important consideration. Many devices are unsuitable for infants and young children because of the respiratory effort required to deliver the medica-tion to the lungs. For this reason the metered dose inhaler plus large volume spacer device, or nebulized therapy is usually the method of choice. These are often the methods of choice for the very elderly too.

Whichever device is chosen, careful education in its use and repeated checks on technique are important. If technique is poor and cannot be improved, then the device should be changed to one that can be used reliably.

Conclusion

Asthma is a common and chronic condition with a wide range of symptoms and effects which vary between individuals and in the same individual. The successful management of asthma involves an increasing awareness by the sufferer and carer of factors in the environment, psychological influences and physiological reasons for their condition. It is dependent on their ability to adapt to and accept these influences. As health professionals we must remember that different people will experience the symptoms of asthma differently, will have different knowledge, attitudes, beliefs and feelings. They will have different work and social functions to carry out and will live in different environments. The key to successful management of this complex condition necessitates an individualized approach. Most patients *do not* die, and for most of the time *do not* have acute attacks, but they *do* have to live with the daily disturbance to their lives of symptoms such as cough, dyspnoea and wheeze, as well as restrictions to their activity levels, work opportunities and environmental concerns.

Useful contacts

British Lung Foundation (Breathe Easy Club)
8 Peterborough Mews
London SW6 3BL
Tel 0171 371 7704

British Thoracic Society
1 St Andrews Place
London NW1 4LB
Tel 0171 486 7766

National Asthma and Respiratory Training
  Centre
The Athenaeum
10 Church Street
Warwick CV34 4AB
Tel 01926 493313

National Asthma Campaign
Providence House
Providence Place
London N1 0NT
Tel 0171 226 2260
(Asthma Helpline: 0345 010203)

QUIT: the charity helping people to stop
  smoking
102 Gloucester Place
London W1H 3DA
Tel 0171 487 2858
Smokers quitline: 0171 487 3000

References

Alderoth E, Rosenhail L, Johansson S A, Linden M, Venge P (1990) Inflammatory cells and eosinophilic activity in asthmatics investigated by bronchoalveolar lavage: the effects of anti-asthmatic treatment with Budesonide or Terbutaline. *American Review of Respiratory Disease* **142**, 91–99

Allen D B, Mullen M, Mullen B (1994) A meta-analysis of the effects of oral and inhaled corticosteroids on growth. *Journal of Allergy and Clinical Immunology* **93**, 967–976

Ayres P, Renvoize T, Robinson M (1995) Clinical guidelines: key decisions for acute service providers. *British Journal of Health Care* **1** (11), 547–551

Barnes P J (1995) Corticosteroids. Cited in: O'Byrne P M, Thomson N C (eds) *Manual of Asthma Management.* Saunders, London

Bergner M, Bobbitt R A, Carter W B (1981) The Sickness Impact Profile: development and final revision of a health status measure. *Medical Care* **19**, 787–805

Bowling A (1995) *Measuring Disease* Buckingham: Open University Press

Bowling A (1997) *Measuring Health* Buckingham: Open University Press

BTS (1997) The British Guidelines on Asthma Management 1995: review and position statement. *Thorax* **52**, S1

Chan Yeung M, Lam S, Koener S (1982) Clinical features and natural history of occupational asthma due to western red cedar. *American Journal of Medicine* **72**, 411–415

Charlton I, Charlton G, Broomfield J, Mullee M A (1990) Evaluation of peak flow and symptoms in self management plans for control of asthma in general practice. *British Medical Journal* **301**, 1355–1359

Coultas B (1998) Passive smoking and risk of adult asthma and COPD: an update. *Thorax* **53**, 381–387

Crompton G K (1982) Problems patients have using pressurised aerosol inhalers. *European Journal of Respiratory Disease* **63** (suppl. 119), 101–104

Crompton G K (1995) Delivery systems. Cited in: O'Byrne P M, Thomson N C (eds) *Manual of Asthma Management.* Saunders, London

Drazen J M (1994) Leukotrienes. In *Asthma and Rhinitis*, pp 838–850. Blackwell Science, London

Edgar D (1995) Hypersensitivity. In: (Phillips J, Murray P, eds) *The Biology of Disease* (Chapter 12). Blackwell Science, Oxford

Fishwick D, D'Souza W, Beasley R (1997) The Asthma Self-Management Plan System of Care: what does it mean, how is it done, does it work, what models are available, what do patients want and who needs it? *Patient Education and Counselling* **32** (suppl. 1), s21–s33

Grimshaw J, Russell I (1993) Achieving health gain through clinical guidelines. 1 Developing scientifically valid guidelines. *Quality in Health Care* **2**, 243–248

Hall I (1996) Common questions on asthma genetics. *Asthma Journal* **2** (2) 65–67

Hill AT, McEntegart A (1995) Which asthmatic patients attend accident and emergency departments (abstract)? *Thorax* **50** (suppl. 2)

Hubbard J (1993) Asthma and allergy. *Community Outlook* 21–24

Hyland M E, Kenyon C A, Taylor M, Morice A H (1993) Steroid prescribing for asthmatics: relationship with asthma symptom checklist and living with asthma questionnaire. *British Journal of Clinical Psychology* **32**, 505–511

Jacobs P, Barnes G (1995) Quality of life in asthma. *British Journal of General Practice* **45**, 270

Jenkinson C (1994) *Measuring Health and Medical Outcomes* London: UCL Press

Joint Health Surveys Unit (1998) *Health Survey for England: the Health of Young People 1995–1997*. HMSO, London

Jones P W (1992) Quality of life, health economics and asthma. *European Respiratory Review* **5**, 279–283. Cited in: Gruffyd-Jones K (1997) Quality of life measures in asthma – do they matter to the GP? *British Journal General Practice* **47**, 312–394

Jones P W (1995) Quality of life measurement in asthma. *European Respiratory Journal* **8**, 885–887

Jorenby D E, Leischow S J, Nides M A (1999) A controlled trial of sustained release bupropion, a nicotine patch, or both for smoking cessation. *New England Journal of Medicine* **340**, 685–691

Juniper E F, Guyatt G H, Epstein R S, Ferrie P J, Jaeschke R, Hiller T K (1992) Evaluation of impairment of health related quality of life in asthma: development of a questionnaire for use in clinical trials. *Thorax* **47**, 76–83

Kumar P, Clarke M L (1990) *Clinical Medicine*, 2nd edn. Baillière, Tindall, London

Lewis S, Britton J, Richards D, Brynner J (1995) A prospective study of risk factors for early and persistent wheezing in childhood. *European Respiratory Journal* **8**, 349–356

Lindgren S B, Formgren H, Moren F (1980) Improved aerosol therapy of asthma: effect of actuator tube size on drug availability. *European Journal of Respiratory Disease* **61**, 56–61

McDowell I, Newell C (1996) *Measuring Health* Oxford: Oxford University Press

Marieb E N (1991) *Essentials of Human Anatomy and Physiology*, 3rd edn. The Benjamin/Cummings Publishing Co Ltd., Wokingham

Marinker M (1998) The current status of compliance. *European Respiratory Review* **8**, 235–238

Meighan-Davies J, Parnell H (1999) Asthma – the community challenge. *Journal of Community Nursing* **13**, 42–46

Meredith S K, Taylor V M, McDonald J C (1991) Occupational respiratory disease in the United Kingdom 1989: a report to the British Thoracic Society and the Society of Occupational Medicine by the SWORD project group. *British Journal of Internal Medicine* **48**, 292–298

Morton P G (1993) *Health Assessment in Nursing* 2nd Edition, F A Davis & Co. Philadelphia

National Asthma Campaign (1996) *Impact of Asthma Survey Results*. Allen and Hanburys, London

National Asthma Campaign (1999) *National Asthma Audit*. National Asthma Campaign, London

O'Byrne P M, Thomson N C (eds) (1995) *Manual of Asthma Management*. Saunders, London

Office of National Statistics (1997) *Mortality Statistics: cause 1997*. Series DH2 No. 24

Pauwels R A, Lofdahl C G, Postma D S *et al.* (1997) Effect of inhaled formoterol and budesonide on exacerbations of asthma. *New England Journal of Medicine* **337**, 1405–1411

Pearson R (1990) *ASTHMA Management in Primary Care*. Radford Medical Press, Oxford

Russell G (1993) Asthma and growth. *Archives of Disease in Childhood* **69**, 695–698

Shrewsbury S, Pyke S, Britton M (2000) Meta-analysis of increased dose of inhaled steroid or addition of salmeterol in symptomatic asthma. *British Medical Journal* **320**, 1368–1373

Strachan D P, Cook D G (1998) Parental smoking and childhood asthma: longitudinal and case control studies? *Thorax* **53**, 204–212

Taylor G W E, Black P, Turner N (1989) Urinary leukotriene E_4 after antigen challenge and in acute asthma and allergic rhinitis. *Lancet* **1**, 584–587

Van Schayck C P, Folgering H, Harbers H, Maas K L, Van Weel C (1991) Effect of allergy and age on responses to salbutamol and ipatropium bromide in moderate asthma and chronic bronchitis. *Thorax* **46**, 355–359

Woolcock A J, Yan K, Salome C M (1988) Effect of therapy on bronchial hyperresponsiveness in the long term management of asthma. *Clinical Allergy* **18**, 167–176

Chapter

8

Chronic obstructive pulmonary disease

Kay Holt

Introduction: patient's perspective

Chronic obstructive pulmonary disease (COPD) is a chronic, slowly progressive disorder characterized by airways obstruction, which does not change markedly over several months. Most of the lung function impairment is fixed, although some reversibility can be produced by bronchodilator (or other) therapy. This clinical description of the disease does not adequately represent the lived experience of COPD. The following is an extract from an interview with a 65-year-old COPD sufferer and it is printed with his permission.

It's one of the most frustrating diseases to have because people look at you and think 'what has he got a sticker in his car for?' Little do they know that I have to be in a wheelchair most of the time because I'm so short of breath. We went out one day when I had a cold – my wife told me not to but I had to get out. We got out of the car but I felt so bad. I felt like I was drowning. For anyone who hasn't suffered from it, it's a very hard thing to describe, but it frightens my wife and myself. I couldn't move, I just had to stand there to try to get some air and I couldn't. I thought this is going to be a hospital job, anyway it passed. You get no sympathy from people, if you are standing there gasping for breath people just look at you. Some people say 'are you all right' others just walk by. I should not have gone out. It was against my wife's wishes. I knew I should not have gone and

it made me feel worse. This is where psychologically you are trying to make yourself better, but at the same time you know that it's not working, and so it's a battle. When you are out you try to act normally, you stop and look in the window or anything while you try and compose yourself and get your breath back. It's very very frustrating when you've been active all your life, as I was in my job. One of the frustrations is you can't help your wife around the house. I don't know what I'd do without my wife, and she's not so well herself. It's one of the frustrations psychologically – it does play on your mind. One of the things with having this is that it makes you short tempered, but the more you lose your temper the tighter your chest gets, it's a catch 22 situation. It's paramount that you don't get a cold – you've got trouble then. So you have to avoid people with colds. I can't even take a shower, it takes your breath away, the arm movements – so I have a bath, even simple things like having a shave – at times I have to stop, lean on the sink until I calm down. If you go shopping it's one way of getting exercise as long as I've got a trolley at least I can walk a bit, at least it keeps my legs moving. Thank the lord that I'm still able to hear and see and watch the sport on television – I couldn't even think of going to a football match anymore. I can't go into any pubs, because of the smoke, so your social life then takes a knock. Fortunately the grandchildren live away, because if they were here, I couldn't lift them or play with them – that's another frustration. There are a lot of people that don't realize what it's like. It's so hard to explain to people who are able to breathe quite freely and take lungs full of fresh air.

Epidemiology

Prevalence of COPD

In Europe COPD is the third leading cause of death after cancer and heart disease (Office of Population, Census and Surveys, 1993). There are about 600 000 people in the UK diagnosed with COPD. The prevalence is around 2% for men aged 45–75 and 7% for men over 75. These figures could be a significant under-estimation as many patients with mild COPD accept symptoms such as dyspnoea on exertion or cough as due to smoking and therefore do not contact their doctor. The prevalence in women is currently lower than in men but is rising due to their increased smoking over the past 20 years. In the UK there is a wide geographical variation in mortality rates for COPD with higher rates in urban areas. In general practice annual consultation rates for COPD are four times the equivalent rates for angina. The direct costs of the disease are estimated at £468 million, however, when the social impact is taken into account the estimate is more like £1.5 billion each year (Calverley and Sondhi, 1998). Nearly half of all COPD costs are hospital admissions.

Genetic and environmental determinants of COPD

Cigarette smoking is the dominant risk factor for COPD, but only about 10–15% of smokers develop the condition (Higgins, 1991; Hanrahan *et al.*, 1996) and cumulative cigarette smoking does not correlate with risk (Higgins, 1991; Dockery *et al.*, 1988). The pathogenesis of emphysema is thought to depend upon excess proteolytic activity in the human serine elastase, which is released from polymorphs as a result of cigarette smoking. There are obviously other factors that predispose a smoker to COPD. Clark *et al.* (1998) explored aspects of smoking behaviour in relation to risk of COPD by measuring depth, duration and quantity of smoke inhalation. They found no relationship between smoke inhalation and airflow obstruction, but found emphysema is associated with high alveolar smoke exposure as measured by carbon monoxide boost (the increment of expired carbon monoxide 5 minutes after smoking a cigarette) and productive coughing is associated with high nicotine uptake, probably from airway smoke particle deposition. The risk of COPD from smoking pipes or cigars is less than those from smoking cigarettes as these smokers do not tend to inhale. Smokers who switch from cigarettes to pipes or cigars may reduce their risks (Wald and Watt, 1997), although those who have previously smoked cigarettes may go on to inhale pipe or cigar smoke. Although it is often assumed that passive smoking predisposes to COPD, there is no evidence to confirm this. In developed countries cigarette smoking increased greatly during the first half of this century. It was several decades before the resulting increase in male deaths from tobacco was evident (Peto, 1994; Doll *et al.*, 1994).

There is increasing evidence that occupational exposure to dust and fumes can lead to the development of airway obstruction (Hendrick, 1996). Some occupations carry a greater risk of COPD than others, for example coal and gold mining, welding, working in the cement and cotton industries, grain handling and farming. There is also a significant correlation between lung function and the degree of occupational dust exposure in COPD patients (Goren and Bruderman, 1989).

There is large variation in individual susceptibility to COPD and there are some beliefs that COPD and asthma result from a common genetic root (Meighan-Davies and Parnell, 1999; and Chapter 7). This theory recognized the common features of chronic bronchitis, emphysema and asthma and the frequent overlap of the conditions (Sluiter *et al.*, 1991). The common genetic root is considered to be an innate predisposition to airway hyperresponsiveness and to allergy. Vermiere and Pride (1991) argue that the differences in the nature of airway inflammation in the two conditions, in respect of eosinophilia, does not support the hypothesis. The only proven genetic link to COPD is alpha-1-antitrypsin deficiency (Hutchinson, 1988). Persons with this deficiency may have no clinical manifestations at all if they are a non-smoker. Cigarette smoking is the major risk factor for people with alpha-1-antitrysin deficiency developing COPD and where most COPD patients do not experience symptoms until their 50s or 60s, patients with this deficiency can present as young as their 20s or 30s.

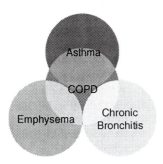

Figure 8.1 Emphysema, chronic bronchitis and chronic asthma may all be features of COPD (reproduced with permission from the National Asthma & Respiratory Training Centre)

Pathophysiology

Emphysema, chronic bronchitis and chronic asthma may all be features of COPD (Figure 8.1). The diagnosis of these three conditions is defined in different ways: chronic bronchitis on symptoms, asthma by lung function testing and emphysema pathologically. In reality, in COPD, the three conditions tend to overlap; some patients have a significant asthmatic element, others may have more of a chronic brochitic element with daily sputum production, and some patients may have a dominant emphasematous element with hyperinflated chest and pursed lipped breathing. Signs and symptoms may vary among individuals, however dyspnoea due to airflow obstruction appears to be the most consistent and also most disabling symptom. The precursor to COPD, before any signs or symptoms are evident, is thought to be small-airway disease involving the small peripheral airways, often less than 2 mm in diameter and known as the silent area of the lung. Usually as a result of cigarette smoke, these small airways become narrowed and distorted, causing airflow resistance. It is thought that COPD patients must pass through a stage in which there is considerable peripheral airway obstruction without a reduction in FEV_1 (Macklem, 1972). FEV_1 (forced expiratory volume in 1 second is fully explained on page 107 – Spirometry). Detecting people with this very early airway obstruction could identify those at risk of COPD who would most benefit from stopping smoking. Spirometry, if performed accurately with appropriate equipment,

can detect this small airway obstruction and could be used as a screening tool to identify smokers susceptible to COPD. Unfortunately, by the time patients present with symptoms of COPD there is considerable airflow obstruction demonstrated by a reduced FEV_1. Most of the airflow limitation is due to pathological changes; narrowing of the bronchioles causing increased airflow resistance and loss of pulmonary elastic recoil due to emphysema with reduction of the alveolar attachments around the airways making them prone to collapse during expiration.

Emphysema

Emphysema is a destructive process characterized by abnormal, permanent enlargement of the air spaces distal to the terminal bronchiole and destruction of the airway walls. In *centrilobular emphysema* damage is limited to the central part of the lobule around the respiratory bronchiole, whereas in *panacinar emphysema* there is a destruction and distension of the whole lobule. Where the air spaces are greater than 1 cm in diameter they are termed *bullae*. This destructive process is largely associated with cigarette smoking. Cigarette smoke causes a low-grade inflammation of the airways and alveoli, attracting macrophages and neutrophils into the airways which produce proteolytic enzymes, the most important being elastase (Janoff, 1985). This enzyme has been found to be important in COPD and many other respiratory conditions as it destroys elastin, the protein that makes up lung tissue. The damage to the airways caused by smoking begins well before the symptoms of emphysema occur. Evidence of damage to the elastic fibre network of the lungs in current smokers without airflow obstruction has been found (Stone *et al.*, 1995) and evidence of elastin degradation, by markers excreted in urine, are around twice as high in smokers and COPD patients than in those who have never smoked. In healthy lungs elastic tissue supports the smaller airways and alveoli keeping them open by the 'guy rope' effect (Figure 8.2).

Loss of elasticity slackens off this elastic tissue (loosening the guy ropes) leading to airway collapse (Figure 8.3).

With the loss of elasticity the lungs become hyperinflated by up to 2 or 3 litres, but most of this extra capacity is inaccessible as the maximum

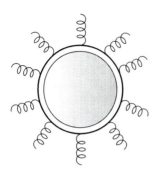

Figure 8.2 Elastic tissue in healthy lungs supports the smaller airways and alveoli (reproduced with permission from the BTS COPD Consortium, UK)

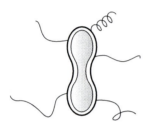

Figure 8.3 In emphysema elastic tissue in the smaller airways slackens (reproduced by permission from the BTS COPD Consortium, UK)

breath size may only about 1 litre. Gas exchange is obviously compromised.

Chronic bronchitis

Chronic bronchitis is characterized by impaired mucociliary clearance due to structural and functional defects of both the cilia and the mucus secreting cells (Wanner, 1990). Chronic bronchitis is defined by the Medical Research Council as *'The production of sputum on most days for at least three months in at least two consecutive years'* (Medical Research Council Working Party, 1981). It may occur in isolation or more commonly coexist with airflow limitation and/or emphysema. Elastase, the 'culprit' enzyme in emphysema, has also been implicated in the development of chronic bronchitis. It has been found to contribute to increasing the number of goblet cells. It is the goblet cells and the mucus glands that are responsible for secreting mucus in the airways, the mucus glands secreting 40 times more mucus than the goblet cells. Cigarette smoking causes an increase in the

size of the mucus glands along with an increase in the number of goblet cells. The combination of mucus hypersecretion and ciliary impairment leads accumulation of secretions in the lower airways. This mucus hypersecretion is associated with a decline in lung function (Vestbo *et al.*, 1996), but it is not certain whether it is causative. This excessive mucus production of chronic bronchitis is unpleasant and distressing for the patient and puts the patient at risk of lower respiratory tract infection. Patients with mucus hypersecretion are more likely to die from pulmonary infection than those without (Prescott *et al.*, 1995).

Chronic asthma

Around 10% of early-onset and 25% of late-onset asthmatics develop permanent structural changes in their airways, associated with a degree of fixed airflow obstruction. The duration and severity of the asthma are important factors along with smoking and long-term asthma control. (See Chapter 7 for further information on asthma.) The main physiological changes seen in patients with irreversible chronic asthma are epithelial disruption, basement membrane thickening and airway smooth muscle hypertrophy. Bronchial hyperresponsiveness, atopy and raised serum IgE levels have all been suggested as risk factors for COPD (Itabashi *et al.*, 1990; Rijcken *et al.*, 1995).

Hypoxia in COPD

COPD, in particular the pathological changes due to emphysema, disrupts the alveolar–capillary interface where gas exchange takes place. Some of the alveoli will be ventilated but will not have a blood supply for gas exchange. Conversely, however, some of the alveoli will have a blood supply to enable gas exchange but will be poorly ventilated as a result of damaged airways. This loss of 'alveolar–capillary interface' leads to an abnormal gas exchange. The respiratory centre in the brain controls the amount of oxygen and carbon dioxide in the blood and in the early stage of the disease the respiratory centre is able to correct abnormalities. This is known as the respiratory drive and whether patients have the ability to continue normalizing the blood gases as the disease progresses appears to depend on their respiratory drive.

In patients with a normal respiratory drive the increased work of breathing causes a decrease in blood O_2 and an increase in blood CO_2 and this combination of hypoxia and hypercapnia stimulates increased output from the respiratory centre in the brain and consequently an increased breathing rate. This fast breathing will normalize the blood gases. Characteristically, these patients tend to expire through pursed lips which causes a back pressure, splinting open the collapsed airways. Patients who breathe in this way were historically known as 'pink puffers'; pink because they are not hypoxic and puffers due to the way they appear to breathe.

For patients with an impaired respiratory drive the increased blood carbon dioxide does not stimulate an increase in breathing rate and the patient becomes hypoxic. The long-term effect of hypoxia is to cause pulmonary hypertension, raised artery pressure and oedema. Historically these patients were known as 'blue bloaters'; blue because of the hypoxia and bloated due to the oedema.

In reality patients do not fit neatly into these two categories but tend to fall somewhere in between. What causes these differences in respiratory drive is unclear, but it has been suggested that there is a genetic tendency towards impaired respiratory drive (Fleetham *et al.*, 1984). These differences in respiratory drive have important implications for oxygen therapy particularly during exacerbations (see page 115 – Oxygen).

Assessment of the patient

Presenting problems

Patients usually present with breathlessness on exertion and cough, with or without sputum. As discussed earlier, by the time patients present with symptoms there is significant loss of lung function. Therefore patients only usually present to health care professionals when the disease is established. People describe breathlessness in different ways and one description from a sufferer of COPD is presented at the beginning of this chapter. Breathlessness is worse on exertion so it may be difficult to assess how breathless a patient is during a consultation as they may have been sat resting in the waiting room for half an hour. The subjective assessment of breathlessness will be discussed later in the chapter (p. 108 – Assessment of dyspnoea). Cough in COPD is usually worse in the morning but, unlike asthma, does not usually occur during the night. Cough is often associated with sputum production especially in those who continue to smoke. Patients may feel better after expectorating during their first coughing episode of the day, often brought on by the first cigarette of the day which they describe as 'clearing their lungs'. When patients with COPD present with a cough it has usually been with gradual onset slowly getting worse over the years. If a patient with a significant smoking history presents with a new cough or cough that has changed then this symptom should be regarded as suspicious. Sputum is usually grey or white but becomes green and purulent with infection. Haemoptysis is not a normal finding in COPD and this also should be taken as a potentially serious sign. In patients who produce an excessive volume of sputum, especially where there are frequent exacerbations, then bronchiectasis should be suspected.

History

An important aspect of the history is the 'smoking history'. It needs to be established how much exposure to smoking the individual has had. This can be objectively assessed in terms of pack years. Smoking 20 cigarettes a day for a year equates to one pack year. The following formula calculates pack years smoked:

$$\frac{\text{Cigarettes smoked per day}}{20} \times \text{Years smoked}$$

The pack years smoked is not always easy to calculate as many peoples smoking habits vary over years. It is thought that smoking for 20 pack years or more is a significant risk factor for developing COPD. When a smoking history is less than 20 pack years then a different diagnosis should be considered, for example asthma. A history of exposure to dust and fumes should also be sought, particularly welding fumes, coal dust, chemicals or paint spray. It is important to take a respiratory history from as far back as possible asking about childhood diseases such as pneumonia, measles, tuberculosis, atopy and childhood wheeze. Patients may describe childhood symptoms of recurrent bronchitis which may in fact have been undiagnosed asthma. This respiratory history can be very helpful when considering differential diagnosis, for example early pneumonia may predispose a patient to bronchiectasis or early asthma symptoms might suggest that there may be an asthmatic element to their COPD. A family history of emphysema is also important especially in patients presenting with symptoms at a relatively young age or with a smoking history of less than 20 pack years. If it is suggested that there may be a possibility of alpha-1 antitrypsin deficiency then the patient should be referred to a respiratory physician. It must also be remembered when taking a history that breathlessness can also be due to cardiovascular disease and a history of heart disease and hypertension must be explored.

Physical examination

This cannot diagnose COPD, but a complete respiratory examination is an important aspect of patient assessment. Physical signs can help demonstrate the severity of the disease. Observing the patient's posture and movements as they walk into the room can be revealing. For a respiratory examination the patient should be stripped to the waist so the full chest is exposed. Patients may find it more comfortable to sit down for most of the examination.

Observation

It is particularly important to notice the shape and symmetry of the chest; the anteroposterior diameter of the chest may increase in COPD and the chest may appear barrel shaped with a decreased cricosternal distance. Observe the neck for supraclavicular retraction and for contraction of the sternomastoid or other accessory muscles of respiration. Note the position of the trachea, which is normally midline. Observe the rate, rhythm, depth and effort of breathing; prolonged expiration suggests airflow obstruction. Pursed lipped breathing is a feature of emphysema. Listen to the patient's breathing; can wheezing or stridor be heard and if so where in the respiratory cycle are they heard? Observe the colour of the patient; are there signs of central cyanosis such as blueness

around the mouth and tongue? The hands should be observed for signs of nicotine staining or finger clubbing (thickening of the tissues at the base of the nail with obliteration of the angle between the nail base and adjacent skin of the finger). If the hands are slightly blue are they cold or warm? Warm, blue hands signify poor oxygen saturation, whereas cold blue hands may mean poor peripheral circulation. Signs of hypercapnia may occur during exacerbations and these include flapping tremor, bounding pulse and drowsiness. Observe for signs of peripheral oedema, which can suggest cor pulmonale among other causes. Signs of pulmonary hypertension include raised jugular venous pressure, loud pulmonary second heart sound or tricuspid regurgitation.

Palpation

Identify any tender areas. Assess respiratory expansion and assess tactile fremitus; fremitus may be decreased or absent as transmission of vibrations from the larynx to the surface of the chest is impaired in COPD.

Percussion

Generalized hyperresonance may be heard over the hyperinflated lungs of a patient with COPD. Unilateral hyperresonance may suggest a large air-filled bulla in the lung. Dullness may suggest an area of consolidation such as lobar pneumonia.

Auscultation

Listen for adventitious breath sounds such as crackles, wheezes or rhonchi and identify in which part of the respiratory cycle the sounds are heard. In COPD where the airflow is decreased breath sounds will also be decreased and there may be very little actually to hear with the stethoscope. Diminished breath sounds are one of the few diagnostic signs in COPD and have been reported as a predictor of moderate COPD (Badgett *et al.*, 1993).

Differential diagnoses

The possibilities for differential diagnoses of COPD include asthma, lung cancer, cardiac causes of breathlessness, anaemia, recurrent

Table 8.1 Differential diagnosis of COPD and asthma

Features	COPD	Asthma
Current or ex-smoker	Yes	Maybe
History of asthma or childhood chestiness	Maybe	Often
Age at diagnosis	Usually over 40	Any age, often young
Productive cough	For many years	In exacerbations only
Breathlessness	Progressively worse over years	During exacerbations only
Variable symptoms	No	Yes
Nocturnal symptoms	Not usually	Yes
Morning symptoms	Short-lived. Often relieved by expectoration	Persist for several hours
Airway obstruction reversible	Not usually	Yes
Peak flow variability	No	Yes

pulmonary emboli, bronchiectasis or restrictive lung disease

It is particularly important to differentiate between asthma and COPD as the treatment strategies are different. Both diseases can present with similar clinical pictures but a careful history and assessment of lung function can confirm the diagnosis. Some diagnostic clues to differential diagnosis between asthma and COPD are shown in Table 8.1.

Assessment of lung function

Peak flow

Unlike in asthma peak flow measurements are not helpful in COPD. In asthma FEV_1 correlates reasonably well with peak flow but in COPD the peak flow can be misleadingly optimistic. In COPD the loss of elasticity in the airways means they are unable to resist compression. As the person breathes out the initial rise in expiratory flow is similar to that of a healthy person but after the peak is reached, there is a rapid reduction in flow and very low flows for the remainder of the expiration. COPD patients will have different degrees of airways collapse, depending on the degree of emphysema, so the relationship between FEV_1 and peak flow will vary. A peak flow variability of more than 15% is suggestive of asthma, but when peak flows are low, the spontaneous variability of the measurement may exceed 15% even in COPD. A normal peak flow (80% of predicted) does not exclude mild COPD.

Spirometry

Spirometry provides us with an objective assessment of respiratory function. The important spirometry measurements involved in COPD assessment are forced vital capacity (FVC), forced expiratory volume in one second (FEV_1) and the FVC/FEV_1 ratio. Basically this measures the total volume of air that can be forcibly expired from the lungs following full inspiration (FVC) and the proportion that can be expired in the first second (FEV_1). In healthy lungs, the airways are fully open and the individual can blow about 75% or more of the air out of their lungs in the first second (Figure 8.4). Where the airways are narrowed due to disease the airflow is much slower so it takes the individual much longer to expire fully (Figure 8.5). In severe obstruction less than 40% of air is expired in the first second.

The British Thoracic Society Guidelines (1997) recommend that spirometry should be performed on all patients with suspected COPD, both to confirm the diagnosis and to plan appropriate treatment. An abnormal FEV_1 (80% of predicted) with an FEV_1/FVC ratio of 70% and little variability in serial peak flow strongly suggests COPD. A normal FEV_1 excludes the

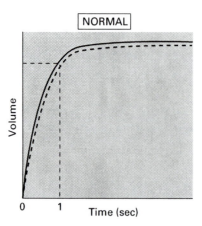

Figure 8.4 A normal volume/time trace (reproduced by permission from the BTS COPD Consortium, UK)

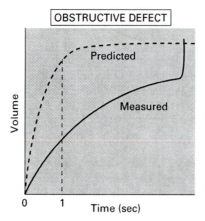

Figure 8.5 Obstructive spirometric pattern (reproduced by permission from the BTS COPD Consortium, UK)

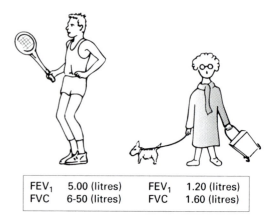

| FEV$_1$ | 5.00 (litres) | FEV$_1$ | 1.20 (litres) |
| FVC | 6-50 (litres) | FVC | 1.60 (litres) |

Figure 8.6 Normal values (reproduced by permission from the BTS COPD Consortium, UK)

spirometry the recommendations of the British Thoracic Society and the Association of Respiratory Technicians and Physiologists guidelines for the measurement of respiratory function should be followed (see Appendix A). For interpretation of spirometry readings, see Table 8.2.

Assessment of dyspnoea

Dyspnoea is probably the most disabling and distressing symptom of COPD, leading to much anxiety. Scales that have been specifically devised to measure this breathlessness have often been found to be inadequate (Mahler and Wells, 1988). Numerous studies have shown that dyspnoea is not strongly correlated with objective measures of pulmonary function (Stark *et al.*, 1982; Shandu, 1986; Schrier *et al.*, 1990; Alonso *et al.*, 1992); however, much of the treatment offered to people with COPD is aimed at reducing dyspnoea and therefore a dyspnoea scale can be a useful measure of the patient's response to treatment. However,

diagnosis (Figure 8.6). Although FEV$_1$/FVC ratio is diagnostic of obstruction, it is the FEV$_1$ measurement that is most useful in assessing severity and prognosis and demonstrating responsiveness to therapy. When undertaking

Table 8.2 Interpretation of spirometry readings

	FEV$_1$	FVC	FEV/FVC ratio
Normal	Greater than 80% predicted	Greater than 80% predicted	Greater than 70%
Obstructive	Reduced	Normal	Reduced
Restrictive	Reduced	Reduced	Normal/high
Combined	Reduced	Reduced	Reduced

Reproduced by permission from the BTS COPD Consortium, UK

Table 8.3 MRC Dyspnoea Scale

Grade	
0	Not troubled by breathlessness except on strenuous exercise
1	Short of breath when hurrying on the level or walking up a slight hill
2	Walks slower than people of the same age on the level because of breathlessness or has to stop for breath when walking at own pace
3	Stops for breath after walking about 100 metres or after a few minutes on the level
4	Too breathless to leave the house or breathless when dressing or undressing

MRC Dyspnoea Scale (Eakin *et al.*, 1993)

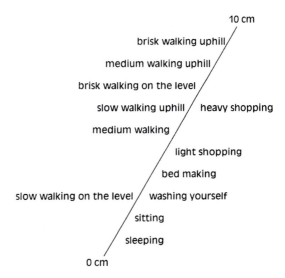

Figure 8.7 Oxygen cost diagram (Durnin and Passmore, 1967)

there is wide variation between individuals in the perceived intensity of dyspnoea in relation to lung ventilation.

In the Medical Research Council (MRC) Dyspnoea Scale (Eakin *et al.*, 1993) (Table 8.3), patients are graded depending on the activity which induces breathlessness.

The MRC scale is a useful tool when assessing the severity of the condition but is not very sensitive to change. Patients can experience improvements in the level of dyspnoea due to an intervention without actually going up a grade in the scale. A scale that is more sensitive to change is the Oxygen Cost Diagram (Durnin and Passmore, 1967) (Figure 8.7). This lists daily activities and the patient is asked to mark a point on a line above which breathlessness would be present. An 'ability score' is given as the distance in centimetres up the line from the zero point.

This test is quite sensitive to change and can help assess the impact of an intervention or measure deterioration in dyspnoea.

Another recognized way of assessing dyspnoea is formally measuring the walking distance with a 6-minute walk which measures the distance a patient can walk in 6 minutes, indoors and on the flat. The facilities need to be suitable, for example a long corridor without doors and free from the interruptions of other people. This unfortunately rules out many primary care settings. The shuttle test may be more appropriate in a clinic setting and in this test the patient performs a paced walk between two points 10 metres apart (a shuttle). The pace of the walk is increased at regular intervals, dictated by 'bleeps' on a tape recording, until the patient is forced to stop because of breathlessness or cannot keep up with the bleeps. The number of completed shuttles is then recorded.

As it is so important to assess dyspnoea before and after a given intervention then it may be necessary to adapt any of the above suggestions to fit the patient and the setting. This can be done by something as simple as asking the patient how many lamp posts they can walk past or how many stairs they can climb at home.

Assessment of health status

Patients are often graded as 'mild', 'moderate' or 'severe' according to their lung function results as recommended by the COPD Guidelines (Summary of British Thoracic Society, 1997) and many outcome measurements focus on pathophysiological measures which often correlate poorly with general quality of life (Jones, 1991). The FEV_1 can be reduced by as much as 50% before the patient notices significant disability due to dyspnoea. Dyspnoea puts a mental and physical strain on the patient and has a major impact on health status. The physical symptoms of COPD significantly affect psychological, social and sexual health and can leave patients feeling socially isolated and depressed. Due to its handicapping and disabling nature 'quality of life' is an important consideration in assessing the impact of COPD. However, there are many determinants of 'quality of life' not directly related to the disease process, for example expectations of life/illness, mood, mental health, coexisting disease, treatments (and side effects), family support and social network. Quality of life is unique to the individual and a more appropriate term to assess health related quality of life is 'health status' which aims to measure the health of the patient in a formal standardized manner. Assessing dyspnoea may give you part of the picture, but assessing health status tells you how dyspnoea is affecting life.

There are a number of validated health status questionnaires that are generic and can be used over a spectrum of diseases and several of these are appropriate to assess patients with COPD. Scales such as 'Sickness Impact profile' (Bergner *et al.*, 1981), the 'Quality of Wellbeing Schedule (Kaplan *et al.*, 1984), and the SF-36 (Ware *et al.*, 1993) have been used with varying success. Some correlate better with lung function, others with dyspnoea. Some are more sensitive to symptoms of severe disease and less useful in mild or moderate disease. Another set of health status questionnaires has been developed that are disease specific and are appropriate only for patients with chronic respiratory disease. Examples of disease specific questionnaires include:

- The Chronic Respiratory Disease Index Questionnaire (Guyatt *et al.*, 1987), a 20 item questionnaire which considers fatigue, mastery (control of the disease), sleep disturbances, social disruption, cognition, anger, depression, anxiety, frustration and irritability. The questionnaire (taking about 15–25 minutes) must be administered by an interviewer who has received training.
- The St George's Respiratory Questionnaire (Jones *et al.*, 1992) is a self-administered questionnaire divided into three parts: symptoms, activity and impact. It contains 76 items and while the impact section covers social and emotional disturbances it does not include anxiety and depression.

Scores are calculated using weights attached to each item.

A shortened version of the SGRQ, with just 20 questions, is available and may be appropriate in some settings.

There are other disease specific questionnaires in use but these two are commonly used in the UK.

Many of the health status questionnaires have been developed in hospital/research settings to measure formal, trial interventions and in many studies a combination of generic and disease specific instruments are needed to demonstrate the impact of the intervention on the health status of the patients. These instruments are not practically suitable for measuring individual interventions in primary care because they are far too complex. There is certainly a need for the development of a simple and effective tool to assess health status routinely. At present it may be more appropriate simply to ask the patient what impact the disease is having on their daily life and recording this at each consultation. It has been demonstrated that by asking patients simple questions such as; 'How do you feel?' correlates well with their health status (Jones and Bosh, 1997). Specifically enquiring about anxiety, depression and frustration should be part of the routine consultation, as when asked how they feel, patients often assume the enquiry is just about physical symptoms. Treating depression can have a significant impact on health status.

Limiting the impact of COPD on the patient

COPD is a complex disease with individual patients responding differently to the treatment options available. Generally in primary care COPD is underdiagnosed and under-treated. In an average GP list of 2500 patients there are likely to be about 100–150 patients with COPD, however, there is wide geographic variation that correlates to smoking rates in the area. The patients with mild to moderate COPD may be unknown to the health professionals and those with more severe disease may be being treated but inappropriately. With the surge of asthma clinics in the 1990s patients who presented regularly with persistent breathlessness and cough tended to be managed along the asthma guidelines (Summary of British Guidelines on Asthma Management, 1997), which means they may have been inappropriately treated. In 1997 the British Thoracic Society published its long awaited COPD guidelines which offered an evidence-based approach to managing this complex condition. The guidelines offer a structured way to differentiate between asthma and COPD, using spirometry, and to patient management. Suggested management differs significantly from the asthma guidelines and guide the management of exacerbations and referral to secondary care. A summary of the guidelines can be found in Figure 8.8.

Regular monitoring of disease impairment in patients with COPD is not as important as some other chronic conditions, e.g. diabetes and ischaemic heart disease. Accurate diagnosis, appropriate therapy trials and of course 'stop smoking advice' are important issues of planned care. With these interventions in mind annual planned monitoring may be enough to manage the stable COPD patient. Spirometry assessment will initially provide the diagnosis and is needed for therapeutic trials, but there is little to gain from performing these tests regularly simply as a monitoring procedure. Ongoing care should consist of what is important to the patient, which is not their FEV_1. Patients need to be seen around times of exacerbations when they may experience fear and a loss of control. They should be encouraged to make appointments when *they* feel it necessary.

Smoking cessation

Stopping smoking is the single most important intervention in COPD and the only thing that significantly alters the natural history of the disease. Whatever stage of COPD, from small airways disease to severe disease, stopping smoking is beneficial. In healthy non-smoking adults FEV_1 declines continuously and smoothly over their lifetime and they almost never develop clinically significant airflow obstruction. Fletcher and Peto (1977) discovered that many smokers are resistant to the effect of smoke on their airways and follow the same pattern as non-smokers, never developing airflow obstruction. Some smokers, however, are susceptible to the effects of smoking and develop varying degrees of airflow obstruction. Stopping smoking may make little difference in the decline in FEV_1 in a non-susceptible smoker (although the individual is still at risk of other smoking related diseases) but can normalize the decline in the susceptible smoker. They will never recover lost FEV_1, but the subsequent rate of loss of FEV_1 will revert to normal. The Fletcher and Peto diagram (Figure 8.9) can help demonstrate to susceptible smokers the benefits of stopping smoking and, in the right situation, can be a powerful tool for the health professional. However, this approach does not work for all smokers and is criticized by some as being too negative. Whichever way smoking cessation is encouraged, the positive benefits of not smoking should always be the primary focus of the advice. Unfortunately, attempts at stopping smoking are commonly unsuccessful. Nicotine is a highly addictive neural stimulant, enhancing concentration and mental agility as well as reducing anxiety and 'calming the nerves'. Reducing the amount of cigarettes smoked or changing to a lower tar often just results in the smoker taking longer and deeper puffs of each cigarette to get the same amount of nicotine.

Nicotine replacement therapy (NRT) doubles long-term abstinence rates (Silagy *et al.*, 1994). A meta-analysis conducted by Petty and Mett (1995) of the effectiveness of nicotine replacement patches in 5098 patients showed abstinence rates after 6 months of 22% among users compared to 9% using placebo. The European CEASE trial found that a higher than average dose of nicotine patch was associated with an increase in long-term success in smoking cessation but continuation of treatment beyond 8–12 weeks did not increase the success rate (Tonnesen *et al.*, 1999).

Bupropion is the first licensed non-nicotine pharmacological therapy for smoking cessation. This drug has been licensed in the USA as an antidepressant and works by inhibiting the neuronal reuptake of dopamine and noradrenaline (Ascher *et al.*, 1995). It was noticed anecdotally that some patients treated with bupropion for depression spontaneously stopped smoking, so further studies have been done to investigate bupropion as an aid to smoking cessation. The first studies (Hurt *et al.*, 1997; Jorenby *et al.*, 1999) demonstrate that point prevalence abstinence rates after 4 weeks and one year were higher in patients treated with bupropion and the results of further studies are awaited.

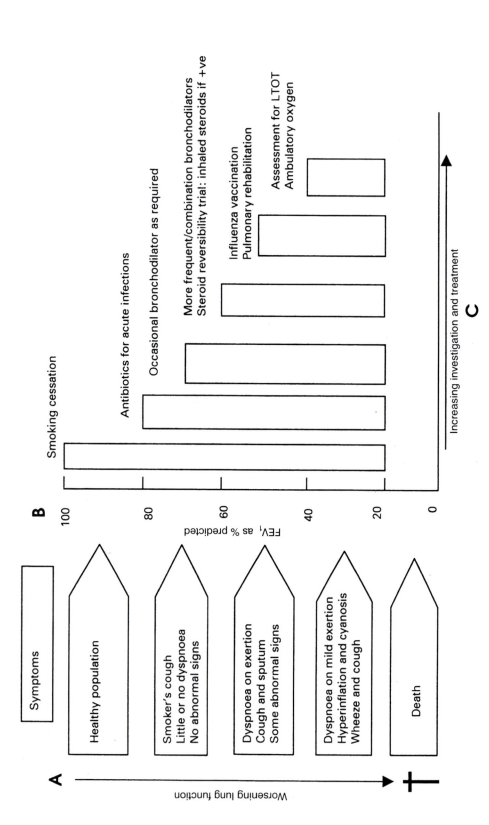

Figure 8.8 The COPD escalator. A, Worsening lung function; B, FEV₁ % predicted; C, increasing investigation and treatment (adapted with permission from BMJ Publishing Group (summary of the COPD Guidelines from the British Thoracic Society – COPD Management Guidelines, *Thorax*, **52** (suppl. 5), S1–S28), 1997)

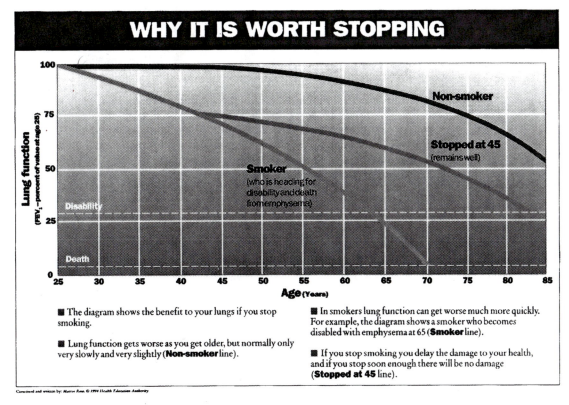

Figure 8.9 Why it is worth stopping (Reproduced by permission from the Health Education Authority, Trevelyan House, London)

These smoking cessation aids, both bupropion and NRT, are not magic cures for nicotine addiction. Stopping smoking needs a great deal of willpower and motivation and the most important way health professionals can limit the impact of COPD is by being fully committed to smoking cessation interventions as early in the disease process as possible. If patients cannot give up all together they should be encouraged to cut down as much as possible to reduce the harmful effect of carbon monoxide. NRT may help them smoke less. Preventative strategies must focus on reducing smoking rates nationwide.

Treatment of infective exacerbations

Because of airway damage patients with COPD are highly prone to bacterial infections which are thought to play an important role in exacerbations. The clinician has the problem of identify-ing which patients have infections caused by bacterial infections and what treatment they should receive. Anthonisen *et al.* (1987) suggest that patients with at least two of the following three symptoms will benefit from an antibiotic:

- Increased breathlessness
- Increased sputum volume
- Development of purulent sputum

A meta-analysis by Saint *et al.* (1995) showed that antibiotics improved patient peak flow rates compared with placebo during an exacerbation, however, not all exacerbations are due to a bacterial organism. Antibiotic prescribing is usually empirical in acute exacerbations of COPD due to the length of time it takes to perform laboratory tests and get the results. The decision on whether and which antibiotic to prescribe should be based on the presenting symptoms, the history and the physical examination. It should be guided by the BTS COPD guidelines (Summary of British Thoracic Society,

1997) and local antibiotic guidelines, where they exist.

Bronchodilators

After smoking cessation and appropriate treatment of acute infections, bronchodilators are the next intervention that can often reduce symptoms. They can be introduced early in the disease process, while the patient shows only mild symptoms and little reduction in lung function. As the disease progresses, more frequent, higher doses may be required and evidence suggests that there is an advantage to combining anticholinergics with $\beta2$ agonists (Sclar *et al.*, 1994). Even when patients show no reversibility to bronchodilators they often benefit from regular bronchodilator therapy. Teramoto *et al.* (1997) suggest that a reduction of air trapping after the inhalation of an anticholinergic (oxitropium bromide) may enhance the ability of the diaphragm to generate pressure resulting in a reduced sensation of dyspnoea during exercise in patients with COPD. Studies have demonstrated that long-acting $\beta2$ agonists are of benefit to some patients with COPD (Ulrik, 1995; Matera *et al.*, 1995; Boyde *et al.*, 1997) and the 1997 BTS guidelines suggest that long-acting $\beta2$ agonists should be used in those patients who demonstrate objective evidence of their benefit.

Steroids

The inflammatory component of COPD is likely to worsen during an exacerbation and this has been the rationale for rescue courses of steroids at this time. There is now evidence to support the early use of oral or parenteral corticosteroids in exacerbations of COPD (Wood-Baker and Walters, 1998). However, there is no firm evidence supporting the use of steroids in stable COPD. The BTS Guidelines (1997) suggest that inhaled steroids should be given to patients who respond to an oral or inhaled steroid trial. About 10% of patients with stable COPD will achieve an improvement in FEV_1 following a steroid trial (Callahan *et al.*, 1991). However, the use of inhaled steroids following a trial of high dose oral steroids has been questioned for some time. Stokes *et al.* (1982) found that even a response to prednisolone 30 mg/day

over 3 weeks was unlikely to be followed by maintenance of this improvement in FEV_1 3 months later when the dose was reduced to a more acceptable level of 10 mg/day. Fenley (1988) questions the need to find out whether there is a response to high dose prednisolone if this cannot be related to the response to a more acceptable long-term maintenance dose and called for the benefit of high dose inhaled steroids to be evaluated. There have since been several clinical trials of inhaled steroids in COPD. The EUROSCOP study (Lofdahl *et al.*, 1998) investigated patients with mild COPD and compared budesonide 800 µg daily with placebo over 2 years. There was no significant change in the rate of decline in FEV_1. The Copenhagen Lung Study (Vestbo *et al.*, 1999) investigated a similar group of patients and also found no benefit from budesonide 800 mg compared to placebo. The ISOLDE study (Burge, 2000) investigated patients with more severe COPD and demonstrated no effect of fluticasone propionate 1000 µg daily on the rate of decline in lung function, although there was a small positive impact on exacerbation rates and quality of life. A meta-analysis of studies (Van Grunsven *et al.*, 1999) showed that there was a preservation of FEV_1 during 2 years of treatment but only with high doses of inhaled steroids. Low dose inhaled steroids do not seem to have a beneficial effect. The use of high dose inhaled steroids in irreversible COPD is not standard practice but may be an appropriate therapeutic option especially in patients who suffer frequent exacerbations.

Influenza and pneumonia vaccination

The Department of Health recommends that patients with chronic lung disease should be vaccinated against influenza and pneumococcal pneumonia. There is yet little evidence to back up pneumococcal vaccination but influenza vaccination has been shown to reduce serious illness and death (Nichol *et al.*, 1994).

Pulmonary rehabilitation

Breathlessness on exertion and the fear related to it often leads the individual to avoid activity and with disease progression patients with

COPD become increasingly less mobile. Their skeletal muscles are underused and there is diminishing exercise capacity. Patients often lose confidence and start to withdraw from social activities. The normal stresses and anxieties of daily life are sometimes enough to induce breathlessness and patients may live within an 'emotional straightjacket' fearing anything that may bring on breathlessness. Rehabilitation aims to restore the individual to the best physical and mental state possible. It does this by a structured programme involving individually prescribed exercise training along with education about managing the disease and psychological support. It has been shown to improve exercise capacity and psychological well-being of patients with COPD (Holle *et al.*, 1988; Celli, 1989). Unfortunately, pulmonary rehabilitation is usually given low priority even though there is good evidence to demonstrate that the intervention optimizes functional capacity and reduces hospital admissions.

When considering a patient for a pulmonary rehabilitation programme, issues such as disease severity, age, cultural background, smoking status and level of hypoxia must be considered. The main barriers to successful rehabilitation are motivation, co-morbidity and geography or transport. Good, accessible rehabilitation programmes are few and far between and the main reason for this is one of funding. Those programmes that are available tend to be hospital based, some being funded through research and trials. There is a great need for community-based pulmonary rehabilitation.

Oxygen

Short-term oxygen may be administered to COPD patients while in hospital for acute exacerbations but long-term oxygen therapy (LTOT) is used quite differently. It is the only intervention, apart from smoking cessation, that can actually increase life expectancy. Studies have shown that LTOT improves survival in patients with COPD and respiratory failure (Medical Research Council Working Party, 1981). To be effective LTOT must be administered for at least 15 h/day. An oxygen concentrator is the most cost-effective way to do this and allows the patient the flexibility to move around the home and garden. LTOT is only usually appropriate for patients with severe

COPD who are hypoxic and have evidence of right ventricular failure and peripheral oedema. The clinical criteria for LTOT are: FEV_1 less than 1.5 litres, PaO_2 less than 7.3 Pa with no hypercapnoea, evidence of peripheral oedema and pulmonary hypertension. The patient should also be living in a non-smoking environment due to the fire hazard of smoking and oxygen. Before LTOT is prescribed a trial of long-term oxygen must establish that oxygen corrects arterial oxygen tension without causing a rise in arterial carbon dioxide as this could increase the respiratory failure.

Nutrition

The act of preparing and eating a meal can induce breathlessness. Chewing a large meal needs a considerable amount of energy and the severe COPD patient and their family need practical advice about preparing small, frequent, easily digestible meals. There is no convincing evidence to support nutritional supplements in COPD. Lewis *et al.* (1987) found no differences in respiratory muscle function between poorly-nourished men with COPD and well-nourished men with a similar degree of the disease. In practice a nutritional assessment is made from body mass index, clinical history, anorexia, breathlessness on eating and difficulty chewing or swallowing. For individual patients with specific problems such as obesity or malnutrition then a dietician referral may be useful.

Organization of care

Historically much of the assessment, diagnosis and management of COPD patients happened in secondary care but, since the BTS COPD Guidelines (1997), there has been an increasing interest in managing COPD in primary care. This is a complex condition occurring often in older patients with other co-morbidity, however, with the right spirometry equipment and adequately trained health professionals, assessment and diagnosis can be undertaken in primary care. Following the recommendations of the guidelines a structured approach of patient management is possible. However, the commitment for individual practices to take this on is considerable and it may be a more consistent option to provide community-based spirometry services through primary care groups. One barrier to effective management of COPD in the community is the low priority the government has placed on respiratory diseases. Where there is a National Service Framework, for example in coronary heart disease, primary care groups are more likely to invest in services for both treatment and prevention. The quality of care offered to COPD patients varies greatly. There are some excellent examples of good practice such as community-based spirometry services for diagnosis and assessment, accessible high quality pulmonary rehabilitation, specialist teams to manage exacerbations at home and prevent hospital admission. One problem is that the provision of these services is inconsistent and the care received may depend on where you live.

Self-help groups can offer support and advice to patients with chronic disease and their carers. The Breathe Easy Group, linked to the British Lung Foundation, offers a wide range of support materials and organizes local, patient-led groups in many localities.

Primary and secondary care collaboration

Whatever the quality of primary care for COPD patients secondary care will be inevitable at times. In practices where full spirometry assessment is not an option then referral may be necessary to establish a diagnosis and recommend treatment. With disease progression admissions for acute exacerbations may become inevitable. Good communication is important to know what tests and treatment the patient has already tried. If a formal steroid trial or other therapeutic trials, using spirometry, have been undertaken in primary care then the results should be relayed to the hospital to ensure patients are not discharged on inappropriate treatment.

Conclusion

COPD is a progressive and destructive lung disease directly linked to cigarette smoking. The only way to reduce the prevalence of the disease is to reduce smoking rates. The British Thoracic Society COPD Guidelines (1997) pro-

vide the benchmark for current best practice and the next anticipated COPD guidelines, the Global Obstructive Lung Disease (GOLD) guidelines, may offer further evidence-based recommendations. Spirometry is needed to make a formal assessment and diagnosis and the results will demonstrate the severity of the disease. However, spirometry will not accurately predict the level of disability and handicap of the individual sufferer. The goals of management must be to reduce that disability and handicap due mainly to dyspnoea. Patient assessment involves much more than lung function measurement and management involves much more than drug therapy. What COPD patients expect and deserve from the health service is accurate diagnosis, appropriate treatment, management by trained health professionals and support to cope with the physical, social and psychological consequences of the disease.

Appendix A

Guidelines for the measurement of respiratory function

(Recommendations of the British Thoracic Society and the Association of Respiratory Technicians and Physiologists – adapted from *Respiratory Medicine* (1994) **88**, 165–194)

Section 1 – Preliminary procedures

1.1 The subject should be correctly prepared for the tests and various subject details recorded.

1.2 The subject's age, height and weight (wearing indoor clothes without shoes) are obtained for later use in the calculation of the reference values. The height should be measured without shoes, with the feet together standing as tall as possible with the eyes level looking straight ahead using an accurate measuring device. For patients with a deformity of the thoracic cage, such as kyphoscoliosis, the arm span from finger tip to finger tip can be used instead as an estimate of height.

1.3 The operator should record the type and dosage of any (inhaled or oral) medication and when the drugs were last administered.

1.4 Ideally the subject should be asked to avoid:

A Smoking for 24 h prior to the test

B Consuming alcohol for at least 4 h prior to the test

C Vigorous exercise for at least 30 minutes prior to the test

D Wearing clothing which substantially restricts full chest and abdominal expansion

E Eating a substantial meal for at least 2 h prior to the test

F Taking short-acting bronchodilator drugs for at least 2 h prior to the test.

These requests should be made at the time of making the appointment. On arrival, all the points should be checked, and any deviations from them recorded. Where possible corrective action should be taken.

1.5 Subjects should be as relaxed as possible before and during the tests, and should be seated for 5–10 minutes prior to testing. This will give time for careful instruction in all the required manoeuvres. The subject should remain seated until all technically acceptable manoeuvres are completed.

1.6 For reasons of safety the patient should not stand during dynamic tests such as PEF and FVC but should sit upright in a chair with arms. The patient should be positioned correctly in relation to the equipment.

1.7 Patients should be asked to loosen tight fitting clothing. Dentures should normally be left in place; if they are loose, they may interfere with performance and are best removed.

1.8 When patients attend for repeat testing, for example at a clinic, then ideally the time of day, the equipment and the operator should be the same.

1.9 Ambient temperature and barometric pressure must be recorded in order to allow BTPS corrections to be made. With most devices, however, temperature and pressure corrections are not required or are done automatically. For greater accuracy ambient temperature and barometric pressure can be recorded in order to facilitate BTPS correction to be made. When using a spirometer, recording the gas temperature within the spirometer would lead to a more accurate correction factor.

Section 2 – Procedures for FEV_1 and VC

2.1 Definitions

2.1.1 Forced expiratory volume in 1 second (FEV_1)

This is the maximal volume of gas that can be expired from the lungs in the first second of a forced expiration from a position of full inspiration.

2.1.2 Vital capacity (VC)

When the term vital capacity is used without further qualification it conveniently refers to a relaxed vital capacity measurement as defined below.

Forced vital capacity (FVC)

This is the maximal volume of gas that can be expired from the lungs during a *forced* expiration from a position of full inspiration.

Relaxed vital capacity (RVC)

This can be measured in two ways:

A Expiratory vital capacity (EVC):
The maximal volume of gas that can be expired from the lungs during a relaxed expiration from a position of full inspiration.

B Inspiratory vital capacity (IVC):
The volume of gas that can be inspired into the lungs during a relaxed inspiration from a position of full expiration.

NB: All these volumes should be expressed in litres at body temperature and pressure, saturated with water vapour (BTPS)

2.2 Equipment

The equipment should be capable of measuring volumes of at least 7.5 l and produce a graphical display of adequate size.

Calibration checks to confirm correct equipment function with regard to volume and time should be carried out on a regular basis. Non-sealed spirometers (e.g. pneumotacograph-based systems) should be calibrated prior to each recording session. Sealed spirometers require regular checking for leaks, and dry bellows spirometers should be checked before each recording session.

Any necessary cleaning and maintenance procedures should also be carried out on a regular basis.

2.3 Procedure

2.3.1 The equipment and the patient are prepared for the test and the purpose and nature of the test are explained to the patient.

2.3.2 For FEV_1 and FVC the patient is instructed to breathe in as deeply as possible (i.e. to full inspiration) before placing the lips tightly around the mouthpiece and then to blow out into the equipment as hard and as fast as possible until no further gas can be exhaled.

The patient should prevent the tongue from occluding the mouthpiece and the teeth should be placed around the outside of the mouthpiece if it is a rigid tube.

Some systems require the patient to insert the mouthpiece and to breathe normally prior to the maximal inspiration.

A nose clip is not essential for measurement of FEV_1 and FVC.

2.3.3 A relaxed VC should be recorded as well as the FVC. A nose clip is required. The patient is instructed to blow out from a position of maximal inspiration at a sustained and comfortable speed until no further gas can be exhaled.

Useful contacts

The National Asthma and Respiratory Training Centre
The Athenaeum
10 Church Street
Warwick
CV34 4AB

British Lung Foundation
New Garden House
78 Hatton Garden
London EC1N 7BE

References

Alonso J, Anto J M, Gonzalez, M, Fiz J A, Izquierdo J, Morera J (1992) Measurement of a general health status of non-oxygen-dependent chronic obstructive pulmonary disease patients. *Medical Care* **30** (suppl.), 125–135

Anthonisen W R, Manfreda J, Warren C P W, Hershfield E S, Harding G K M (1987) Antibiotic therapy in exacerbations of chronic obstructive pulmonary disease. *Annals of Internal Medicine* **106**, 196–204

Ascher J A, Cole J O, Colin J N *et al.* (1995) Bupropion: a review of its mechanism of antidepressant activity. *Journal of Clinical Psychiatry* **56**, 395–401

Badgett R G, Tanaka D J, Hunt D K (1993) Can moderate chronic obstructive pulmonary disease be diagnosed by historical and physical findings alone? *American Journal of Medicine* **94**, 188–196

Bergner M, Bobbitt R A, Carter W B, Gibson B S (1981) The Sickness Impact Profile: development and final revision of a health status measure. *Medical Care* **19**, 787–805

Boyde G, Morice A H, Pounsford J C, Siebert M, Peslis N, Crawford C (1997) An evaluation of salmeterol in the treatment of chronic obstructive pulmonary disease. *European Respiratory Journal* **10**, 815–821

Burge P S (2000) Randomised, double blind, placebo controlled study of fluticasone propionate in patients with moderate to severe chronic obstructive airways disease: the ISOLDE trial. *British Medical Journal* **320**, 1297–1302

Callahan C, Dittus R S, Katz B P (1991) Oral corticosteroid therapy for patients with stable chronic obstructive pulmonary disease: a meta analysis. *Annals of Internal Medicine* **114**, 216–223

Calverley P M A, Sondhi S (1998) The burden of obstructive lung disease in the UK – COPD and Asthma. *Thorax* **52** (suppl. 4), A83 and poster presented at the BTS meeting 1998

Celli B R (1989) Pulmonary rehabilitation. *Pulmonary Critical Care Update* **4**, 2–8

Clark K D, Warfrobe-Wong N, Elliott J J, Gill P T, Tait N P, Snashall P D (1998) Cigarette smoke inhalation and lung damage in smoking volunteers. *European Respiratory Journal* **12**, 395–399

Dockery D W, Speizer F E, Ferris B G Jr (1988) Cumulative and reversible effects of lifetime smoking on simple tests of lung function in adults. *American Review of Respiratory Disease* **137**, 286–292

Doll R, Peto R, Wheatley K *et al.* (1994) Mortality in relation to smoking: 40 years' observation on male British doctors. *British Medical Journal* **309**, 901–911

Durnin J G V A, Passmore R (1967) *Energy, Work and Leisure.* Heinemann, London

Eakin E G, Kaplan R M, Reis A L (1993) Measurement of dyspnoea in chronic obstructive pulmonary disease. *Quality of Life Research* **2**, 181–191

Fenley D C (1988) Chronic obstructive pulmonary disease. *Disease-a-month.* Year Book Medical Publishers, Chicago

Fleetham J A, Arnup M E, Anthonisen N R (1984) Familial aspects of ventilatory control in patients with chronic obstructive pulmonary disease. *American Review of Respiratory Disease* **129**, 3–7

Fletcher C, Peto R (1977) The natural history of chronic airflow obstruction. *British Medical Journal* **1**, 1645–1648

Goren A I, Bruderman I (1989) Effects of occupational exposure and smoking on respiratory symptomatology and PFT in healthy panellists and COPD patients. *European Journal of Epidemiology* **5**, 58–64

Guidelines for the Measurement of Respiratory Function: Recommendations of the British Thoracic Society and the Association of Respiratory Technicians and Physiologists (1994) *Respiratory Medicine* **88**, 165–194

Guyatt G H, Berman L B, Townsend M *et al.* (1987) A measure of quality of life for clinical trials in chronic lung disease. *Thorax* **42**, 773–778

Hanrahan J P, Sherman C B, Bresnitz E A, Emmons K M (1996) Cigarette smoking and health. *American Journal of Respiratory and Critical Care Medicine* **153**, 861–865

Hendrick D J (1996) Occupation and chronic obstructive pulmonary disease (COPD). *Thorax* **51**, 947–955

Higgins M (1991) Risk factors associated with chronic obstructive lung disease. *Annals of the New York Academy of Sciences* **624**, 7–17

Holle R H, Williams D V, Vandree F C *et al.* (1988) Increased muscle efficiency and sustained benefits in an outpatient community-based pulmonary rehabilitation program. *Chest* **94**, 1161–1168

Hurt R D, Sachs D P L, Glover E D *et al.* (1997) A comparison of sustained-released bupropion and placebo for smoking cessation. *New England Journal of Medicine* **337**, 1195–202

Hutchinson D C S (1988) Natural history of alpha-1-protease inhibitor deficiency. *American Journal of Medicine* **84** (suppl. 6A), 3–12

Itabashi S, Fukashima T, Aikawa T *et al.* (1990) Allergic sensitization in elderly patients with chronic obstructive pulmonary disease. *Respiration* **57**, 384–388

Janoff A (1985) Elastases and emphysema. Current assessment of the protease-antiprotease hypothesis. *American Review of Respiratory Disease* **132**, 417–433

Jones P W (1991) Measurement of quality of life in chronic obstructive pulmonary disease. *European Respiratory Journal* **1**, 445–453

Jones P W, Bosh T K (1997) Quality of life changes in COPD patients treated with salmeterol. *American Journal of Respiratory and Critical Care Medicine* **153**, 1283–1289

Jones P W, Quirk F H, Baveystock C M *et al.* (1992) A self-complete measure of chronic airflow limitation: the St George's questionnaire. *American Review of Respiratory Disease* **147**, 832–838

Jorenby D E, Leischow S J, Nides M A *et al.* (1999) A controlled trial of sustained-released bupropion, a nicotine patch, or both for smoking cessation. *New England Journal of Medicine* **340**, 685–691

Kaplan R M, Atkins C J, Times R *et al.* (1984) Validity of quality of well-being scale as an outcome measure in COPD. *Journal of Chronic Diseases* **37**, 85–95

Lewis M I, Belman M J, Dorr-Uyemura L (1987) Nutritional supplementation in ambulatory patients with chronic obstructive pulmonary disease. *American Review of Respiratory Disease* **135**, 1062–1068

Lofdahl C G, Postma D S, Laitinen L A *et al.* (1998) The European Respiratory Society study on chronic obstructive pulmonary disease (EUROSCOP): recruitment, methods and strategies. *Respiratory Medicine* **92,** 467–472

Macklem P T (1972) Obstruction in small airways – a challenge to medicine. *American Journal of Medicine* **52**, 721–724

Mahler D A, Wells C K (1988) Evaluation of clinical methods for rating dyspnoea. *Chest* **93**, 580–586

Matera M G, Cazzola M, Vinciguerra A *et al.* (1995) A comparison of bronchodilating effects of salmeterol, salbutamol and ipratropium bromide in patients with chronic obstructive pulmonary disease. *Pulmonary Pharmacology* **8**, 267–271

Medical Research Council Working Party (1981) Long-term domiciliary oxygen in chronic hypoxic cor pulmonale complicating chronic bronchitis and emphysema. *Lancet* **1**, 681–686

Meighan-Davies J, Parnell H (1999) Asthma – the community challenge. *Journal of Community Nursing* **13**, 42–46

Nichol K L, Margolis K L, Wuorenma J, Von Sternberg T (1994) The efficiency and cost effectiveness of vaccination against influenza among elderly persons living in the community. *New England Journal of Medicine* **331**, 778–784

Office of Population, Census and Surveys (1993) *Mortality statistics cause – England and Wales*. Series DH no 19. HMSO, London

Peto R (1994) Smoking and death: the past 40 years and the next 40. *British Medical Journal* **309**, 937–939

Petty T L, Mett L M (1995) How to help your patients stop smoking – what works and what doesn't. *Seminars in Respiratory and Critical Care Medicine* **16**, 92–98

Prescott E, Lange P, Vestbo J (1995) Chronic mucus hypersecretion in COPD and death from pulmonary infection. *European Respiratory Journal* **8**, 1333–1338

Rijcken B, Schouten J P, Xu X, Rosner B, Weiss S T (1995) Airway hyperresponsiveness to histamine associated with accelerated decline in FEV1. *American Journal of Respiratory and Critical Care Medicine* **151**, 1377–1382

Saint S, Bent S, Vittinghoff E, Grady D (1995) Antibiotics in chronic obstructive pulmonary disease exacerbations: a meta-analysis. *Journal of the American Medical Association* **273**, 957–960

Schrier A C, Dekker F W, Kaptein A A, Dijkman J H (1990) Quality of life in elderly patients with chronic non-specific lung disease seen in family practice. *Chest* **90**, 894–899

Sclar D A, Legg R F, Skaer T L, Robinson L M, Nemic N L (1994) Ipratropium bromide in the management of chronic obstructive pulmonary disease: effect on health service expenditures. *Clinical Therapeutics* **16**, 595–601

Shandu H (1986) Psychosocial issues in chronic obstructive pulmonary disease. *Clinics in Chest Medicine* **7**, 629–642

Silagy C, Mint D, Fowler G, Lancaster T (1994) Meta-analysis on efficiency of nicotine replacement therapy in smoking cessation. *Lancet* **343**, 139–142

Sluiter H J, Koeter G H, deMonchy J R G, Postma D S *et al.* (1991) The Dutch Hypothesis (chronic non specific lung disease) revisited. *European Respiratory Journal* **4**, 479–489

Stark R D, Gambles S A, Chattergee S S (1982) An exercise test to assess clinical dyspnoea: estimation of reproducibility and sensitivity. *British Journal of Diseases of the Chest* **76**, 269–278

Stokes T C, Shaylar J M, O'Reilly J F *et al.* (1982) Assessment of steroid responsiveness in patients with chronic airflow obstruction. *Lancet* **2**, 345–348

Stone P J, Gottlieg D J, O'Conner G T *et al.* (1995) Elastin and collagen degradation products in urine of smokers with and without chronic obstructive pulmonary disease. *American Journal of Respiratory and Critical Care Medicine* **151**, 952–959

Summary of the Asthma Guildelines from The British Thoracic Society (1997) COPD management guidelines. *Thorax* **52** (suppl.) S1–S28

Summary of the BTS Guidelines for the Management of COPD from The British Guidelines on Asthma Management (1997) *Thorax* **52** (suppl.) S1–S34

Teramoto S, Suzuki M, Matsus T *et al.* (1997) The effect of inhaled anticholinergic drug on dyspnoea and on the physiologic function of respiratory system in patients with chronic obstructive pulmonary disease. *Nippon Kyobu Skikkan Gakkai Zasshi* **35** (11), 1209–1214

Tonnesen P, Paoletti P, Gustavsson G (1999) High dose nicotine patches increases on year smoking cessation rates: results from the European CEASE trial. *European Respiratory Journal* **13**, 238–246

Ulrik S (1995) Efficacy of inhaled salmeterol in the management of smokers with COPD: a single-centre, randomised, double blind placebo-controlled, crossover study. *Thorax* **50**, 750–754

Van Grunsven P M, Can Schayck C P, Derenne J P *et al.* (1999) Long term effects of inhaled corticosteroids in chronic obstructive pulmonary disease: a meta-analysis. *Thorax* **54**, 7–14

Vermiere P A, Pride N B (1991) A 'splitting' look at chronic nonspecific lung disease (CNSLD): common features but diverse pathogenesis. *European Respiratory Journal* **4**, 490–496

Vestbo J, Prescott E, Lange P (1996) Association of chronic mucus hypersecretion with FEV1 decline and chronic obstructive pulmonary disease morbidity. Copenhagen City Heart Group. *American Journal of Respiratory and Critical Care Medicine* **153**, 1530–1535

Vestbo J, Sorensen T, Lange P *et al.* (1999) Long term effects of inhaled budesonide in mild and moderate chronic obstructive pulmonary disease: a randomised controlled trial. *Lancet* **353**, 1819–1823

Wald N J, Watt H C (1997) Prospective study of effect of switching from cigarettes to pipes or cigars on mortality from smoking related disease. *British Medical Journal* **314**, 1860

Wanner A (1990) The role of mucus in chronic obstructive pulmonary disease. *Chest*, Feb (suppl.), 11S–15S

Ware J E, Brook R H, Davies-Avery A (1993) *SF-36 Health Survey: Manual and Interpretation Guide*. The Health Institute, New England Medical Center, Boston

Wood-Baker R, Walters E H (1998) The role of corticosteroids in acute exacerbations of chronic obstructive pulmonary disease. *The Cochrane Library* Issue 4, Oxford, Update Software

Chapter

9

Continence

Wendy Colley and Ian Pomfret

A patient's perspective

I was in my late 30s when I was diagnosed as being incontinent following hysterectomy. My whole day, every day, is planned around the keeping of my condition a secret. I feel, if I am watchful and keep dry and clean, the sight and smell of an 'accident' does not pervade my daily life and that of others. No spontaneous acts for me!

The dictionary tells me that incontinence is 'an inability to control the evacuation of urine and faeces'. The medical profession explain to me that this is a common condition affecting many thousands of people. Why then do I feel dirty, isolated and alone?

In the Middle Ages leprosy sufferers were made, by law, to ring a handbell in public and cry 'Unclean'. I feel this is how incontinence is viewed among non-sufferers today; something which only affects the old and senile and which is not discussed in 'polite society'.

Visits to places outside my home must be meticulously planned by means of 'Toilet Routes' both public loos and the bathrooms of sympathetic friends who have become used to my urgent need to 'go'.

My body and home have become shrines to plastic, with catheters and drainage bags, bed and chair covers, all geared to the protection of skin and furniture against the effects of ammonia and smell.

Making new relationships, especially ones of a sexual nature, are almost impossible because of the fear of rejection and ridicule once the condition is known.

A common condition yes, but one that condemns the long-term sufferer to a 'half life' ruled by it . . .

More from a patient

So many factors rule my life with regard to my incontinence, that each day is different and 'a typical day' doesn't apply. The weather, my mood, if I need to leave the house, or my daily tasks, all affect how I deal with my condition day-to-day.

When I get up in the morning my first task is to check that my sheets are still dry. I have sheets and blankets because they are easier to wash, being less bulky than heavy duvets when wet. I have protective mattress and pillow covers on my bed (so no electric blankets for me even in winter), but sometimes urine leaks down the side of my night/Foley catheter, or the joint between night catheter and drainage bag becomes disconnected due to my sleep movements. Consequently I never sleep well . . .

The second thing I do on rising is turn off my 'Flip Flo' valve which connects the catheter to the drainage bag so that I can separate them safely and carry the filled bag down my steep staircase to the bathroom below, to empty and dispose of it. Before I used the catheter valves I fell over the trailing tubing whilst coming downstairs in the early hours, as I was half asleep. Fortunately I did myself no serious damage . . .

Prevalence

Incontinence is not a disease; it is a symptom of an underlying disorder (see Aetiology) and it may be defined in differing ways. Thomas, in her seminal study on the prevalence of incontinence, defined regular urinary incontinence as 'an involuntary excretion or leakage of urine in an inappropriate place or at an inappropriate time, twice or more a month' (Thomas *et al.*, 1980).

With regard to the definition of incontinence, the International Continence Society (ICS) in 1988 took a more holistic view, including the social problems associated with incontinence and defined the problem as 'an involuntary loss of urine which is objectively demonstrable and a social or hygienic problem' (Andersen *et al.*, 1988).

More recently in Britain, two major reports, *Incontinence – Causes, Management and Provision of Services* (Royal College of Physicians of London, 1995) and *Commissioning Comprehensive Continence Services* (The Continence Foundation, 1995), stated that around three million people in the UK are regularly incontinent, which accounts for a prevalence of around 40 per 1000 adults. In real terms this means that an average Health Care Trust of 250 000 population may have 10 000 adults and 1000 children who are incontinent with many of them unknown to health and social care services.

The Department of Health (DoH) review of *Good Practice in Continence Services* (Department of Health, 2000a) stated that it is difficult to measure accurately the prevalence of incontinence because the definitions of differing degrees of incontinence are subjective and people under-report their problems because of embarrassment. The report took a combination of the Thomas and the ICS definition, and stated that incontinence is 'the involuntary or inappropriate passing of urine and/or faeces that has an impact on social functioning or hygiene' and it also included nocturnal enuresis (bed-wetting).

The prevalence of urinary incontinence is as follows.

For people living at home:

- Between 1 in 20 and 1 in 14 women aged 15–44
- Between 1 in 13 and 1 in 7 women aged 45–64
- Between 1 in 10 and 1 in 5 women aged 65 and over
- Over 1 in 33 men aged 15–64
- Between 1 in 14 and 1 in 10 men aged 65 and over.

For people (both sexes) living in institutions:

- 1 in 3 in residential homes
- Nearly 2 in every 3 people in nursing homes
- one-half to two-thirds in wards for the elderly and elderly mental infirm.

The information relating to prevalence of faecal incontinence is less reliable, but the Department of Health report states that the prevalence for adults at home is about 1%, rising to 17% in the very elderly and with approximately 25% of people in residential care experiencing regular problems with faecal incontinence. The DoH report does, however, acknowledge that prevalence rates for incontinence are notoriously difficult to determine.

Children also have problems with urinary incontinence, with an estimated half million children in the UK experiencing nocturnal enuresis (persistent bed-wetting). The prevalence decreases with age as follows:

- 1 in 6 of children aged 5
- 1 in 7 of children aged 7
- 1 in 11 of children aged 9
- 1 in 50 of teenagers.

Children also have problems with faecal incontinence, as follows:

- 1 in 30 of children aged 4–5
- 1 in 50 of children aged 5–6
- 1 in 75 of children aged 7–10
- 1 in 100 of children aged 11–12.

In addition to adults and children there are groups within society who tend to experience problems with incontinence. It is usually associated with women and the elderly, but significant problems may be experienced by people with learning difficulties, physical and neurological disabilities, people from ethnic minorities, homeless people and people in institutional care, for example prisons.

Aetiology

Aetiology in a medico/nursing sense is a scientific study of the causes of disease, but incontinence is not a disease as seen from the definitions given in the section on epidemiology.

If incontinence were to be defined as a disease, it would mean that all babies are born diseased, based upon the current ICS definition!

Therefore, what is incontinence?

Given the definitions described in the section on epidemiology, incontinence, both urinary and faecal, can be due to four primary causes: physical, mental, social and environmental. These may be present individually, or more commonly as a combination of two or more, with any aspect predominant.

Incontinence is often identified as a healthcare need, but it has an equal, if not greater, effect on the social care needs of the individual. The ICS definition, for example, recognizes the social, rather than the medical aspects of the condition and this was reinforced by Sanderson (1991) who stated, 'The maintenance of continence is a health matter which, as well as affecting the health of the individual, has tremendous consequences for people. It is a major quality of life issue, which, if unchecked, frequently leads to social isolation and high stress rates in both sufferers and carers.'

Physical storage problems

Both the bladder and bowel have dual functions – storage and expulsion of waste material, i.e. urine and faeces. With regard to the bladder, physical urine storage problems include stress, urge and mixed incontinence.

Stress incontinence

This is defined as leakage of urine on exertion, in the absence of a bladder contraction (Andersen *et al.*, 1988). The cause is an incompetent urethral closure mechanism and is more common in post-menopausal, multiparous women, though it may also affect men post-prostatectomy.

Urge incontinence

This is the loss of varying amounts of urine following a strong, uncontrollable desire to void. Contributory factors may include urinary tract infection, poor mobility and/or dexterity, anxiety, diuretics, fluid restriction or drinks containing caffeine or alcohol.

Mixed incontinence

Mixed incontinence usually describes the presence of symptoms of both stress and urge incontinence. Causes of faecal storage problems would include diarrhoea and anal sphincter incompetence.

Voiding problems

These may be due to an outflow obstruction, for example an enlarged prostate, or faecal impaction causing pressure on the urethra. Alternatively, it may be due to a hypotonic or acontractile bladder, which is unable to expel urine. The most common cause of faecal expulsion problems is constipation.

Neurogenic bladder dysfunction

Problems of urine storage and efficient bladder emptying may be due to underlying neurological damage and symptoms vary with the site of the damage within the nervous system. One example is that of voiding problems which may be caused by detrusor sphincter dyssynergia, which occurs when the detrusor (bladder) muscle contracts but the sphincter mechanism fails to relax and open to allow complete bladder emptying. This is often seen in patients suffering from multiple sclerosis.

Reflex incontinence is due to detrusor hyper-reflexia in neuropathic absence of sensation, for example in paraplegia.

Mental, social and environmental causes of incontinence

These may also be described as functional incontinence, when the individual's inability to cope with society's demands for 'normal' continent behaviour is restricted, resulting in an inability to get to a toilet or other socially acceptable place to void or defaecate. Functional difficulties may include poor mobility, poor environmental facilities, confusional states, dementia, lack of motivation and depression.

The causes of incontinence are complex and multifactorial, requiring skilled, professional assessment and intervention if they are to be resolved.

Assessment of urinary incontinence

All patients presenting with incontinence should be offered an initial assessment by a suitably trained individual (Department of Health, 2000a). The purpose of assessing bladder function is to identify the underlying dysfunction, which can then be treated to effect a cure or an improvement. This may be relatively straight-forward or much more complex. Compare the following two examples:

Patient 1

A 35-year-old woman with two children presents to her general practitioner complaining of urinary leakage when attending her aerobics class. She also occasionally leaks urine if she suddenly sneezes. She does not complain of undue urinary frequency, urgency or nocturia, passes urine in a good flow and feels she is emptying her bladder. She is a non-smoker and her body mass index is considered 'healthy' at 25. On vaginal examination the bladder and urethra are well supported and there is no uterine descent or rectocoele. The Oxford Scale is used by trained health care professionals to estimate the strength of the pelvic floor muscle contraction during digital vaginal examination and in this patient the pelvic floor contraction, is estimated as grade 1, on a scale of 0–5 (Laycock, 1994). Routine urinalysis shows no abnormality, blood pressure is normal and she is otherwise fit and well. The patient is referred for advice and a course of pelvic floor exercises. Six months later she reports that she is now able to carry out her aerobic exercise without leakage and the pelvic floor contraction is estimated at grade 4.

Patient 2

A 35-year-old married man presents to his general practitioner with back pain, some changes to his gait and occasional episodes of sudden spontaneous bladder emptying over the previous 6 months. He also feels incomplete bladder emptying and has experienced several urinary tract infections. The urinary tract was investigated and showed hydronephrosis, dilated upper tracts and on cystoscopy the bladder was found to be trabeculated. This patient was found to have previously undetected spina bifida. Following urological investigations, bladder management is now achieved using intermittent self-catheterization.

These two patients are examples of two extreme cases, however, the challenge of assessment of incontinence and planning effective treatment and management is equally essential to both patients to maintain a healthy urinary tract and ensure quality of life for the sufferer.

Who should carry out the assessment?

Assessment is ideally multiprofessional and several members of the health care team can be involved. Examples include the practice nurse, GP, district nurse, occupational therapist and health visitor all of whom have a role to play. Further advice is available from the local continence adviser, who may be a nurse or physiotherapist and referral to a urodynamic clinic, a urologist, gynaecologist or urogynae-cologist or other consultant should be available in severe or complex cases.

The use of a single assessment tool or method should ensure that unnecessary repetition is avoided when the patient is seen by more than one member of the health care team (Button *et al.*, 1998).

What should be considered during assessment?

The *Good Practice in Continence Services* (DoH, 2000a) document suggests the key components of an initial assessment as:

● review of symptoms and their effect on quality of life
● assessment of desire for treatment alternatives

- examination of abdomen for palpable mass or bladder retention
- examination of perineum to identify prolapse and excoriation and to assess pelvic floor contraction
- rectal examination to exclude faecal impaction (not to be carried out in children)
- urinalysis to exclude infection
- assessment of manual dexterity
- assessment of the environment, e.g. accessibility of toilet facilities
- use of an 'Activities of daily living' diary
- identification of conditions that may exacerbate incontinence, e.g. chronic cough.

History

The history should at least include:

- Description of problem as perceived by the patient
- Onset – is it sudden, gradual, or related to an event, for example childbirth, bereavement, surgery
- Symptoms, which will describe:
  - frequency of micturition
  - urgency
  - nocturia
  - nocturnal enuresis
  - leakage of urine if present, how much, how often
  - urine stream – normal or reduced
  - pain or discomfort on micturition
  - urine – odour, presence of blood
  - female – any symptoms of prolapse
- Medical history
- Medication. It is essential to review the current medication of the patient as the side effects of many drugs can cause or contribute to incontinence.

Urinalysis

Testing the urine should be carried out as a matter of routine as a urinary tract infection or previously undiagnosed diabetes may be a contributing factor for the patient's symptoms.

- If the urine is obviously infected or blood-stained, send a clean specimen for culture and microscopy

- If the urine is clear, test with a urine reagent strip
- If the results are negative to blood, protein, nitrite and leucocytes, discard and report as no evidence of infection
- If any of the above are positive, send for culture and microscopy (Bayer Diagnostics, 1993).

Urine cytology

Urine cytology should be performed in the presence of incontinence and haematuria or when red cells are seen on urine microscopy, in order to exclude urothelial neoplasia (Shah and Leach, 1998).

Volume/frequency charting

It is very useful to ask the patient to chart information to aid diagnosis and to act as a baseline to compare the effect of interventions. The patient may be asked to keep a bladder diary in which they will be asked to record fluid intake and to measure urine volumes when voiding. Episodes of incontinence may also be recorded. Often, charts are available from companies (Figure 9.1), but it is very easy for the patient to make their own chart if ready printed charts are not available.

Usually information is collected for one week where practical and once the chart is complete, the following baseline data can be collated:

- Frequency – the number of voids each 24 h. The parameters quoted are the least and highest number of voids, for example frequency of 6–13 times in 24 h. Passing urine between 4 and 7 times in 24 h can be considered normal for someone with a reasonable fluid intake
- Maximum functional bladder capacity – this is the highest single void during charting and the normal bladder should be able to hold around 500–600 ml of urine
- Nocturia – the number of times the patient wakes needing to void during the night. Make sure that waking does not occur for other reasons, such as pain or to feed a baby. Waking to void once a night can be considered normal.

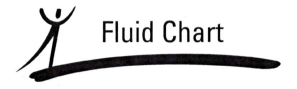

Fluid Chart

Please enter the amount you drink.

	Monday	Tuesday	Wednesday	Thursday	Friday	Saturday	Sunday
Midnight							
1am							
2							
3							
4							
5							
6							
7							
8							
9							
10							
11							
Noon							
1pm							
2							
3							
4							
5							
6							
7							
8							
9							
10							
11							
Totals							

= 150ml   = 200ml

Provided as a service to medicine by Pharmacia & Upjohn Limited

Figure 9.1 Example of chart available for patients (reproduced with kind permission from Pharmacia)

- Total output of urine in 24 h.
- Fluid intake in 24 h – the type of drinks should be recorded, as caffeinated drinks, tea, coffee and alcohol, can exacerbate symptoms of frequency and urgency in some people. A fluid intake of around 2 litres in 24 h is reasonable.
- Number of incontinent episodes – counting the number of episodes of incontinence provides a baseline for comparison after treatment. Make sure that the patient is not compromised at this time, for example a woman with stress incontinence who has a chest infection may leak urine more often than is usual, therefore counting incontinent episodes at this time would give false comparisons.

Physical examination

The physical examination is carried out by a competent professional. This may be a nurse, doctor or physiotherapist. Included in the physical examination will be:

- Abdominal examination – for palpable bladder, loaded colon, operation scars and any abnormalities
- Genitalia – to assess the condition and integrity of the skin, also tightness of the foreskin in male patients
- Vaginal examination – for the presence of cystocoele, urethrocoele, rectocoele, enterocoele, uterine descent and atrophic vaginitis, also to assess the strength of the pelvic floor contraction. During vaginal examination when observing the urethral opening, the patient may be asked to cough and the assessor will record whether or not urine leakage occurs
- Rectal examination – to assess anal tone and the presence of faeces. Rectal examination of the male patient will include assessment of the size and texture of the prostate gland by a professional trained to carry out digital rectal examination (DRE). It may be appropriate to measure the prostate specific antigen (PSA).

Neurological examination

A neurological examination must be included in all patients presenting with urinary incontinence.

Bowel function

Constipation, leading to faecal impaction, can cause direct pressure on the urethra, so preventing bladder emptying. Chronic straining at stool can contribute to the development of stress incontinence (Bayliss, 1996). Constipation can also be troublesome in patients using an indwelling catheter, resulting in by-passing of urine around the catheter.

Voiding flow rate and bladder emptying

How well urine is expelled from the bladder and whether or not bladder emptying is being achieved are important considerations. Urinary flow rate may be decreased due to outflow obstruction, such as prostatic disease, direct pressure from a full rectum, or due to a decreased or absent detrusor contraction. Absent or ineffective spinal cord nerve pathways affected by spinal injury, neurological disease such as multiple sclerosis or spina bifida, or damaged by diabetes will affect bladder function to some extent. Hesitancy, straining to pass urine and terminal dribble may also be present in patients with voiding difficulty.

Voiding normally results in complete bladder emptying, however, when obstruction to the outflow, neurological damage or detrusor failure is a factor, incomplete emptying may occur, resulting in a residual urine which can vary from 50 ml or so, to several litres. The consequence of a large residual urine is that the patient is at risk from urinary tract infection and reflux to the kidneys causing infection and eventually kidney damage and failure.

If there is any doubt regarding bladder emptying, a post-void in/out catheterization should be done or an estimate using an ultrasound Bladderscan machine if one is available.

Other factors

Other factors which may be relevant for some patients when assessing their incontinence include:

- Mobility
- Manual dexterity
- Cognitive function
- Environment
- Psychological state.

When the underlying cause of the bladder dysfunction has not been identified or a mixed picture of symptoms emerges, then referral for further investigation and advice may be indicated. Throughout the country, service provision varies, however, local services should include a continence advisory service and acute service provision should offer a urodynamic facility with appropriate consultant input.

Investigations

Urodynamic studies

Urodynamic evaluation of bladder function becomes critically important when other, simpler methods of investigation have not provided a concrete clinical diagnosis. Urodynamic investigations study the pressure and flow relationships in the bladder and urethra. There are several investigations that may be carried out, the most frequently undertaken are uroflowmetry, cystometry and videourodynamics.

Uroflowmetry

Urinary flow can be measured easily and non-invasively by use of a flow meter, which should be available in all urological units. Flow studies should be performed in all patients with voiding dysfunction and incontinence (Shah and Leach, 1998). The patient is asked to void urine onto the flowmeter (in a private room), once the bladder feels reasonably full. Flow rate is expressed in millilitres of urine passed per second. A series of several separate flow studies may be done for comparison, as variations in flow rates do occur and a single

test should not be used as the basis of a firm clinical diagnosis.

Abrams and Torrens (1979) suggested that with voided volumes greater than 200 ml, the free peak flow rates for normal patients are:

- Males under 40 years: >22 ml/s
- Males 40–60 years: >18 ml/s
- Males over 60 years: >13 ml/s
- Females under 50 years: >25 ml/s
- Females over 50 years: >18 ml/s

The above data should be used as a guideline only as male patients with outflow obstruction may appear to have a normal flow rate which is maintained at the expense of a very high voiding pressure (Shah, 1984).

Cystometry

Cystometry is the urodynamic test carried out to measure the pressure within the bladder during filling and emptying, the presence of any residual urine and the urinary flow rate. The investigation takes approximately 30 minutes and the patient can eat and drink normally prior to the test. A small diameter catheter is passed urethrally and used to fill the bladder with sterile normal saline at room temperature, usually at a medium-fill rate of 30–60 ml/minute. The urethral catheter may incorporate a sensor to measure the pressure or a separate fine bore catheter is passed at the same time as the filling catheter to measure the pressure in the bladder. Abdominal pressure is measured simultaneously using a sensor inserted rectally (or vaginally) to identify pressure changes which are due to talking, coughing and so on, so these can be deducted from bladder pressure to give true intravesical pressure when interpreting the results.

Videourodynamics

Videourodynamics, which combines cystometry using contrast medium with simultaneous radiological screening of the bladder and urethra, is currently the gold standard of urodynamic investigation. It is more helpful in the diagnosis of more complex cases of incontinence than cystometry alone (Shah and Leach, 1998).

Other investigations

Plain radiography

In patients with suspected urological abnormality, a plain abdominal X-ray should be used to eliminate calculi, soft tissue masses and faecal impaction.

Ultrasonography

As an aid to diagnosis and management, ultrasonography can detect abnormalities in the kidneys and bladder.

Intravenous urography

Ultrasound scanning has largely replaced the routine use of intravenous urography. It may be appropriate if renal obstruction is suspected, following ultrasonography.

Cystoscopy

Referral to the urologist should be made for assessment and possible cystoscopy in those presenting with haematuria, voiding difficulties and recurrent cystitis.

Diagnosis

Once a diagnosis has been reached then it is possible to plan a positive treatment regimen or make an appropriate specialist referral. It is essential that all patients are reviewed and reassessed at regular intervals and treatment regimens are adjusted accordingly.

Stress incontinence

- Leakage of urine with cough, sneeze or any activity which raises intra-abdominal pressure
- The leakage may be described as slight, moderate or severe
- More common in women, especially after childbirth and at the menopause
- Can occur in men post-prostatectomy
- The patient does not *usually* complain of undue frequency, urgency or nocturia. If the patient does complain of frequency and

urgency, this may be a mixed stress/urge problem.

Treatment options for stress incontinence

Complete baseline information which can be used to measure progress, for example the strength of the pelvic floor contraction and number of wet episodes over one week.

Weight management
If overweight, advise on a healthy low-fat diet. Although the association between weight and incontinence is not proven, obese patients requiring surgery may be more at risk and surgery may be more difficult.

Smoking cessation
If a smoker, advise on the benefits of cessation (see Chapter 8). A chronic cough will increase pressure on the pelvic floor and, if already weak, can result in considerable urine leakage.

Bowel care
Give advice on bowel care if prone to constipation. Straining at stool or chronic constipation can lead to nerve damage to the pelvic floor.

Exercise
Advise to stop exercise (during treatment) such as 'sit-ups', which put extra strain on the pelvic floor, also to avoid lifting heavy weights.

Management of atrophic vaginitis
Treat atrophic vaginitis if present. Around the menopause, stress incontinence may increase as the oestrogen level decreases. The vagina may appear dry and the tissues pale and easily damaged. The urethra, being oestrogen sensitive will be affected in that the folds of the urethra will not effect as efficient a closure as a well-oestrogenized urethra. Hormone replacement therapy or topical oestrogens should be prescribed, unless contraindicated.

Pelvic floor exercises
Plan an individual pelvic floor exercise programme (male or female). As there can be vast differences between patients in the ability to contract the pelvic floor, the strength of the contraction and the ability to lift and hold the contraction, it is essential that an individual pelvic floor exercise programme is planned. It is

vital to motivate the patient, as this and other treatments for incontinence rely on patient commitment. Many different pelvic floor exercise sheets are available, some of questionable value, and some women may be causing more damage if following inappropriate and outdated advice. See Appendices A and B for examples of female and male pelvic floor exercise sheets which have been developed by a multidisciplinary group, who believe that these instructions can be used by professionals after digital estimation of pelvic floor contraction, but should do no harm if the patient uses the sheet without professional advice.

Electrical stimulation treatment
Electrical stimulation treatment may be available from the physiotherapist or the continence adviser. There is an ever increasing number of different stimulators on the market and access to such treatment is through a physiotherapy department or continence service with a professional trained in their use.

Vaginal weighted cones
Vaginal weighted cones are cone-shaped, graded weights which may be a helpful addition to pelvic floor exercise. By gradually increasing the weight of the cone the strength of the pelvic floor may be increased (Peattie *et al.*, 1988). The cone is introduced into the vagina by the patient and should be retained by contracting the pelvic floor muscles during standing, walking and coughing. Use of the vaginal cones is contraindicated in the presence of prolapse or vaginal infection. Vaginal cones may be available through the physiotherapy department or continence services or can be bought by mail order or at a large retail pharmacy chain.

Internal prosthetic devices
Currently there are two main internal prosthetic devices available either by mail order or over the counter for women with mild stress incontinence. Before recommending the use of such products the clinician must be aware of possible contraindictaions and be accountable for any advice given regarding the purchase of such devices. The Association for Continence Advice (ACA) has issued 'Notes of Good Practice' regarding the use of internal prosthetic devices for female stress incontinence.

Surgery
There are a number of different surgical techniques used to treat stress incontinence. Which operation is recommended, is a matter for the consultant to decide after full investigations into the cause of the incontinence and anatomical deficits. There are alternatives to open surgical procedures, such as injectables, for example collagen, which may be considered for some patients. Finally, an artificial urinary sphincter may be implanted which Shah and Leach (1998) consider to be the optimum method of treatment for intractable post-prostatectomy stress incontinence in men with normal bladder pressures during filling. The most common complications following this type of surgery are infection, erosion and mechanical problems affecting the artificial sphincter.

Urge syndrome. Frequency, urgency and nocturia with or without the symptom of urge incontinence

Factors associated with urge syndrome include detrusor instability and hypersensitivity. Detrusor instability or unstable bladder, describes the occurrence of involuntary detrusor contractions during bladder filling, which give rise to the feeling of severe urgency, which may be accompanied with urine leakage (urge incontinence). It may underlie overt neuropathy, can occur in association with bladder neck obstruction, but often is idiopathic. Hypersensitivity of the bladder or urethral sensory nerve endings can give similar symptoms, which may be due to conditions diagnosed endoscopically, such as bladder tumours or stones, or those which have no demonstrable urodynamic explanation.

If a patient is suffering from urge syndrome they may complain of frequency, urgency or nocturia.

Frequency

The number of times urine is voided in 24 h depends on fluid intake, and therefore a 'normal' frequency is subjective, however, voiding between 4 and 7 times in 24 h may be considered normal, providing the total volume voided is around 1600–2000 ml.

Urgency

Undue urgency is not normal. Urgency may occur in the normal bladder if the urge to void has been deferred several times. Drinking coffee, tea and other fluids known to be irritant to the bladder in some individuals can increase urgency and caffeinated drinks will increase urine output and make the detrusor muscle contract more powerfully. Cutting down on fluid intake will also increase urgency as concentrated urine appears to irritate the sensory bladder receptors.

Nocturia

Having to rise several times during sleeping hours to void is a nuisance and may be a symptom of detrusor instability. Most people do not usually need to rise during the night to void, unless having taken more fluid than usual during the hours before retiring to bed. If a poor sleeper or waking due to pain or anxiety, an individual may decide to empty the bladder while awake. This is not true nocturia. In those under 60 years of age, rising once during sleeping hours to void may be considered normal. With increasing age, the physiological effects of ageing on the kidneys result in a disturbed diurnal rhythm of urine production compared with young adults, who produce most urine by day and very little when asleep. Older people often produce urine at the same rate day and night, or even produce more at night (Swaffield, 1996).

Other symptoms that may be associated with urge syndrome include leakage of urine associated with an urgent desire to void and stress incontinence.

Treatment options for urge syndrome

- Complete baseline information which can be used to measure progress, for example a volume/frequency chart, the strength of the pelvic floor contraction (if appropriate) and number of wet episodes over one week
- Test the urine and treat urinary tract infection if present
- If the patient is female and there are menopausal symptoms, for example atrophic vaginitis, then consider hormone replacement therapy or topical oestrogen

- Review the patient's medication as many drugs have side effects which can affect bladder function
- Ensure that the patient has a fluid intake of about 2 litres a day, unless pre-existing medical conditions contraindicate this. Some fluids have a diuretic effect and some appear to have an irritant effect on the bladder in some people. These include tea, coffee, cola and alcohol. The caffeine in drinks has a diuretic effect and can make the bladder contraction stronger
- Assess the patient's mobility and environment. Involve the physiotherapist and occupational therapist where indicated
- Plan an individual pelvic floor exercise programme as contracting the pelvic floor muscles helps the detrusor muscle to relax
- Plan a bladder retraining programme around the baseline chart. Times for voiding are planned according to the individual's pattern. The time between voidings is gradually increased as progress is made
- Anticholinergic medication may be added in an attempt to control unstable detrusor contractions, where appropriate
- It is important to see the patient regularly to offer support and encouragement during bladder retraining.

Urinary voiding problems

The patient may complain of some or all of the following:

- Frequency
- Urgency
- Nocturia
- Nocturnal enuresis
- Recurrent urinary tract infection
- A feeling of incomplete bladder emptying
- Voiding difficulties such as hesitancy, poor stream and post-micturition dribble
- Urinary leakage sometimes without the sensation of needing to void.

Treatment options for urinary voiding problems

- Examine to exclude enlarged prostate gland (or refer to prostate assessment clinic)
- Exclude constipation as a cause of symptoms

- Exclude urinary tract infection
- Review medication
- Estimate post-void residual urine by use of a Bladderscan machine if one is available, or do an in/out catheterization to measure residual urine
- It may be appropriate to take blood for urea and electrolytes and also prostate specific antigen (PSA).

Referral to the urologist may be indicated for treatment and advice for future management. Surgery may be indicated or the use of medication. The bladder may be managed using an indwelling catheter or intermittent self-catheterization.

Functional incontinence and inappropriate voiding

Functional incontinence and inappropriate voiding can occur as a result of severe physical disability, impaired manual dexterity, poor environment, mental health problems, confusion, learning difficulties, dementia and short-term memory loss.

Treatment options for functional incontinence and inappropriate voiding

- It is important to exclude any underlying bladder dysfunction for the incontinence
- Improve the environment where possible
- Ensure that supporting agencies are involved.

Plan an individualized toileting programme with carers around the behaviour of the individual and the voiding pattern.

More from a patient

When I was first diagnosed, I lived with my late mother who helped me keep the 'secret' that, at such a young age (in my late 30s) I wet myself constantly, something her generation found 'not quite nice' and 'not to be talked about' or if it was, it was called 'woman's troubles'. She also helped with the constant large amount of washing when I had 'accidents'. At that time I tried to manage with just a regime of intermittent self-catheterization and, by using an alarm clock set to wake me every two and a half to three hours at night, so as to try to stay reasonably dry.

With the help of sanitary pads and the pelvic floor exercises I had been taught, I thought it only a matter of time until the medical profession would find me an operation or at least a tablet solution to my problem and make my bladder react normally again . . .

Management options

The primary aim of health and social care professionals involved in continence care should be to promote continence whenever that is achievable. When true social continence is not achievable by the individual, the aim should be to provide the highest standard of available health and social care and management to ensure an optimum quality of life, independence and personal dignity.

There is a wide range of incontinence aids available, The Continence Products Directory, published by The Continence Foundation, lists over 2500 aids available in the UK (The Continence Foundation, 2000). The role of all incontinence aids is to absorb or collect and contain urinary and/or faecal loss effectively, enable the individual to conceal and manage that loss and thereby preserve the user's dignity and self-respect.

With regard to incontinence management options in chronic diseases, incontinence aids have two main functions:

- To promote continence by managing temporary episodes of incontinence and thereby providing confidence until continence is regained or achieved
- To promote confidence, when continence is not achievable, by managing irreversible incontinence effectively.

This relationship between confidence and continence is important. The best aid, whether it is being used to promote continence or manage incontinence by the individual user, is that one which works efficiently and effectively every time, is acceptable to the user and the carer and is suitable for that individual's lifestyle.

There is no single aid or type of aid that is suitable for all patients' needs as these vary from patient to patient. That which may be ideal to one person may be totally unacceptable to another, indeed the needs of the individual may change during the course of the disease process, necessitating review and reassessment for alternative aids on an ongoing basis.

The key to successful management of incontinence in chronic disease is accurate, objective, professional assessment of individual continence needs combined with an empathetic understanding of the use and performance of the aids available. Some continence specialists evaluate products on themselves, not a prerequisite for the role, but certainly a way of understanding the problems their patients experience.

The range and types of incontinence aids is continually increasing, necessitating research based evaluation of these products. This is currently provided by the Continence Product Evaluation Network, a Department of Health funded research body reporting via the Medical Devices Agency. This agency evaluates continence products, using test centres across the UK and produces scientific reports on respective product performance. Health care professionals can use these when advising patients on selection and use of aids.

Equipment to aid continence

There is such a wide range of aids available it is impossible, in this context, to describe them all and their respective uses. There are also many extrinsic factors that affect our ability to be continent, i.e. meet society's demands to conform to social norms and etiquette. An attempt to group aids according to their generic types and give general advice regarding selection and usage follows. In a broad allocation of usage, aids may be classified as continence or incontinence aids.

Continence aids may be defined as those which enable the user to toilet in a socially acceptable manner. In order to maintain the complex social and physical skills required to be continent, the environment has to be conducive to individual needs and in order to be independently continent, a person must have the skills to recognize the need to void, identify a socially acceptable place and reach/use that place in time to prevent incontinence.

Aids to continence may include environmental adaptations to toileting facilities, e.g. raised toilet seats, support rails and personal cleansing aids. It should be remembered that aids which

enable one person to use a toilet can prevent another from using it; this can be especially important when assessing patients in residential care. Other alternative aids for toileting may include commodes, chemical toilets and hand-held urinals, providing that they are acceptable to the user and carer.

Incontinence aids include body-worn absorbent and collection aids which enable the achievement of social continence, i.e. absorption/collection of incontinence loss. Their use should be questioned if personal/environmental adaptations would promote social continence.

Though there are thousands of incontinence aids available, they can be classified in three broad groups:

- Absorbent or containment aids
- Collection or conduction aids
- Occlusion aids, which restore the storage function of the bladder by internal or external pressure upon the urethra. For faecal incontinence, an example would be anal plugs.

It is difficult to obtain accurate national costs of incontinence aids. The Royal College of Physicians report (1995) stated that, 'The direct cost of pads and appliances used in UK hospitals and long term care in 1986 was over £50 million, with a further £18 million in prescription items in England and Wales.'

The Royal College of Nursing stated that 'The substantial rise in the numbers of (people) over the age of 65 years within the next 30 years will have a financial impact on many budgets and many organisations. The overall cost of continence care and management is set to rise substantially. With 48% of all NHS spending on the over 65 year old age group, the cost of incontinence is estimated to rise to at least £2 billion by the year 2020 without adjustment for inflation' (Royal College of Nursing, 1995).

The most recent report on Good Practice in Continence Services (Department of Health, 2000b) does not provide an update in expenditure figures, but does recommend that, 'Pads should be provided in quantities appropriate to the individual's continence needs. Arbitrary ceilings are inappropriate. It is unacceptable to have waiting lists for pads as a means of rationing the service.'

Many health care trusts currently ration supplies of absorbent incontinence aids, as described in the document, this guidance if implemented, will of course dramatically increase the cost of such supply.

Absorption/containment aids, which include body-worn pads, fixative and incontinence garments are available in a huge variety of styles, both disposable and washable (re-usable). Individual assessment is essential to ensure the correct size, style and absorbency. While the rapid development in this aspect of incontinence management has provided a far greater choice for users, it has also created difficulties in ensuring that the optimum product is selected for the individual user.

This is further compounded by the widely varying rules and regulations surrounding the supply by NHS Trusts, again as described in the DoH Continence Services report (Department of Health, 2000a). This showed a variation of between two and seven pads per day supplied by Trusts in the study. With more and more patients having to purchase their own pads or supplement the supply from their Trust, the role of the health care professional is changing from that of supplier to adviser in self-purchase. There are numerous suppliers of absorbent incontinence aids and local availability varies with most retail pharmacists now offering at least a limited selection of aids. Mail order services are developing and some products are advertised on prime time television. This is a radical change in public attitude to continence awareness.

In general patients will want to know the advantages and disadvantages of disposable versus reusable aids (Table 9.1) and advice on the most care and cost effective aids.

Absorbent incontinence aids

As incontinence has a wide range of causes, it is important that people obtain professional advice from their doctor, nurse or continence adviser before buying absorbent incontinence aids.

In order to ensure optimum performance of any absorbent product, it is important that the correct style and size are selected. The ten tips on fitting pads are given in Table 9.2.

Collection aids

These can be divided into internal and external devices. External devices include penile sheaths, of various designs and fixation methods, also urinary and faecal collection appliances. Internal collection aids are urinary catheters, intermittent or indwelling, urethral and suprapubic.

Urinary catheters

Urinary catheterization is the insertion of a hollow tube into the bladder to allow drainage of urine or instillation of fluids. Over 12% of hospital patients (Crow *et al.*, 1986) and 4% of people on district nursing case loads having an indwelling catheter *in situ* (Roe, 1989).

Table 9.1 The advantages and disadvantages of disposable versus reusable aids (Philp *et al.*, 1992)

Reusables advantages	*Reusables disadvantages*
Can't be torn apart	Require washing
Retain shape better	High (initial) capital outlay
Don't break up	Concept may be unacceptable to users
Potential for more design options	(especially during menstruation and if faecally
Facilitate independence from supply system	soiled)
Eliminate need for constant disposal	
Reduce storage requirements	
Can be reused if remain dry	
Disposables advantages	*Disposables disadvantages*
Flexibility for experimentation to match user requirements	Tendency for pulp compression
No need to launder	Tendency for pulp to break up
	Can be torn apart

Table 9.2 Ten tips on fitting pads

1. Always make sure that the correct size of pants are worn with pads
2. Measure around the waist to decide size of pants required
3. Ensure that the correct absorbency of pad is selected, never 'double' pad, i.e. put one pad inside another – this is both ineffective and expensive
4. Fold pad lengthways prior to fitting, to create a natural 'bowl' shape
5. Ensure pants are put on with seams on the outside and pull up to mid-thigh area
6. Insert pad from front to back – make sure you put wider end of pad to the back
7. Pull pants and pad up, ensuring pad is smoothed out both front and back
8. Check pad is as close to the body as possible and that the 'bowl' shape has been maintained
9. Ease pant legs up into crease of groin to prevent skin marking and to ensure pad is held securely
10. Take time to check pad is well-fitted and comfortable – a badly fitted pad will leak and create more work!

Reproduced with permission from SCA Hygiene Products UK Ltd.

Types of catheters

There are two types of catheters, intermittent and indwelling.

Intermittent catheters are single channel, hollow tubes inserted into the bladder intermittently via the urethra or continent stoma. As with absorbent aids, there is a wide range of intermittent catheters available but they can be divided into single use, hydrophilic or gel-coated catheters and reusable PVC, non-coated and metal catheters.

Indwelling catheters remain in place once they have been inserted. The most commonly used indwelling catheter is the Foley catheter. This is a hollow, flexible tube retained in the bladder by a balloon, inflated with sterile water following insertion of the catheter. The catheter may be inserted via the urethra (urethral catheterization) or through an incision in the lower abdominal wall (suprapubic catheterization).

Urinary catheters can provide an effective method of urinary incontinence management for patients with intractable incontinence. In chronic disease management urinary catheters, both intermittent and indwelling, can offer a valuable management option. For many patients with chronic diseases, long-term catheterization is an aid to daily living and the catheter is a prosthesis which, like spectacles, hearing aids and dentures, enables the individual to perform a normal body function, i.e. void urine in a socially acceptable manner.

Unfortunately, urinary catheters also cause significant hazards to health, therefore the decision to catheterize, or to be catheterized, should only be undertaken after careful consideration of the possible complications and effects of the procedure (Pomfret, 2000).

External urinary collection devices

These are devices designed to be attached externally for the purpose of collecting urinary and faecal loss and channel it into an external reservoir which can be emptied or disposed of, when socially acceptable. There is a wide range of external urinary collection devices and systems available for men (most of which are on prescription) but, at present, none are suitable for women. External faecal collectors include stoma appliances and anal collection bags, which are on prescription.

The most commonly used external urinary collection devices for men are penile sheaths, also known as condom urinals, incontinence sheaths, and external male catheters. A penile sheath is a soft, flexible sleeve that fits over the penis and attaches to a urine collection system to facilitate collection and storage of urine.

The use of such devices has a long history, possibly starting with the use of 'Pauls Tubing', soft latex tubing, rolled over the penis, draining into a suitable receptacle and modified contraceptive sheaths glued to the penis with skin adhesive, as described by Evelyn Pearce in 1971.

The Drug Tariff for England and Wales (Department of Health, 2000b) lists sixteen manufacturers and distributors of penile sheaths with 13 companies offering fixing strips and adhesives which are available separately from the sheaths. With such a wide range of products available, it is not surprising that confusion may arise when choosing the optimum system for individuals.

There are too many sheaths available to describe individual types but they may be divided into two broad groups:

- One size, lightweight latex sheaths, gathered distally into a rigid outlet tube. These are now used less often, and are modifications of the 'contraceptive type' sheaths. They are prone to twisting and kinking, resulting in back-flow of urine with consequent leakage. Internal or external fixation may be used.
- Multisized, semi-rigid, re-usable sheaths and single use, multisized sheaths with pre-formed outlet. These are the most commonly used types of sheaths and are now available in latex and non-latex designs. They are available in a wide range of sizes and have a variety of design features. As with the other incontinence aids described, it is important to seek skilled, professional advice regarding selection, fitting and use of these aids. No one type of sheath will suit all men and it may be necessary to try several types, in order to find the most suitable.

General points for use of penile sheaths
In order for a penile sheath to be suitable for the management of urinary incontinence in chronic disease management, the patient must:

- Be male and have moderate to severe urinary incontinence
- Have adequate penile length and girth to enable fixation of the sheath
- Be able to affix and manage the sheath and urinary drainage system, or have a carer able and willing to do it
- Not be confused or likely to try to pull the sheath off as this can result in severe trauma
- Not be in retention of urine, if so, penile sheaths are not the appropriate method of management and further investigations/ alternative treatments, e.g. catheterization, either intermittent or indwelling would be more appropriate.

Fitting penile sheaths
This is a skill, which may be learned by social and informal carers, but should be taught by health care professionals who are themselves skilled and experienced in the selection, fitting and care of these devices. Penile sheaths can cause severe trauma if inappropriately used or fitted incorrectly.

Male patients with insufficient penile size are not suitable for this type of management and should be assessed for urinary collection devices, e.g. pubic pressure flanges and urinals. These are specialist devices and referral to an incontinence appliance practitioner should be made if the assessor is not skilled in the use of these aids.

In conclusion, penile sheaths and urinary collection devices are a valuable method of managing male urinary incontinence which may be summarized by the mnemonic:

C Cost-effective control of urinary incontinence
O Odour-proof method of management
N Non-invasive and noiseless
D Disposable and discreet
O On prescription
M Male image
S Sexuality preserving

Occlusion devices
The aim of occlusion aids is to restore the storage function of the bladder by internal or external pressure on the urethra. These aids are not commonly used and require expert assessment, fitting and advice on their use. Devices include, penile clamps and vaginal tampons or pressure appliances. Advice should be sought from the local continence adviser, or incontinence appliance practitioner.

Conclusion

Continence and incontinence aids have an invaluable role to play in both the promotion of continence and the management of intractable incontinence, but incontinence is not a disease and aids are not a cure; however, aids can put confidence back into incontinence!

Appendix A

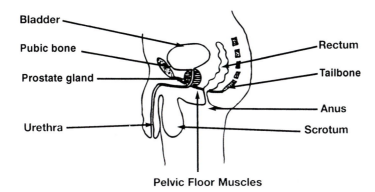

(Reproduced with permission from the West Cumbria Continence Care 2000 Working Group – sponsored and produced by Paul Hartmann Ltd)

Pelvic floor exercises (male)

Why?

The pelvic floor muscles pass from the pubic bone to the tailbone and provide the floor to your pelvis. Various things, including trauma, constipation, coughing, sneezing and some surgical procedures, can affect these muscles.

The urethra (bladder tube) and anus (back passage) open through the pelvic floor. They are controlled by muscles which relax when you pass water. The rest of the time they should be contracted and tight.

If they are weakened, then bladder and bowel problems may occur.

In males the prostate gland sits just below the neck of the bladder and surrounds the bladder tube. In later life the prostate gland may enlarge, causing constriction of the bladder tube.

The aim is to increase the tone and strength of your pelvic floor muscles – this will help to control your bladder and bowel.

How?

- Pull up and tighten your pelvic floor muscles, as if you were trying to stop yourself passing water.
- Pull up and tighten around your back passage as though trying to stop yourself passing wind. Keep your buttocks relaxed.

The aim is to be able to tighten both at the same time. **This is a Pelvic Floor Contraction.**

When?

There are *two* types of exercise you should aim to do *every hour.*

Fast contraction

Contract your pelvic floor muscles as quickly and tightly as you can, then relax. Repeat this 2 to 3 times (these exercises should be done *a minimum of 6 times a day*). As the muscle gets stronger the number of contractions should increase (aim for a maximum of 10 times a day).

Appendix A continued on next page

Slow contractions

Contract your pelvic floor muscles as tightly as you can and hold for as long as you are able. Repeat this 2 to 3 times (minimum of 6 times a day). As the muscle gets stronger, the length of hold time and number of contractions should increase (aim for a maximum of 10 times a day). The exercise will be easier earlier in the day when the muscles are less tired.

It may take up to 3 months before you start to see results.

Where?

When able, these exercises should be practiced in all positions progressing from lying – sitting – standing – walking – running.

Points to remember

Some men may experience a problem with after-dribble (it can affect all ages). This is the loss of a few drops of urine after the main stream has finished, which may produce a wet patch on your clothes and can happen a few minutes after leaving the toilet. This occurs because there is still some urine left in the bladder tube.

To empty the bladder tube completely, apply firm pressure behind the scrotum (which should be directed upwards and forwards), whilst standing at the toilet. Any residual urine will then be passed. This procedure may be repeated if required.

Additional information/instruction

Patient Name: Date

Appendix B

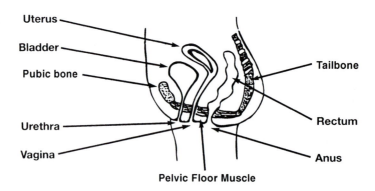

(Reproduced with permission from the West Cumbria Continence Care 2000 Working Group – sponsored and produced by Paul Hartmann Ltd)

Appendix B continued on next page

Pelvic floor exercises (female)

Why?

The pelvic floor muscles pass from the pubic bone to the tailbone and provide the floor to your pelvis. Various things, including childbirth, constipation, coughing and sneezing can strain these muscles.

The urethra (front passage), vagina (birth canal) and anus (back passage) all open through the pelvic floor. They are controlled by muscles which relax when you pass water. The rest of the time they should be contracted and tight.

If they are weakened, then bladder and bowel problems may occur.

Weakened pelvic floor muscles can also allow the bladder, bowel or womb to bulge into the vaginal passage – this is known as a prolapse.

The aim is to increase the tone and strength of your pelvic floor muscles – this will help to control your bladder and bowel.

How?

- Pull up and tighten around your vagina as if you were trying to stop yourself passing water.
- Pull up and tighten around your back passage as though trying to stop yourself passing wind. Keep your buttocks relaxed.

The aim is to be able to tighten both at the same time. **This is a Pelvic Floor Contraction.**

When?

There are *two* types of exercise you should aim to do *every hour.*

Fast contraction
Contract your pelvic floor muscles as quickly and tightly as you can, then relax. Repeat this 2 to 3 times (these exercise should be done *a minimum of 6 times a day*). As the muscle gets stronger the number of contractions should increase (aim for a maximum of 10 times a day).

Slow contractions
Contract your pelvic floor muscles as tightly as you can and hold for as long as you are able. Repeat this 2 to 3 times (minimum of 6 times a day). As the muscle gets stronger, the length of hold time and number of contractions should increase (aim for a maximum of 10 times a day). The exercise will be easier earlier in the day when the muscles are less tired.

It may take up to 3 months before you start to see results.

Where?

When able, these exercises should be practised in all positions progressing from lying – sitting – standing – walking – running.

Caution

Whilst doing these exercise you should get the sensation of pulling up and in from below NOT straining to push down and out.

STOP TEST – stopping and starting whilst passing water. **This should not be performed more than once a week as it may eventually prevent the bladder from fully emptying.**

Additional information/instruction

Patient Name: Date

Useful contacts

Association for Continence Advice
102a Astra House
Arklow Road
New Cross
London SE14 6EB
Tel: 020 8692 4680 www.aca.uk.com

Enuresis and Information Centre (ERIC Advice
    on paediatric enuresis and encopresis)
34 Old School House
Britannia Road
Kingswood
Bristol BS15 8DB
Tel: 0117 960 3060 www.eric.org.uk

Incontact
United House
North Road
London N7 9DP
Tel: 020 7700 7035 www.incontact.org

PromoCon 2001 (Continence Product
    Information)
Disabled Living
4 St Chad's Street
Cheetham
Manchester M8 8QA
Tel: 0161 834 2001

The Continence Foundation (Continence
    Information)
307 Hatton Square
16 Baldwins Gardens
London EC1N 7RJ
Tel: 020 7404 6875; helpline 0845 345 0165
www.continence-foundation.org.uk

West Cumbria Continence Forum
www.wccf.co.uk

References

Abrams P H, Torrens M (1979) Urine flow studies. Symposium on clinical urodynamics. *Urologic Clinics of North America* **6**, 71–79. Cited in: Shah P J R (1984) The assessment of patients with a view to urodynamics. In: (Mundy A R, Stephenson T P, Wein A J, eds) *Urodynamics. Principles, Practice and Application* **5**, 57. Churchill Livingstone

Andersen J, Abrams P, Blavias J G, Stanton S L (1988) The standardisation of terminology of lower urinary tract function. *Scandinavian Journal of Urology and Nephrology* Suppl. 114, 5–19

Bayer Diagnostics (1993) *Urinary Tract Infection Testing Pathway*. Diagnostic Division, Bayer House, Strawberry Hill, Newbury, Berks. RG14 1JA

Bayliss V (1996) Female urinary incontinence In: (Norton C, ed.) *Nursing for Continence*, 2nd edn, **6**, 129. Beaconsfield Publishers Ltd, Beaconsfield

Button D, Roe B, Webb C, Frith T, Colin-Thome D, Gardner L (1998) *Continence: Promotion and Management by the Primary Health Care Team – Consensus Guidelines*. Whurr Publishers Ltd, London

Crow R, Chapman R, Roe B, Wilson J (1986) *Study of Patients with Indwelling Urethral Catheters and Related Nursing Practice*. Nursing Practice Research Unit, University of Surrey, Guildford

Department of Health (2000a) *Good Practice in Continence Services*. Department of Health, London

Department of Health (2000b) *Drug Tarriff*. HMSO, London

Laycock J (1994) Clinical evaluation of the pelvic floor. In: (Schussler B, Laycock J, Stanton S, Norton P, eds) *Pelvic Floor Re-education: Principles and Practice*, pp 42–48. Springer-Verlag, London

Pearce E (1971) *A General Textbook of Nursing*. Faber and Faber, London

Peattie A B, Plevnik S, Stanton S L (1988) Vaginal cones: a conservative method of treating genuine stress incontinence. *British Journal of Obstetrics and Gynaecology* **95**, 1049–1053

Philp J, Cottenden A, Ledger D (1992) *A Study of Reusable Body worn Absorbent Incontinence Products from the UK Consumers' Perspective*. DoH, London

Pomfret I (2000) Urinary catheters: selection, management and prevention of infection. *British Journal of Community Nursing* **5**, 6–13

Roe B H (1989) Catheters in the community. *Nursing Times* **84**, 43–44

Royal College of Nursing (1995) *A Briefing Paper on the Cost of Continence*. Royal College of Nursing, London

Royal College of Physicians of London (1995) *Incontinence – Causes, Management and Provision of Services*. RCP, London

Sanderson J (1991) *An Agenda for Action on Continence Services*. Department of Health, London

Shah J, Leach G (1998) *Fast Facts – Urinary Continence*. Health Press, Oxford

Shah P J R (1984) The assessment of patients with a view to urodynamics. In: (Mundy A R, Stephenson T P, Wein A J, eds) *Urodynamics. Principles, Practice and Application* **5**, 57. Churchill Livingstone, Edinburgh

Swaffield J (1996) Continence in older people. In: (Norton C, ed.) *Nursing for Continence*, 2nd edn, **11**, 261. Beaconsfield Publishers Ltd, Beaconsfield

The Continence Foundation (1995) *Commissioning Comprehensive Continence Services, Guidance for Purchasers*. The Continence Foundation, London

The Continence Foundation (2000) *Continence Products Directory*. The Continence Foundation, London

Thomas T M, Egan Plymat K R, Blannin J, Meade T W (1980) Prevalence of urinary incontinence. *British Medical Journal* **281**, 1243–1245

10

Epilepsy

Gillian Armitage

A patient's perspective

At school I faced prejudice not only from children who did not understand, but also from teachers. At school I tried hard but was always at the bottom of the class. I also tried night school but still couldn't get on. I started work but worried about my education and my epilepsy became worse. My parents took me to see a specialist and I was taken to a colony. None of my family visited and I later found out they were afraid of my seizures.

The most difficult part was coming to terms with my illness and understanding what was happening to me. At a young age, not understanding epilepsy led to feelings of anger. Like many other people in similar situations, lies were told and a lot of feelings held inside. Coming to terms with my epilepsy was not aided by the medical profession, which I found of little help in advising me about everyday living.

There is always the fear of having another seizure. I spend most of my time now sitting around at home, as I never know when I'm going to have another seizure. I'm 25 years old and only occasionally go out to visit my family. I used to drive and now I feel very uneasy about travelling by bus in case I have a seizure.

Introduction

Epilepsy is a common medical condition, defined as the occurrence of transient paroxysms of uncontrolled electrical discharges from nervous tissue in the brain, which leads to epileptic seizures. The seizures must recur to constitute epilepsy. Epilepsy is not an illness but a symptom of many diseases with different causes. Seizures may occur at any age but are more common in the first 20 years of life and in elderly people.

Since epilepsy is a symptom, rather than a specific condition and the underlying cause is often obscure, the study of epilepsy has largely focused on defining and classifying seizures. Classification of seizures and epilepsy syndromes are numerous, most nurses in practice will have little experience of epilepsy and may have actually witnessed few, if any, seizures ever. Words such as 'grand mal' and 'petit mal' seizures convey an idea of fits being 'big and bad' or 'small and not so bad'. Other confusing terms such as temporal lobe epilepsy, Jacksonian fits and juvenile myoclonic epilepsy all add further to the feelings of the nurses' inadequacy in helping to deal with their patients.

Classification of epilepsy

The classification of epilepsy (Table 10.1) is now more clearly related to seizure experience and parts of the brain involved than the older classifications. Generalized seizures are those in which epileptic discharges involve both hemispheres simultaneously from the onset, and partial seizures those in which epileptic activity starts in a focal area of the brain, where it remains confined or may spread to become generalized.

Categorizing epilepsy into further syndromes (Table 10.2) provides better guidance on prognosis and the choice of treatment than seizure

Table 10.1 Classification of epilepsy

Classification of seizures	Old term
Partial seizures (local onset)	
• Simple partial (no impairment of consciousness)	Jacksonian
May involve: motor symptoms	
Sensory/somatosensory symptoms (auras)	
Autonomic symptoms	
Psychic symptoms	
• Complex partial (impairment of consciousness)	
Either simple partial evolving to complex partial	Psychomotor
Or impairment of conscious from onset (abnormal behaviour/ sensation: automatisms, chewing, lip smacking)	Temporal lobe epilepsy
• Both simple and complex partial seizures may evolve to become secondary generalized seizures	
Primary generalized seizures (bilateral symmetrical, no focal onset)	
Tonic–clonic	Grand mal
Tonic	
Clonic	
Absences	Petit mal
Myoclonic	Absence
Infantile spasms	
Atonic	Drop

Taylor, 1996

type alone#. Most epilepsy syndromes are age-related, occurring in childhood. Although it is not necessary to have an in-depth understanding of the epilepsy syndromes, a broad awareness is helpful.

Aetiology

The possible causes of epilepsy (Table 10.3) are numerous covering most cerebral pathology, for example genetic causes, congenital malformations, infections, tumours, vascular disease and severe head injury. In practice, no specific cause can be found in 60–70% of people, though this is changing with the introduction of magnetic resonance imaging (MRI). The National General Practice study of newly diagnosed epileptic seizures undertaken by Sander *et al.* (1990) found the commonest remote symptomatic causes were vascular disease (15%) and tumour (6%). In patients over 60 years of age,

cerebrovascular disease accounted for 49% of cases. Tumour was rare under the age of 30 years, but reached 19% between 50 and 59 years.

The potential for preventing epilepsy currently rests with improvements in the treatment of vascular disease and infection, and the avoidance of trauma, alcohol and other toxic substances. Improved prenatal and perinatal care might reduce the incidence of congenital causes of epilepsy, although in most cases, the nature of pre- or perinatal abnormality resulting in epilepsy is not fully understood.

Incidence and prevalence

Epilepsy is the most common serious neurological condition; more than 300 000 people in the UK have epilepsy. Studies undertaken by Sander and Shorvan (1987) and Lesser (1996) examined the number of people affected by

Table 10.2 Epilepsy syndromes

Localization-related (partial) epilepsies and syndromes

Idiopathic	Benign focal motor epilepsy
Benign occipital epilepsy of childhood	
Symptomatic	Simple partial epilepsies
Complex partial epilepsies	
Cryptogenic (presumed symptomatic but aetiology unknown)	

Generalized epilepsies

Idiopathic	Childhood absence
Benign myoclonic epilepsy	
Tonic–clonic awakening epilepsy	
Juvenile myoclonic epilepsy	
Symptomatic	Infantile spasms (West's syndrome)
Lennox-Gastaut syndrome	
Early myoclonic epilepsies	

Unclassified epilepsies and syndromes
Neonatal seizures
Undetermined epilepsies

Specific epileptic syndromes
Situation-related seizures
Febrile convulsions
Acute symptomatic seizures, e.g. metabolic, drugs, alcohol
Reflex epilepsy

Taylor, 1996

epilepsy. Difficulties in diagnosing the condition, together with the sometimes poor identification of people with epilepsy, have led to variations in the reported rates and prevalence. Sander (1997) suggests the world-wide prevalence of epilepsy is between 0.5% and 1%, with the number of new cases per year, or incidence, being 40–70 per 100 000 population. Translated to general practice, this means that an individual GP, with a list of about 2000 patients, can expect to have between 10 and 15 patients with active epilepsy on his or her list and to see one or two new cases each year.

Camfield *et al.* (1994) and Hauser *et al.* (1993) suggest the incidence of epilepsy is greatest at the extremes of life, i.e. in childhood and in the elderly. In 50% of cases epilepsy begins in early childhood or adolescence. Rates are lowest in early adult life but rise again in the elderly. Willmore (1996) states that patients over 75 years have a higher incidence of epilepsy than children under the age of 10. The percentage of people aged 75 years and older is expected to become the most rapidly growing segment of the population and future increases in elderly patients with epilepsy can be expected, presenting yet another challenge to general practice.

Prognosis

The prognosis of epilepsy may be defined as the prospect of attaining terminal remission once the patient has established a pattern of recurrent epileptic seizures. Seventy to 80% of people developing epilepsy will achieve this, while the remaining 20–30% will continue having seizures despite optimum drug treatment. Remission usually occurs within the first 5 years. Thus, for most people, epilepsy is a short-lived condition. A good prognosis is associated with seizures precipitated by alcohol, drugs and metabolic disturbances, benign syndromes, or adult-onset

Table 10.3 Causes of epilepsy

Genetic propensity

Ante- and perinatal injury – anoxia, intracerebral haemorrhage, infarction

Effects consequent to prolonged febrile convulsions

Infections – bacterial meningitis, cerebral abscess, viral encephalitis

Immunization – pertussis vaccine

Vascular causes – infarction, hypertensive encephalopathy, cerebral venous thrombosis, arteriovenous malformations, post-anoxic encephalopathy

Toxic causes – alcohol ingestion and withdrawal, chronic alcohol encephalopathy, heavy metals, particularly lead

Metabolic causes – hypoglycaemia, hyperglycaemia, hypoxia, hypocalaemia, hypercalaemia, hyponatraemia, hypernatraemia

Uraemia – deficiency of pyridoxine

Degenerative causes – Alzheimer's disease

Hopkins, 1993

idiopathic seizure. A poor prognosis is likely where there is evidence of diffuse cerebral disorder (intellectual or behavioural disturbance), onset of seizure in the first year of life, severe epilepsy syndromes or progressive neurological disorders. Seizure type is of major importance in determining outcome, and childhood epilepsy is more likely to remit than adult-onset epilepsy.

In primary care, Sander (1997) shows that only 50–60% of patients with epilepsy are seizure free. Direct comparisons are difficult, as secondary care results suggest that 30–40% more patients could be seizure free. A recent study undertaken by the Epilepsy Task Force (1999) states that there may be a treatment gap. Not all patients who could become seizure free are actually achieving this.

Mortality

There is often an assumption among healthcare professionals that epilepsy is a benign condition with a low mortality. There is, however, increased mortality in patients with epilepsy, which is relatively high among younger patients and those with severe epilepsy. The cause of death is usually subdivided into different categories: status epilepticus, seizure-related, suicide, accident or sudden unexpected death. Deaths are highest in the first year, usually asso-

ciated with stroke or tumour. Newly diagnosed patients without serious underlying pathology can be reasonably reassured that, although there is a risk of premature death, it is quite small.

It is worthwhile noting that sudden unexpected deaths in epilepsy (SUDEP) are common in people with chronic epilepsy. The term 'seizure-related death' is used when the patient dies during or shortly after a seizure, when there is no evidence for status epilepticus and when, after autopsy, no other explanation is found. The Epilepsy Bereavement group has been set up to provide support for relatives. (See Useful addresses at the end of the chapter.)

Management in general practice

Over the past 40 years, numerous government-sponsored reports have dealt specifically with service provision for people with epilepsy and their families. Each report provides a careful evaluation of existing practice, highlights current shortcomings and makes recommendations for future service development. The extent to which recommendations have been implemented over the years is disappointing, probably due to very limited financial backing and the lack of enthusiasm from professional groups involved in the care of epilepsy.

Government-sponsored reports specifically dealing with service provision for people with epilepsy and their families

1. Ministry of Health National Assistance Act 1948.
2. Central Health Services Council – the Cohen Committee (1956) Report of the Sub-Committee on the medical care of Epileptics. HMSO, London. This report emphasized the importance of the general practitioner in the management of epilepsy.
3. Central Health Services Council (1969) People with Epilepsy: Report of the Joint Sub-Committee of the Standing Medical Advisory Committee and the Advisory Committee on the Health and Welfare of Handicapped Persons. HMSO, London. This report became known as the Reid Report.
4. Kurtz Z, Morgan J D (1987) Special services for people with epilepsy in the 1970s. HMSO, London. The Bennett Report consisted of two parts, which considered adult and children's services, which were completed in 1980 and 1981 respectively but were not published until 1987.
5. Department of Health and Social Security (1986) Report of the working group on services for people with epilepsy. HMSO, London. This report was commissioned in 1983 by the DHSS to consider the recommendations of the Reid Report in the light of the findings of the Bennett Report.
6. Brown S, Betts T, Chadwick C *et al.* (1993) An epilepsy needs documemt. *Seizure* **2**, 91–103.

A British Epilepsy Association (BEA) survey undertaken by Nelson (1994) illustrates dramatically the extent to which poor management of epilepsy can have a lasting and devastating effect on the patient's life. The sample consisted of members from the BEA and a total number of 4500 adults (response rate 30%) returned a questionnaire, which examined quality of life issues surrounding epilepsy and its treatment. Although the sample was not representative of the total adult epilepsy population in the UK, the survey is one of the largest and most in-depth pieces of research carried out into epilepsy and the issues surrounding the condition.

Thapar (1996) examined the management of epilepsy in the NHS and found that patients with epilepsy are seldom managed in a systematic and structured way. He highlights doctors' poor overall control of the condition, their inappropriate prescribing and their poor communication with people with epilepsy. Patients' unsatisfactory understanding of their condition was also reviewed. Scambler (1989) commented that it has been frequently reported that doctors lack the motivation, training or time to elicit and address the patient's own perspective of epilepsy since an individual GP will only have 20 patients with active epilepsy and see only one to two new cases each year. These small numbers make it difficult for a GP easily to develop expertise, or understand the role of the newer drugs.

Aims of epilepsy management

The aim of epilepsy management is to prevent further seizures. A single seizure is not usually treated in the UK and before commencing therapy a definite diagnosis of epilepsy needs to be confirmed, with a classification of seizure type and epilepsy syndrome. The underlying cause also needs to be elicited (see Table 10.3), although 60–70% of all cases have no clear identifiable cause. The patient should be referred to a neurologist, physician or paediatrician with an interest in epilepsy (the maximum wait for an appointment should be 4 weeks) and, in most cases, the patient's history and detailed seizure description will provide the seizure classification and often the syndrome.

About 80% of patients are well controlled on monotherapy. Poor understanding of medication to be taken and incorrect diagnosis should be considered if monotherapy fails. If polytherapy is needed, it is best approached systematically, as it can lead to poor compliance, drug interactions, increased teratogenicity and increased long-term toxicity. An holistic approach to epilepsy is needed to meet the needs of the patient and carers. They require support and counselling of the nature, dangers and consequences of epilepsy.

Management of initial presentation

When a patient has their first seizure, he or she usually presents to the general practitioner, whose task is to take a history from the patient and any eye witness account. The GP provides the patient with information, regarding dealing with further seizures, avoidance of danger and makes a referral to an epilepsy specialist. GPs should not normally initiate treatment themselves unless the patient faces a long delay in seeing a specialist.

Misdiagnosis commonly results from failure to distinguish epileptic seizures from syncope or other cardiovascular causes of loss of consciousness. Useful clues to diagnosis are:

- Abruptness of onset
- Genuine loss of awareness
- Attacks are usually brief
- An individual's attacks tend to be stereotyped.

The patient with a suspected seizure should be advised not to drive a motor vehicle until a diagnosis is established and they can be given definitive advice. Patients with a diagnosis of epilepsy are required to notify the Driving Vehicle Licensing Centre and are required to surrender their licence until they have been seizure free for 1 year.

History taking

Epilepsy is primarily a clinical diagnosis, therefore, a good clinical history is the most important aspect of assessment, to determine whether a patient has epilepsy and also the underlying cause.

History must include:

- Perinatal insults and complications
- Early development and developmental milestones
- History of meningitis, encephalitis or head injury
- Presence or absence of febrile convulsions
- Family/medical history
- Medication
- History of alcohol or drug abuse
- Detailed history of seizures.

Investigations

Possible investigations include:

- Routine bloods, for example full blood count, erythrocyte sedimentation rate, electrolytes, liver function, calcium and glucose.

- Electroencephalogram (EEG) plays an important role in the assessment and classification of epilepsy, and in localizing seizure origin. The routine EEG is often misinterpreted and minor abnormalities may be used to support an unsatisfactory diagnosis of epilepsy when there is clinical uncertainty. Non-specific EEG abnormalities can occur in 10–15% of the normal population and patients with undoubted seizures may have normal interictal EEGs. EEG plays an important role in the assessment and classification and in localizing the seizure origin.
- Sleep EEG combined with repeated routine EEG increases sensitivity to above 90%.
- EEG can also be carried out with video monitoring (telemetry); the EEG is recorded while the patient is videoed as an inpatient, usually for several days. Video telemetry is used routinely to define accurately the point of initiation of a seizure in presurgical assessment and in the diagnosis of epilepsy, especially where pseudoseizures are suspected.
- Intracranial EEG is used in presurgical assessment when scalp EEG is unable to provide adequate information for the localization of the epileptic focus.
- Ideally, patients with epilepsy should have magnetic resonance imaging (MRI) or computerized tomography (CT). It is particularly indicated where there is evidence of focal onset, for example adults presenting with partial seizures with or without focal neurological signs and/or focal abnormality on the EEG. Other indications are epilepsy unresponsive to anti-epileptic drugs (AEDs), epilepsy increasing in severity and new or progressive neurological signs and/or symptoms. MRI is far more sensitive than CT but is also more expensive.

Anti-epileptic drugs (AEDs)

Seizure type is the most important factor in determining the choice of medical treatment and further identification of a syndrome, if possible, is also important. A guide to the choice of AEDs related to seizure types and syndromes is given in Table 10.4. In the past, first line drugs for treating partial and primary generalized seizures were phenobarbitone, phenytoin, carbamazepine and sodium valproate. Over the

Table 10.4 Choice of anti-epileptic drugs related to seizure type

Partial seizures	First line drug
Simple,	
Complex partial	Carbamazepine/sodium
Secondary generalized	valproate
Generalized seizures	
Tonic–clonic	
Absence	Sodium valproate
Myoclonic	
Syndromes	Sodium valproate

years, phenobarbitone and phenytoin have fallen into disuse because of their side effects. Carbamazepine and sodium valproate have established themselves as effective drugs with fewer side effects. Three new drugs, vigabatrin, lamotrigine and gabapentin, were initially used as add-on therapy and now lamotrigine and gabapentin have been licensed for mono-therapy.

Regular AED treatment is usually recommended after two or more unprovoked seizures have occurred, with an interval between seizures of less than 12 months. Some patients with only occasional seizures, particularly if these are minor events, such as simple partial seizures or brief absences, may elect not to take regular AEDs. If therapy is commenced, it should be a single drug. The combination of two or more drugs often exacerbates any side effects and poor compliance.

Polytherapy is best approached systematically (see Figure 10.1). The effectiveness of an AED should be assessed by measuring seizure frequency. Patients should be encouraged to keep a seizure diary. They should learn to discern and record different types of seizures and perceived seizure severity (many patients may have a useful therapeutic response to an AED, which does not necessarily involve the reduction in seizure frequency). Patients should also record their use of medication in the diary because side effects or lack of efficacy are often the result of patients misunderstanding the drugs and dosage they should be taking.

Provided that the clinical control is satisfactory it is not normally recommended that serum levels should be estimated regularly once an initial dose is established. The exception to this is during the growth period of children when doses will need to be altered according to the increased body weight. It is probably worth checking on initial interview with an established sufferer to determine a baseline and any cases of overdosing. Otherwise serum levels are only of value if a normally stable patient exhibits a seizure pattern outside of their normal.

Surgery and other non-drug treatment

It has been realized that some patients will never become seizure free on currently available AEDs and surgery is an important treatment option. About 50% of carefully selected patients with seizures originating in the temporal lobe will become seizure free after surgery. However, the assessment needed is complicated and requires a multidisciplinary team, which is only available at a few neurosciences centres in the UK. Multiple subpial transections, corpus callo-sotomy and hemispherectomy may be of value in the severe intractable seizure disorders.

Other new therapies include vagal nerve stimulation. The stimulator device is placed under the skin to the left side of the chest and is connected to the vagus nerve. The device sends out a signal at regular intervals (typically for 30 seconds every 5 minutes) and this stimulation has an inhibiting effect on seizure activity. It is effective across a broad spectrum of epilepsies for both adults and children.

Management strategy

The first step in review of the patient with epilepsy in general practice is to undertake an audit of past management.

Areas to examine could include:

- Record the last fit
- Named diagnosis
- Driving status
- Last seen regarding epilepsy.

A practice register could be compiled from repeat prescriptions and regular follow up undertaken to discuss the patient's condition, medication and the effects of both upon their lives. A checklist produced by Epilepsy Association of Scotland ensures that all the important

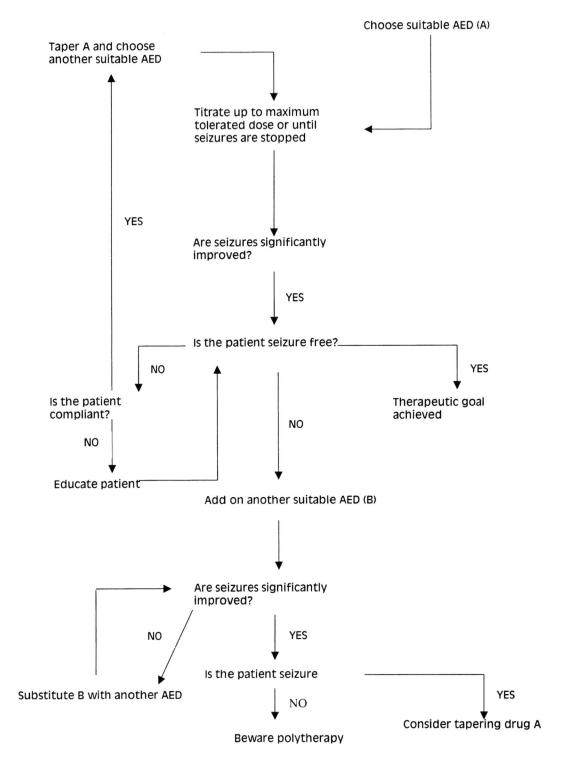

Figure 10.1 Managing epilepsy (Walker, 1996)

basic areas of information are covered (see Figure 10.2). In those not willing to avail themselves of the service, an open invitation should be left with them.

Guidelines of essential topics to cover during an interview

- Current status of seizures, last one, prodromal period, type, duration, post fit state, quality and duration
- Medication taken and compliance, last serum estimation
- Effects upon lifestyle, family, friends, school, job, driving, use of machinery, leisure and sporting pursuits, pregnancy, contraception
- Any intercurrent illness
- Advice or counselling to the patient and relatives or friends
- Further action (if any), for example referral to consultant, community services, school, work and possibly the DVLA.

The practice needs to establish an agreed standard of care. Points to consider are criteria for:

- Potential new diagnosis
- Preconceptual review
- Re-referral if seizures persist for 5 years
- Annual review
- Special situations, such as the elderly with epilepsy
- Referral to hospital.

Epilepsy in children

The incidence of epilepsy is greatest at the extremes of life, i.e. childhood and in the elderly; 70% of all epilepsy starts before the age of 20 and approximately half begins before the age of 16. The epilepsies of childhood are much more variable in expression and outcome than those in adults and the features can change with age. The clinical expression is also often atypical in infants and young children because of the incomplete cerebral development.

Children with epilepsy should be encouraged to live normal lives, once the seizures are under control, although it would be wise to exercise precautions with swimming and climbing. Parents should be encouraged not to be overprotective, as this is common in children whose seizures are not controlled. The vulnerable child may become withdrawn and avoid competition while the overprotected may become angry and manipulative. Siblings must not be ignored, their attitudes and fears need attention, as the child with epilepsy can become the focus of the family.

Most paediatricians continue to see children until treatment is stopped or they reach the age of 15 or 16 years old. This can be a difficult transition period between the world of paediatrics and the world of adult epilepsy. The change of care becomes patient centred and not parent centred. The adolescent, who is now a young adult, has to take control of the medication regimen, completing the seizure diary and is involved in decision making. Taking medication at the prescribed time can become a problem because of busy lifestyles, school and work and here the new controlled release formulations may be useful.

AEDs are the mainstay of treatment in children and monotherapy should be the aim, in the lowest dose that controls the seizure without producing effects. If a single drug produces a significant improvement but still does not give complete seizure control at the maximum tolerated dose, a second one is added because the first one is obviously doing some good. After a few months, provided the seizures are well controlled, discussion with the family about stopping the first drug and keeping on with the second can be agreed.

Routine blood tests are rarely performed before initiating AEDs. In the past, liver function and blood counts were monitored in children on sodium valproate or carbamazepine, but they have little predictive value for serious complications. Similarly, the place of serum AED levels is controversial. The therapeutic range for AEDs differs between patients and some will be well controlled below, while others experience no side effects above the 'normal' range. Most paediatricians monitor their patients clinically, judging efficacy by seizure control and side effects by parental and child report and examination. However, if there are questions about compliance or toxicity, or if polytherapy is being used, levels are measured.

Other treatments for children

The ketogenic diet has been successfully used in refractory epilepsy of childhood for over 70 years,

Epilepsy Association of Scotland
EPILEPSY CHECKLIST

This Checklist aims to assist GP's, other doctors and community teams in meeting the information needs of epilepsy patients and their carers.

THE DIAGNOSIS   Does the patient/carer understand...
- ★   that the diagnosis is epilepsy?
- ★   what epilepsy is?
- ★   what their own seizures are like?
- ★   what their own seizures are called?

THE MEDICATION   Does the patient/carer know...
- ★   the purpose of the medication?
- ★   the importance of compliance?
- ★   about possible drug side effects?
- ★   about drug interactions (e.g. antiepileptic medication and oral contraceptives)?
- ★   what to do if
  - a dose is missed?
  - vomiting occurs?
  - a trip abroad is planned?
- ★   that the medication is free?

BASIC INFORMATION   Has the patient/carer had...
- ★   a basic information booklet?
- ★   a chance to see an epilepsy video?
- ★   first aid instruction/demonstration?
- ★   information on legal restrictions for driving and certain jobs?

LIFE-STYLE   Has guidance been given on...
- ★   leading a full and active life?
- ★   adopting a moderate approach to alcohol?
- ★   having regular and sufficient sleep?
- ★   safety in the home (consider for each individual fires/radiators, bathing/showering, stairs, pillows, cookers, locked doors, etc.)?
- ★   safety/risk for sport and recreation (consider for each individual swimming, cycling, riding, etc.)?
- ★   implications of epilepsy (e.g. for relationships and parenthood)?

ONGOING DIALOGUE   Has the patient/carer been encouraged to...
- ★   return to questions?
- ★   keep a record of seizures?
- ★   report changes in seizure pattern and general health to GP?

FURTHER HELP   Is the patient/carer aware...
- ★   that additional support and information on all the above topics can be obtained from

THE EPILEPSY ASSOCIATION OF SCOTLAND
NATIONAL HEADQUARTERS
48 GOVAN ROAD, GLASGOW G51 1JL, TEL 041 427 4911

Figure 10.2 Epilepsy checklist (reproduced with permission from the Epilepsy Association of Scotland)

although the mechanism of action is unknown. It is based on carbohydrate restriction and a high fat diet, making it unpalatable and difficult to comply with. It requires the supervision of an experienced dietician to make up micronutrient deficiencies and the diet is given in addition to AEDs rather than as an immediate substitute. If successful AEDs can be withdrawn.

Steroids are often used in severe syndromes, such as West syndrome, Lennox-Gastaut syndrome and continuous spike wave discharges in slow sleep. They are potentially hazardous because of immune suppression, especially if the patient has not been exposed to chicken-pox, which can be fatal. Weekly monitoring is advised during treatment and if long-term use is prescribed growth should be monitored.

Surgery is now an available option for children with refractory epilepsy. Results depend greatly on patient selection, but the prognosis for seizure freedom is up to 70% for temporal lobectomy and about 50% for hemispherectomy.

Withdrawal of medication can be attempted in most children who have been seizure free for 2 years (at 2 years after stopping 75% will be seizure free). Juvenile myoclonic epilepsy is an exception and relapse is likely, so treatment is best continued. As previously stated the paediatrician undertakes the care of these children, but contact with the general practice team should be encouraged to offer support and advice, to make the transition from paediatric to adult care.

Special issues in children

At least 25% of children with epilepsy will have some form of special educational needs and at least 20% will have moderate to severe learning difficulties. It is therefore important that the difficulties experienced by children with epilepsy at school are clearly identified and addressed. It is also recognized that children with epilepsy frequently underachieve at school; 50% achieve less than would be predicted from their Intelligence Quotient (IQ) and extensive evidence informs us that seizures interfere with cognitive ability.

Liaison between consultant-led paediatrician services, educational authorities and school staff is often less than ideal. When the medical contribution to an educational assessment is being written, this should contain relevant information about seizure type, syndrome and aetiology, together with an account of the effect the epilepsy and its treatment are having in the classroom. This will require liaison between the community paediatrician, the epilepsy team and health visitor and community nursing services.

Epilepsy in patients with learning disabilities

Fifteen per cent of people with epilepsy have learning disabilities posing special problems. The central feature of learning disability is a reduction in the patient's ability to communicate with those around. Behaviour replaces language as the patient's link to the outside world and the doctor may need to analyse behavioural changes to guide him or her towards a diagnosis and to assess the affects of treatment that he or she prescribes. Epilepsy tends to be more refractory in this group, difficult to diagnose and treat, hence patients need ongoing contact with the specialist services. The important points with these patients are to make sure that they know they are valued and that you are doing the best things for them. When a carer says that a patient is worse that statement really means a great deal and you must take it seriously and find out what lies behind it.

Within the limits imposed by their severe disability the management of these patients has enormous potential to make their lives better or worse. Medication changes are problematic but small steps can be taken to improve the quality of their epilepsy management, for example adjusting their drug dosage to prevent drowsiness. That drowsiness might have prevented them from going out.

These individuals count in society and they can make a useful contribution to the world around them. Remember that the small changes that you make can help to bring enormous benefits to these men, women and children, many of whom are hugely disadvantaged.

Epilepsy and women

Epilepsy and treatment with AEDs poses many problems for women of childbearing age. In some women with epilepsy, seizures cluster at particular times during the menstrual cycle, which may require tailoring therapy. There are problems with drug interactions, side effects and the majority of AEDs are teratogenic. These problems are usually considered when a female becomes of childbearing age as AEDs during childhood may influence adult life. Treatment with sodium valproate can have long-term effects on fertility and increases the incidence of polycystic ovary syndrome.

Carbamazepine, phenytoin and barbiturates are all liver enzyme inducers and therefore increase the metabolism of the oral contraceptive pill making contraception unreliable. This problem can be overcome by using a higher dose contraceptive pill – 50 μg, and if breakthrough bleeding occurs, 80–100 μg. Alternatively treatment can be changed to sodium valproate, which does not interact.

The management of pregnant women with epilepsy is becoming increasingly important as the risk factors for adverse outcome of pregnancy are becoming more clearly delineated. Most women with epilepsy who do become pregnant will have a normal pregnancy and delivery, unchanged seizure frequency and a 90% chance of delivering a normal baby. However, some AED combinations administered in early pregnancy may significantly increase the risk of a malformed infant and without consultation prior to pregnancy, these drugs could be administered unknowingly in the first trimester. As a consequence, women of childbearing age need to be counselled to:

- discuss the risks of fetal abnormality
- reduce therapy preferably to monotherapy
- emphasize the importance of compliance and the dangers of clonic–tonic seizures
- take folic acid (5 mg) supplements.

The most common abnormality in infants born to mothers with epilepsy is cleft palate (30% of abnormalities), and specific syndromes have been described for different AEDs. Fetal anticonvulsant syndrome (FACS) is the best known. The risk of spina bifida is highest with sodium valproate (1–2%) and carbamazepine (0.5–1%). The Scottish Obstetric Guidelines (1997) provide an excellent tool for the management of pregnant women. Women on AEDs should have fetal ultrasound and alpha-fetoprotein measurement to detect neural tube defects early. For women on enzyme inducing AEDs, Vitamin K 20 mg daily from 36 weeks can be used to prevent haemorrhagic disease of the newborn. Once the child is born, breastfeeding should be encouraged, as AEDs are low in excreted breast milk.

Epilepsy in the elderly

Contrary to popular belief, epilepsy is not only common in the elderly, but its prevalence actually increases with age. The seizure pattern changes with age and partial or focal seizures become much more common with advancing age because of the concurrent rise in structural cerebral pathology. A partial seizure may not betray its focal origin if it quickly becomes secondarily generalized. Under these circumstances all that is visible clinically is a generalized tonic–clonic seizure, making diagnosis more difficult to recognize. The precise diagnosis and effective control of seizures is extremely important. For instance, in an old person with fragile osteoporotic bones, a tonic–clonic seizure may well lead to severely reduced mobility. A lengthy post-ictal state could be dangerous for people living alone.

Cerebrovascular disease is the commonest cause of epilepsy in the elderly and between 10 and 15% of patients who have a stroke go on to develop seizures. Any elderly patient with an unexplained seizure should be screened for cerebrovascular risk factors and consideration given to providing long-term treatment with aspirin. Cerebral tumours are associated with seizures in 5–10% of cases.

Many medical conditions, such as dementia, uraemia, hepatic failure, cardiac disease and metabolic disorders, may be complicated by seizures. Treating elderly patients with epilepsy involves numerous challenges, in addition to the presence of concomitant disease. The consequences of epilepsy can be severely disabling to the lives of elderly people. The stigma of the diagnosis for the elderly can lead to withdrawal and isolation. Loss of their driving licence may greatly reduce their independence and leave them housebound.

The general belief was that epilepsy in the elderly had a rather poor prognosis because of the high incidence of patients with structural abnormalities. This has been found not to be the case as the majority of patients do remarkably well. This raises the question of the potential value of treatment in some patients. It is important to question for example, if it is worth using an anticonvulsant that might produce side effects to prevent one or two minor seizures a year. Moreover, the incidence of side effects from AEDs is significantly higher in the elderly due to the increased pharmacodynamic sensitivity in old age.

Management of these patients consists of a positive outlook but anticipating the possibility of loss of confidence. Most people need time to express their feelings and to discuss the practical impact of their condition. The social workers, health visitors and occupational therapists should be contacted to provide support and review the home situation.

There is often concern about patients whose epilepsy was diagnosed in early life and are taking phenobarbitone and whether they are at risk of developing osteomalacia because of drug-induced vitamin D deficiency. Elevated levels of alkaline phosphatase are common in such patients because of hepatic enzyme induction but frank osteomalacia is rare. These patients are usually well controlled, and withdrawing a barbiturate can be problematic, so they are best left alone or the clinician can reduce the drug slowly to the lowest acceptable dose.

Specific issues – driving, generic prescribing, photosensitive epilepsy

Driving

To be prevented from driving can have devastating effects on the person with epilepsy and their family. Legislation attempts to balance the risks of a person with epilepsy driving, against the psychological and social disadvantages to that person if prevented from doing so. The law requires anyone experiencing a seizure or developing epilepsy to inform the DVLA, since continuing to drive is illegal and may void insurance cover. The current driving regulations state that an ordinary driving licence will be granted to those with epilepsy who have been free from any seizures for 1 year, with or without treatment, or have only had attacks during sleep over 3 years. The DVLA suggests that a person does not drive while treatment is being reduced or for 6 months after stopping treatment. If a person has a seizure when trying to come off therapy or afterwards, they need to inform the DVLA and may not drive for 1 year. Advice about driving and epilepsy is available from the Driving and Vehicle Licensing Agency, Swansea SA99 1TU.

Generic prescribing

Epilepsy poses special problems making it an exception to the rule of generic prescribing. People with epilepsy require careful dose titration of their AED to optimize control. Some AEDs have a narrow therapeutic window, therefore minor changes in bioavailability could translate into breakthrough seizures and increased toxicity. Treatment switches can cause problems and these can be minimized by prescribing consistently.

Photosensitive epilepsy

Seizures sometimes can be triggered by flashing or flickering lights, or even geometric shapes or patterns. A standard EEG can be undertaken with photic stimulation which would usually confirm diagnosis. The condition is relatively rare and unnecessary constrictions on people's lifestyles must be avoided. Photosensitivity usually responds to sodium valproate. Advice regarding using remote controls to change TV channels, consider using a high frequency TV, and avoiding poorly tuned channels and using sunglasses help to prevent glare are helpful. Excessive tiredness may increase the risk of a seizure. It is rare for seizures to be triggered by film in a cinema although stroboscopic lights can cause seizures. It is advisable not to use a computer for more than 30–40 minutes without a break and antiglare screens are useful.

Conclusion

Theoretically, there has never been a better time for people with epilepsy, with advances in imaging techniques, drug treatments, surgery and complementary medicine. Yet, as the report *An Epilepsy Needs Document*, undertaken by Brown *et al.* (1993), states, provision of epilepsy services in the UK is poorly organized, fragmented, patchy and often of unacceptable quality. Successive attempts to address these shortcomings by published recommendations, even with government assistance, have not led to major improvements. Raising the profile of epilepsy, through government strategies and increasing the number of neuroconsultants could help to improve this situation and, of course, epilepsy requires a multidisciplinary team in general practice to move forward. GPs need support from other members of the health-care team, if services are to improve. There is one example of a general practitioner who has developed an Epilepsy Liaison Service which provides a high standard of epilepsy care within a structure that includes comprehensive specialist epilepsy services (Taylor, 1987). In the hospital setting, the introduction of hospital liaison nurses has shown they can improve care and promote links between primary and secondary care. In the modern NHS, with primary care groups and primary care trusts supporting general practice, it is time that we gave the care of people with epilepsy a higher profile in an attempt to provide the highest possible standard of care to this group of people.

Useful addresses

British Epilepsy Association
New Anstley House
Gateway Drive
Yeadon
LS19 7XY
Tel 0133 210 8800
Helpline 0808 800 5050

The Joint Epilepsy Council
PO Box 16696
London
WC1A 2PD
Tel 0171 300 6300

The National Society for Epilepsy
Chesham Lane
Chalfont St Peter
Bucks
SL9 ORJ
Tel 01494 601300
Helpline 01494 601400
www.epilepsynse.org.uk

Epilepsy Bereaved
PO Box 1777
Bournemouth
BH5 1YR

Epilepsy Action of Scotland
48 Govan Road
Glasgow
G51 1JL
Tel 0141 4274911
Helpline 0141 4275225
www.epilepsyscotland.org.uk

Brainwave
The Irish Epilepsy Association
249 Crumlin Road
Dublin 12
Tel 00 35314 557500
www.epilepsy.ie
e-mail info@epilepsy.ie

Epilepsy Wales
15 Chester St
St Asaph
Denbighshire
Wales
LL17 0RE
Tel 08457 413774

National Fetal Anticonvulsant Syndrome
    Association
PO Box 10035
Newton of Brux
Alford
AB33 8YT
Tel 019755 71430
e-mail facsline@aol.com

References

Brown S, Betts T, Chadwick D (1993) An epilepsy needs document. *Seizure* **4**, 207–210

Camfield P, Camfield C, Gordon K, Dooley J (1994) What types of epilepsy are preceded by febrile seizures? A population-based study. *Developmental Medicine and Child Neurology* **36** (10), 887–892

Central Health Services Council – the Cohen Committee (1956) *Report of the Sub-Committee on the medical care of Epileptics*. HMSO, London

Epilepsy Task Force (1999) Service Development Kit GEN 25957–BP London

Hauser W A, Annegers J F, Kurland L T (1993) Incidence of epilepsy and unprovoked seizures in Rochester, Minnesota: 1935–1984. *Epilepsia* **34** (3), 453–468

Hopkins A (1993) *Clinical Neurology: a Modern Approach.* Oxford University Press, Oxford

Lesser R (1996) Psychogenic seizures. *Neurology* **46**, 1499–1507

Nelson (1994) *A Patient's Viewpoint.* British Epilepsy Association

Sander J W (1997) The epidemiology of the epilepsies: future directions. *Epilepsia* **38**, 614–618

Sander J W, Shorvan S D (1987) Incidence and prevalence studies in epilepsy and their methodological problems: a review. *Journal of Neurology, Neurosurgery and Psychiatry* **50**, 829–839

Sander J W, Hart Y M, Johnson A L, Shorvan S D (1990) National General Practice Study of Epilepsy: recurrence after first seizure. *Lancet* **336**, 1271–1274

Scambler G (1989) *Epilepsy.* p. 32. Routledge, London

Scottish Obstetric Guidelines and Audit Project (1997) The management of pregnancy in women with epilepsy

Taylor M P (1987) Epilepsy in a Doncaster practice: audit and change over eight years. *Journal of the Royal College of General Practitioners* **37**, 116–119

Taylor M P (1996) *Managing Epilepsy in Primary Care.* Blackwell Science, Oxford

Thapar A K (1996) Care of patients with epilepsy in the community: will the new initiatives address old problems? *British Journal of General Practice* **46**, 37–42

Walker M (1996) *MIMS – Guide to Epilepsy.* Medical Imprint, London

Willmore L J (1996) Management of epilepsy in the elderly. *Epilepsia* **37** (suppl. 6), 23–33

Chapter

11

Coronary heart disease

Judith Lawrence

Introduction

There has recently been a huge focus on the prevention and management of coronary heart disease (CHD) in the UK. The Department of Health (DoH) in 1999 published *Our Healthier Nation: Saving Lives* (DoH, 1999) which outlined the government's commitment to reduce the death rate from CHD. This has been followed by the National Service Framework (NSF) for coronary heart disease in England and Wales (DoH, 2000). It is vitally important that health care professionals do not lose sight of the patient in the process of implementing government directives.

A patient's perspective

I was first diagnosed with angina when I was fifty-six, and it should not have surprised me, since both my parents had suffered the condition since their mid-fifties. But I did not care to believe it, and desperately tried to prove to myself that it was mere unfitness. Having for years prided myself on my fitness it seemed painfully ironic, and the recognition of my age and mortality.

Eighteen months later the pain could no longer be lived with. I was prescribed increasing amounts of medication, each one cutting me off further and further from normal life. I looked at people far older than myself who smoked, drank excessively and ate large quantities of animal fats and who were still able to break into a run, and felt all the bitterness of an unjust fate.

Eventually, after several hospital visits, each one repeating with a different doctor the previous visit's routine of detail-taking, I was given an angiogram and told that I required bypass surgery. My life was now on hold, waiting 'up to eleven months' for the operation. However much I was assured that the procedure is now 'routine', it could not appear routine to me. I had not undergone any surgery since a tonsillectomy in childhood which I still remembered with fear and confusion, and while for much of the time I put off the prospect, there were occasions in the early hours in the morning when I lay awake and felt that finally I was completely alone. My fears centred on the idea of losing consciousness and never wakening again to my wife and children. Such fears are no less real for being irrational. Your own experience can never be 'routine' – it is absolutely unique, for you only, this time and no other.

Epidemiology

Coronary heart disease is the most common cause of death within the UK. In 1998, there were 135 000 deaths, representing one in four men and one in five women dying from CHD (British Heart Foundation, 2000a). There has been a drop of 42% in the mortality figures over the last 10 years for adults between the ages of 16 and 64. This is, in the main, due to medical research and advances in biotechnology, improving the management of patients with CHD. However, morbidity rates are rising, particularly in the older population. This is reflected in the demographic profile with life expectancy increasing in the UK. It is estimated that 270 000 people have a myocardial infarction each year and 1.5 million people have angina. The incidence of heart failure is increasing, with the prevalence estimated at between 3 and 20 people per 1000. This figure increases to over 80 people per 1000 in those aged over 75 years (DoH, 2000).

Geographical variances in mortality and morbidity rates are well recognized, with the incidence of CHD in Belfast and Glasgow among the highest in the world (Tunstall-Pedoe *et al.*, 1999). Men in Scotland having a 60% higher risk of premature death from CHD in comparison with East Anglia (British Heart Foundation, 2000a).

Inequalities in health and socioeconomic status are recognized as being risk factors for CHD, with a 58% higher premature mortality rate among manual workers, as opposed to non-manual workers. Within the UK, each year, 47 000 working years and 5000 lives are lost from CHD in men between the ages of 20 and 64. It is estimated that one in three deaths from CHD under the age of 65 is related to socioeconomic differences (British Heart Foundation, 2000a).

Pathophysiology

Coronary heart disease (CHD) is due to the partial or total occlusion of the coronary arteries by atherosclerotic plaques. This leads to the myocardium being damaged due to an inadequate supply of oxygenated blood. CHD usually presents as angina, myocardial infarction, heart failure, or sudden death. Ischaemic heart disease (IHD) is a term sometimes used interchangeably with CHD, however, it should be noted that IHD can develop without the involvement of the coronary arteries, for example, in severely anaemic patients.

Atherosclerosis develops slowly, sometimes over many years and the plaques can vary in size from a few millimetres to several centimetres in diameter. The process involves the lumen of the artery becoming narrowed by the formation of atherosclerotic plaques. Macrophages (foam) cells migrate into the lining of the arteries, the intima. It may be that the endothelium lining has been damaged in some way, be it mechanical, chemical, toxic, viral or immunological, for example smoking, inflammation or hypertension. It is thought that these lipid laden foam cells, rich in oxidized low density lipid proteins, especially cholesterol and triglycerides, break down and deposit their lipid and cytoplasmic contents within the intima. Intercellular lipid pools are formed, which are then infiltrated by smooth muscle cells which proliferate within the plaque (Lorimer, 1997).

Some arteries, like the coronary arteries, are more at risk from this disease than others. The internal mammary artery and radial artery are, in the main, spared, which allows for the internal mammary to be considered for use in coronary artery bypass grafts (Boon *et al.*, 1999). Atherosclerosis affects other blood vessels in the body and this can lead to peripheral vascular disease and cerebrovascular accidents. Figure 11.1 demonstrates the development and progression of atherosclerosis.

Cholesterol and lipid proteins

Dyslipidaemia influences the development of atherosclerosis and therefore is a risk factor for CHD.

Essentially there are three main classes of lipids:

- Triglycerides – this is the main form in which fat is stored in the adipose tissue. They are a vital source of cellular energy and can be broken down into fatty acids. Triglycerides are synthesized in the liver
- Phospholipids – they are an important constituent of cell membranes and the only lipid that is partially soluble in water
- Cholesterol – is an essential component of human-cell membranes.

Fats from a person's dietary intake are transported from the intestinal tract to the liver for metabolism. However, as they are insoluble in water, they are combined with proteins to allow for transportation around the body. There are specialized proteins within the lipoproteins and these are called apoproteins. Apoproteins aid the structural stability of the lipoprotein and also ensure that each lipoprotein connects with the correct receptors in the cell walls. The transport of lipoproteins from the liver to the tissues is via the systemic circulation. Cholesterol is excreted from the body in bile either as cholesterol or bile salts (Tortora and Grabowski, 2000).

Development of atherosclerosis

Foam cells — Intercellular lipid

Early lesion or fatty streak

Smooth muscle cell — Fibrous tissue

Lipid core — Foam cells

Advanced lesion or fibrous plaque

Thrombosis ulceration — Haemorrhage

Calcification

Complicated lesion, with ulceration, calcification or haemorrhage

The progression of atherosclerosis

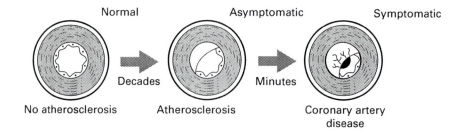

Normal   Asymptomatic   Symptomatic

Decades   Minutes

No atherosclerosis   Atherosclerosis   Coronary artery disease

Figure 11.1 Development and progression of atherosclerosis

Injury hypothesis of atherogenesis

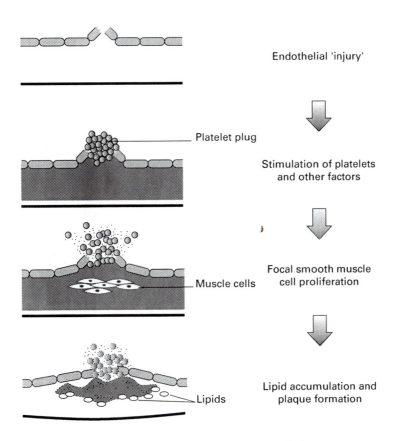

Endothelial 'injury'

Platelet plug

Stimulation of platelets
and other factors

Muscle cells

Focal smooth muscle
cell proliferation

Lipids

Lipid accumulation and
plaque formation

The initiating stimuli could be mechanical,
chemical, toxic, viral or immunological
(e.g. hypertension, smoking)

Figure 11.1 (cont)

The five main classes of lipoproteins are listed below:

1. Chylomicrons are the largest of the lipoproteins. They appear briefly in the blood after a meal. They are removed from the blood quickly and cannot be detected after a 12-h fast. They are formed in the intestines and their role is to transport triglycerides obtained from dietary intake to the liver for metabolism.
2. Very low-density lipoproteins (VLDL): their synthesis is affected by a person's body weight and alcohol intake. Therefore the levels of VLDL-cholesterol tend to be high in obese people and in people who have a high alcohol intake correction. Their composition is made up of 50% triglycerides, approximately 20% cholesterol and 20% phospholipid. Their main function is to transport triglycerides around the body. However VLDLs obtain their triglyceride content from the liver. The liver synthesizes triglyceride when levels of free fatty acids and glycerol rise.
3. Intermediate low density lipoproteins (ILDL), again are an important means of cholesterol transportation.
4. Low-density lipoproteins (LDL) are the main way in which cholesterol is transported from

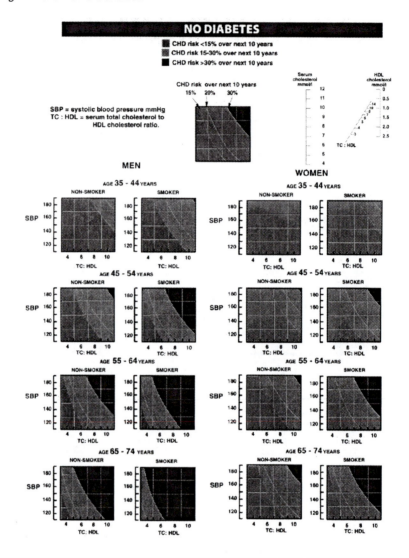

How to use the Coronary Risk Prediction Chart for Primary Prevention

These charts are for estimating coronary heart disease (CHD) risk (non fatal MI and coronary death) for individuals who have not developed symptomatic CHD or other major atherosclerotic disease.

The use of these charts is not appropriate for patients who have existing disease which already puts them at high risk. Such diseases are:

- CHD or other major atherosclerotic disease
- Familial hypercholesterolaemia or other inherited dyslipidaemia
- Established hypertension (systolic BP > 160 mmHg and/or diastolic BP > 100 mmHg) or associated target organ damage
- Diabetes mellitus with associated target organ damage
- Renal dysfunction

- To estimate an individuals absolute 10 year risk of developing CHD find the table for their gender, diabetes (yes/no), smoking status (smoker/non smoker) and age. Within this square define the level of risk according to systolic blood pressure and the ratio of total cholesterol to HDL cholesterol. If there is no HDL cholesterol result then assume this is 1.0mmol/l and then the lipid scale can be used for total cholesterol alone.

- High risk individuals are defined as those whose 10 year CHD risk exceeds 15% (equivalent to a *cardiovascular* risk of 20% over the same period). As a minimum those at highest risk (≥ 30% red) should be targeted and treated now, and as resources allow others with a risk of > 15% (orange) should be progressively targeted.

Figure 11.2 Joint British Recommendations on Prevention of Coronary Heart Disease in Clinical Practice. (a) No diabetes; (b) diabetes (Wood *et al.*, 1998). Reproduced with permission from Professor Dorrington, Manchester University

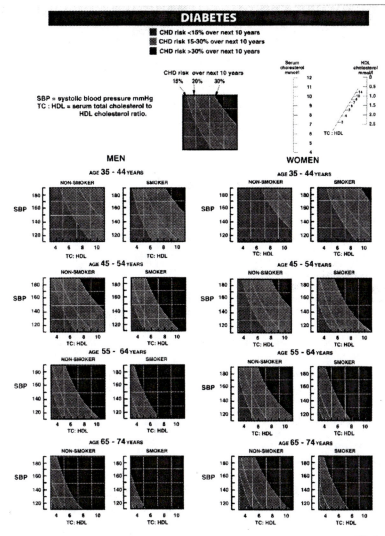

This chart is available in a poster format.

- Smoking status should reflect lifetime exposure to tobacco and not simply tobacco use at the time of risk assessment.
- The initial blood pressure and the first random (non fasting) total cholesterol and HDL cholesterol can be used to estimate an individual's risk. However, the decision on using drug therapy should be based on repeat risk factor measurements over a period of time. The chart should not be used to estimate risk after treatment of hyperlipidaemia or blood pressure has been initiated.
- CHD risk is higher than indicated in the charts for
  - Those with a family history of premature CHD (men <55 years and women <65 years) which increases the risk by a factor of approximately 1.5.
  - Those with raised triglyceride levels.
  - Those who are not diabetic but have impaired glucose tolerance.
  - Women with premature menopause.

- As the person approaches the next age category. As risk increases exponentially with age the risk will be closer to the higher decennium for the last four years of each decade.
- In ethnic minorities the risk chart should be used with caution as it has not been validated in these populations.
- The estimates of CHD risk from the chart are based on groups of people and in managing an *individual* the physician also has to use clinical judgement in deciding how intensively to intervene on lifestyle and whether or not to use drug therapies.
- An individual can be shown on the chart the direction in which the risk of CHD can be reduced by changing smoking status, blood pressure or cholesterol.

Coronary Risk Prediction Chart reproduced (and modified) with permission from Heart 1998; 80: 51-529. © The University of Manchester

Figure 11.2 (continued)

the liver, where it is synthesized, to the tissues. Over 50% of the content of LDL is cholesterol with a small component being triglyceride. Because LDL have such a high cholesterol content there is particular concern if a patient has a high LDL level, as this is associated with CHD.

5. High-density lipoproteins (HDL) are made of mainly apoproteins and phospolipids with only a small proportion of cholesterol being present. HDL is responsible for the transport of cholesterol away from the cells to the liver – this is known as reverse cholesterol transport. High levels of HDL are associated with reduced risk of atherosclerosis and therefore a reduced risk of developing CHD. Exercise is known to increase the level of HDL. Oparil (1996) highlighted that HDL levels were generally higher in women, especially younger women, and this may contribute to the lower incidence of CHD. Frequently, laboratories calculate a total cholesterol (TC)/HDL ratio, this provides information about the proportion of the protective HDL against the total cholesterol.

Risk factors

Epidemiological studies, most notably the Framingham Study undertaken in a small community in Framingham, USA (Dawber *et al.*, 1951, as cited in Lindsay, 1997), have produced research which has been the basis of our knowledge on the identification of CHD risk. The Framingham Study is still ongoing and is one of the few studies to include women in the cohort.

Table 11.1 Non-modifiable and modifiable risk factors

Non-modifiable	Modifiable
Age	Smoking
Gender	Elevated plasma cholesterol
	Elevated BP
Family history of CHD	Diabetes mellitus
Personal history of CHD	Obesity
Ethnic origin	Physical inactivity
Excess alcohol	
Stress	

The most important associated risk factors for CHD are diabetes mellitus, hypertension, smoking and raised cholesterol (hyperlipidaemia). Individuals who have a significant risk of going on to develop CHD should be identified within the population. Figure 11.2a and b is the Joint British Recommendations on Prevention of Coronary Heart Disease in Clinical Practice (Wood *et al.*, 1998). This can be used by the health care professional to assess an individual's risk for the development of CHD. Patients with a risk prediction >15% of having a cardiac event over the next 10 years should be targeted and risk factors treated. However, it is recognized that initially the emphasis should be to target those whose risk is >30%.

Risk factors can be classified as modifiable and non-modifiable and the key to long-term management of CHD is to work with patients to identify risk factors and develop strategies to reduce the harmful effects.

The *major* risk factors are summarized in Table 11.1. Consideration should also be given to other risk factors like low plasma HDL, elevated triglycerides and thrombogenic factors.

Non-modifiable risk factors

CHD increases with age and is more prevalent in men than women, under the age of 60. However, after the age of 60 the incidence of CHD increases substantially in women and it is estimated that, by the age of 70, the rate is the same as for men (British Heart Foundation, 2000a).

It is suggested that women are protected against CHD while they are premenopausal but after the menopause they have reduced circulating oestrogen and therefore their risk of CHD is increased. This fact should not exclude premenopausal women from having a comprehensive risk assessment undertaken as strategies can be put in place for the long-term prevention of CHD by addressing modifiable risk factors.

A family history of CHD is recognized when a first degree relative has presented with CHD before the age of 60 (Lindsay, 1997). Often a genetic predisposition coupled with environmental factors like social class, employment status and geographical area tend to make it difficult to pinpoint exactly what in the family history makes an individual prone to CHD.

However, a clear link has been made to hypercholesterolaemia and when this risk factor is identified in the patient other family members should be screened.

Ethnic origin is a definite causal factor in the progression of CHD. South Asians (Indians, Bangladeshis, Pakistanis and Sri Lankans) have a higher premature mortality rate from CHD (British Heart Foundation, 2000a). Between 1971 and 1991 mortality rates dropped in the Caucasian population by 29% in men and 17% in women between the ages of 20 and 69. The overall reduction in mortality rates from CHD within the UK has not declined as rapidly within the South Asian population. This group only experienced a 20% reduction in men and 7% reduction in women (Wild and McKeigue, 1997). It is sometimes argued that diabetes should be classed as a non-modifiable risk factor. However, it is possible to control the blood glucose level and the blood pressure in people with diabetes and this can lead to a reduction in the risk of developing CHD.

Modifiable risk factors

Smoking

In patients who already have CHD, the risk of a recurrent coronary event or premature death can be reduced by 50% if they stop smoking (US Department of Health and Human Services, 1990; DoH, 1998). It is estimated that CHD can be attributed to smoking in 20% of men and 17% in women. Currently smoking is more prevalent in Scotland and Northern Ireland in comparison with England and Wales. A higher proportion of men smoke in comparison with women but this gap is narrowing. However, in the younger age groups, the percentage of girls smoking is higher than boys. In 1998, 9% of boys aged between 11 and 15 smoked in comparison with 11% of girls. Smoking is also more prevalent in the manual workers and within the male Bangladeshi and Caribbean populations (British Heart Foundation, 2000a).

The effects of smoking on the body are wide ranging. There are around 4000 different chemicals in tobacco smoke and these include carbon monoxide and nicotine. Carbon monoxide reduces the capability of red blood cells to carry oxygen in the blood by attaching itself to the haemoglobin. Other chemicals within the tobacco smoke appear to cause damage to the lining of the coronary arteries leading to the formation of atherosclerotic plaques. Nicotine stimulates an increase in the production of adrenaline which, in turn, increases the heart rate and raises blood pressure.

Exercise

It is recognized that people who are physically active have a lower risk of CHD (British Heart Foundation, 2000a). The optimum level of exercise is 30 minutes of moderate activity on 5 days of the week (DoH, 1996). Unfortunately, only 37% of men and 25% of women exercise at an optimum level. It is estimated that 9% of deaths from CHD could be avoided if activity could be increased to a moderate level within the population.

The benefits of regular exercise include a reduction in heart rate and blood pressure at rest and during exercise. This in turn results in a reduction in oxygen demands on the myocardium. Maintaining an exercise regimen will increase the HDL level, thereby reducing the TC/HDL ratio. If the patient has diabetes, improved glucose tolerance can be achieved, which may allow for a reduction in the dosage of insulin or oral hypoglycaemic medication. An increase in coronary collateral circulation can be achieved, and this leads to an improvement in myocardial perfusion. Fibrinolysis is enhanced, thereby preventing thrombosis formation over atherosclerotic plaques (Armstrong, 1997). Weight reduction can be achieved through the combination of exercise and maintaining a healthy diet, thereby tackling obesity, another known risk factor for CHD.

Hypertension

CHD risk is linked to raised systolic and diastolic blood pressure. Elevated blood pressure accounts for 14% of deaths from CHD in men and 12% in women (British Heart Foundation, 2000a). It is recognized that a reduction in salt and alcohol intake, an increase in physical activity and weight loss can all reduce blood pressure. Current recommendations advocate that blood pressure should be below 140/85, and if the patient has diabetes, then it should be below 140/80 (Ramsay et al., 1999). The exact underlying pathological changes that are attributed to the development of hypertension are unclear,

Table 11.2 Body mass index (BMI)

BMI	Weight
Under 20	Underweight
20–24	Health: desirable weight
25–29	Overweight; should lose weight
30–39	Obese: needs to lose weight
Over 40	Very obese: must lose weight

however, it is thought to be influenced by larger arteries losing their elasticity, leading to an increase in peripheral arteriole resistance. This in turn can accelerate the development of atherosclerotic plaque formation, especially in the smaller arteries, and therefore the lumen of the blood vessel becomes narrower (Boon *et al.*, 1999). It is important to consider secondary causes of hypertension, which include renal disease, primary hypothyroidism or drug induced (for example, corticosteroids).

Cholesterol

Cholesterol is a major contributory factor in the development of atherosclerosis. Current recommendations advise a total cholesterol level of below 5 mmol/l (LDL 3 mmol) or an overall reduction of 30%, whichever is the greater (Scandinavian Simvastatin Survival Study Group, 1994; Sacks *et al.*, 1996). The same reduction in cholesterol is recommended for patients without a diagnosis of CHD but who have a CHD risk of greater than 30% over 10 years (Wood *et al.*, 1998). Cholesterol management will be discussed later in the chapter.

Obesity

It is well recognized that there is a link between obesity and CHD. Obesity also has an influence on other risk factors like diabetes, hypertension and hyperlipidaemia. Obesity is a common condition, especially in affluent countries (Boon *et al.*, 1999). It is important to investigate the possible causes of obesity, which may be due to a consequence of heredity or environmental factors, endocrine dysfunction or it may be due to a variety of drugs, for example, steroids or the oral contraceptive. Obesity is calculated by measuring the person's height and weight to determine their body mass index (BMI). If the

BMI is greater than 30, premature death is increased by 5% in men and 6% in women.

Table 11.2 outlines the current guidelines on body mass index. Population trends indicate that there is an increase in the number of individuals who are overweight and obese, irrespective of age.

Diabetes

Men who live with type 2 diabetes mellitus have a two to fourfold increased risk of developing CHD. There is a three to fivefold increased risk in women with type 2 diabetes (British Heart Foundation, 2000a). The underlying pathological changes that take place that increase the risk of CHD in people with diabetes is unclear, however, it is thought that the effects are related to an alteration in the lipid profile and the increase in atherosclerotic changes. See Chapter 6 for a more detailed discussion on the macrovascular complications of diabetes mellitus.

Coronary heart disease: clinical manifestations

Myocardial infarction

Myocardial infarction (MI) is invariably due to the occlusion of a coronary artery by a thrombus formation or platelet aggregation at the site of an atherosclerotic plaque. In addition, haemorrhage into the plaque can compromise the lumen of the artery. This leads to myocardial ischaemia (insufficient supply of oxygenated blood to the myocardium) and if this continues for a sufficient length of time necrosis of the cardiac muscle can ensue. Sudden, severe hypotension can also reduce cardiac output and result in an insufficient blood supply to meet the needs of the myocardium resulting in ischaemia.

Signs and symptoms of an acute myocardial infarction include central prolonged chest pain, which can radiate to the throat, arms, epigastrium and back, associated with breathlessness, nausea, vomiting, syncope, cold sweating and collapse. Chest pain associated with myocardial infarction is usually described as crushing and constricting. Patients report it being one of the worst pains they have experienced. It may be that breathlessness is the only symptom experienced by the patient. Therefore taking an accurate history is vital to distinguish it from breathlessness caused by a respiratory disease. Syncope is often a result of arrhythmias or severe hypotension. Vomiting and sinus bradycardia are usually the result of vagal stimulation and are common in patients who have inferior myocardial infarctions (Boon *et al.*, 1999).

Sometimes a myocardial infarct can lead to a sudden death and this is usually attributed to a cardiac arrhythmia, such as ventricular fibrillation. Advances in the management of acute coronary events and the increased availability of defibrillators has resulted in a reduction of the mortality rates post-MI. Sometimes a patient may have a myocardial infarction that is not detected. This is particularly common with elderly or diabetic patients and is referred to as a 'silent' MI.

Angina

It is estimated that within the UK each year 20 000 people develop angina (DoH, 2000). Angina is a symptom of an inadequate supply of oxygenated blood to the myocardium muscle. Atherosclerotic plaques are the most probable cause for the impaired supply of blood to the myocardium. Angina is characterized by a heaviness, tightness or restricting pain in the centre of the chest, which may radiate to the jaw, neck or arms. It can be precipitated by physical exertion. Patients will often report symptoms appearing when they walk up an incline, up stairs or when exposed to cold weather or wind. It can also develop after a heavy meal or when the patient becomes emotionally stressed. Vivid dreams can bring on nocturnal angina, but this is less common (Boon *et al.*, 1999).

Unstable angina is characterized by a worsening of the condition, with symptoms at rest or on minimal exertion. Taking an accurate and detailed history is the key to the diagnosis and effective management of angina. Sometimes patients develop a life style that avoids any situation which may bring on the anginal symptoms. It is vital that an understanding of the patient's lifestyle is explored as they may have restricted their activities to a bare minimum. Other contributing diseases or conditions like anaemia, thyrotoxicosis, aortic value disease, aortic stenosis and hypertrophic cardiomyopathy should be considered.

Heart failure

Heart failure occurs when the heart is unable to maintain an adequate cardiac output to meet the demands of the body and thereby ensure the oxygenation of the tissues. The most common causes of heart failure are coronary heart disease, prolonged hypertension and mitral and aortic valve disease. It is important to note that heart failure may present and be unrelated to coronary heart disease, for example, in thyrotoxicosis and anaemia.

The symptoms of left ventricular failure (LVF) include fatigue, dyspnoea, orthopnoea, paroxysmal nocturnal dyspnoea, nocturnal dry cough, giddiness, exhaustion, cold hands and feet, palpitations, loss of weight leading to loss of appetite, muscle wasting and cachexia. Right ventricular failure (RVF) presents with symptoms such as peripheral oedema, abdominal oedema, nausea, fatigue and wasting. Biventricular heart failure can develop with the failure of both the right and left ventricles due to coronary heart disease and cardiomyopathy.

Heart failure can be aggravated by drug therapies such as beta-blockers or short-acting calcium channel blockers (not amlodipine). In addition, excess salt and alcohol in the diet have been linked to aggravating the condition.

Arrhythmias

The contraction of the myocarduim is achieved by electrical impulses travelling from the SA node through the conduction fibres of the heart. Any alteration in the pattern of electrical impulses has the potential to cause serious problems. It is important that consideration is given to heart rate and rhythm when taking a detailed history and do not expect the patient to volunteer information regarding irregularities as they may see them as common place.

Examples of the common arrhythmias, atrial fibrillation, atrial flutter, tachycardia and heart block can be found in the ECG strips in Figure 11.3.

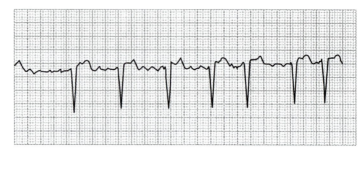

(a)

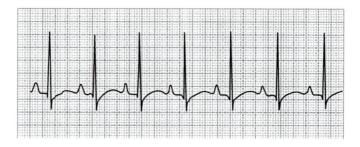

(b)

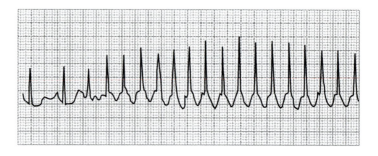

(c)

(d)

Figure 11.3 ECG strips. (a) Atrial fibrillation (note the irregular rhythm and absence of normal P waves); (b) atrial flutter (note regular rhythm – P waves, but ventricular rhythm depends on conduction pattern); (c) paroxysmal supraventricular tachycardia (note development from normal sinus rhythm). Heart block: (d) first degree (note lengthened P–R interval); (e) second degree (occasional dropped beat); (f) second degree (2:1 conduction); (g) third degree (P wave and QRS complex not related) (reproduced with kind permission from Walsh *et al.*, 1999)

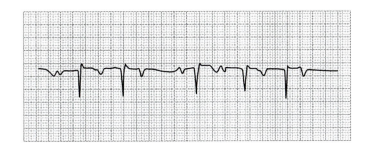

(e)

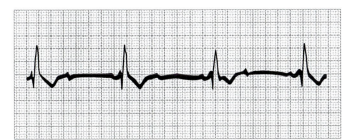

(f)

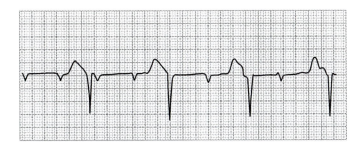

(g)

Figure 11.3 (continued)

Assessment of the patient

The assessment includes taking a detailed history and carrying out a systematic clinical examination. The key to the assessment is to ascertain to what degree the symptoms of CHD are impacting on the patient's quality of life. It may be that the patient's condition is deteriorating and medication needs to be reviewed and altered accordingly. New symptoms may have developed or side effects from medication may be present which need to be explored. The patient may not always realize or acknowledge that there has been an alteration in their physical and/or psychological state and therefore it is vital that the practitioner does not presume that the patient will voluntarily report the infor-mation required to inform the assessment. It is essential for the patient to feel relaxed and be given the opportunity and time to ask questions and express their concerns. No consultation should be viewed as routine. Simply informing the patient at the beginning of the consultation how long it will last and what it will entail can ease the tension. Reducing anxiety levels will ensure that blood pressure and pulse readings are more accurate. Likewise if the patient is relaxed they are more likely to give a fuller detailed history.

Work load pressures are a huge problem within the NHS, but patients with CHD need the time to express fears and anxieties. Failure to recognize these could lead to the patient's physical or mental health deteriorating further.

If it is not possible to give the patient the time they need within the consultation you may need to recognize that another member of the health care team will be more able to support the patient. It is also important to recognize that the patient may benefit from the skills of another health care professional.

History

The key components of a history include:

Past medical history
Current health problems and symptoms
All modifiable risk factors
Family history of CHD
Psychological health
Medication and concordance.

Chest pain, breathlessness, palpitations and intermittent claudication are key symptoms of CHD and therefore attention must be made to exploring these issues with the patient. The prompt and accurate assessment of chest pain is vital, and when this symptom is reported by the patient it should be taken seriously until proven otherwise. Differentiating between cardiac pain and non-cardiac pain can be difficult and therefore it is vital that the relevant information is gained.

Often patients with COPD and asthma associate their breathlessness with their respiratory condition and therefore do not use their cardiac medication appropriately or report the symptom to the health care practitioner. Systematic symptom analysis is aided by using a formal structure like PQRST (Morton, 1993).

P: Provocative/palliative
Q: Quality
R: Region/radiation
S: Severity
T: Timing.

Provocative/palliative

The practitioner needs to explore what brings on the symptom and what relieves it. In relation to all the key cardiac symptoms it is important to explore if a change in position, climate or temperature or the use of over-the-counter medication exacerbates or alleviates the symptom. Ask the patient if exercise exacerbates the problem and if resting relieves the pain.

Quality

The quality of the pain is assessed on the patient's description and by observing their non-verbal communication when they describe the pain. Patients experiencing or describing cardiac pain tend to clench their fist over the affected area or move their whole hand over the central chest area moving over to the left upper arm. It is always important to allow the patient to describe their pain using their own words, however, some patients have difficulty with this. McCaffery *et al.* (1994) suggest that the practitioner may need to use the following words to assist the patient in their description:

* sharp
* dull
* localized or does it spread over the chest
* tightness
* heavy
* burning
* gnawing pain
* stabbing.

Region/radiation

It is important to ascertain where exactly the pain is situated and if it radiates anywhere. Often cardiac pain radiates up into the jaw, down the left or both arms and across the upper shoulder. Again watch for the non-verbal clues presented by the patient.

Severity

A pain scale of 0–10 can be used, with 0 representing no pain and 10 the worst pain imaginable. It is also useful to explore if and by how much their activities of living are impeded by the symptom.

Timing

Useful information can be gained by exploring the timing of presentation. Key questions include:

* How long have you had it for?
* Is it constant, or does it come and go?
* How frequent is it?
* How long does the pain last for?
* Does it wake you up at night?
* When does it occur?

Table 11.3 Differential diagnoses

	Angina	Gastrointestinal	Musculoskeletal	Respiratory
Provocation	Exercise – especially if they walk up an incline or stairs Emotional upset Cold weather and wind After a heavy meal	Related to food consumption	Related to trauma, physical effort	Increases with inspiration or trunk movement
Palliation	Rest GTN	Antacids	Mild analgesics, heat and rest	Little relief
Quality	Tightness. Stops patients activity	Burning, discomfort, wind. Patient can carry on activity	Ache. Patient can carry on activity	Sharp, grabbing (pleurisy, pneumothorax or pulmonary embolism) or dull, aching as in pneumonia. Lower chest, sometimes bilateral
Region	Retrosternal	Epigastric/ retrosternal	Intercostal	Pneumothorax on entire side of the chest
Radiation	Arm, wrist, hand, jaw	Unlikely, though possibly through to the back	Backache	Pneumothorax radiates to the back
Severity	Moderate	Variable	Moderate, though variable	Moderate to severe
Timing	Often related to a trigger such as exercise	Vague onset, though may waken patient from sleep	Shortly after physical effort	Sudden onset and then continual pain

Reproduced with permission from Walsh *et al.* (1999)

Chest pain

Chest pain can present for a variety of reasons, hence the practitioner should always be aware of the potential for a differential diagnosis. The clinical history, examination and investigations are the key to diagnosis and it is vital that the practitioner remains vigilant to conditions like a dissecting aneursym, respiratory malignancy, tuberculosis, anxiety or injury. Table 11.3, using the PQRST format, outlines the key features that can give an indication to the origin of the chest pain. It should only be used as a guide because it is not always possible to neatly categorize where chest pain originates.

Breathlessness

Breathlessness due to impaired cardiac function, for example heart failure or atypical angina, is characterized by dyspnoea on exertion and orthopnoea (breathlessness when the patient is lying flat). There is evidence that orthopnoea is caused by the stimulation of the fine nerve endings in the lungs as a consequence of a rise in pulmonary capillary pressure which is caused by a redistribution of fluid between peripheral tissues and the lungs when the patient lies flat. Sometimes the patient will wake up in the night extremely breathless. This may be accompanied by a cough and the production of white frothy sputum, this is known as paroxysmal nocturnal dyspnoea. A differential diagnosis of pulmonary embolism, pulmonary oedema, lung diseases or severe anaemia should be considered and a full respiratory examination undertaken.

It is important to ask if the patient ever feels short of breath and when does this happen. Using the respirator scale, outlined in the COPD chapter (Chapter 8), can assist in determining how much the patient can do before they get breathless. Check for orthopnoea by asking about night time waking. Is the patient wakening up gasping for breath, necessitating sitting up or getting out of bed, or do they have a cough or wheeze at night? Check how many pillows are being used for sleeping, if the patient is using more than is normal for them you may want to suspect paroxysmal nocturnal dyspnoea.

Palpitations

Palpitations have been defined as an abnormal awareness of the heart beat. It may be that the heart rate is beating abnormally fast or is irregular in nature. It could also be that the impulse is stronger as a result of vasodilation. The key is to find out exactly what the patient means. Ask them to tap the beat with their fingers on a surface as this can help you to understand what is happening. It is also important to find out the frequency and severity of the episodes; are they a mild inconvenience or does the patient have to stop what he/she is doing and lie down? Ask if there is anything that can terminate the attack. Often patients who experience paroxysmal tachycardia take specific actions to stop the palpitations, such as valsalva manoeuvre or drinking ice cold water. Some patients will report that specific foods can precipitate the palpitations, like chocolate, tea, coffee or red wine, however, diet has not been conclusively proved to be an aggravating factor. Specific medications like decongestants which contain sympathomimetic drugs may also precipitate palpitations.

Syncope

This can be a very frightening experience for a patient, especially if they live alone. It may be that the history given by the patient is aug-

mented with information from a relative or friend. Key points to ascertain are whether the attack was sudden or if there was a warning and what were the circumstances or events around the time of the attack. Ask how long it took for the patient to recover and what colour the patient turned during the attack. Enquire whether any medication had been taken prior to the attack and recheck current medication.

Claudication

Intermittent claudication is an early sign of atherosclerotic changes in the arteries of the legs. The key question to ask is whether the patient experiences pain in the calf, thigh or buttock when exercising which eases on rest (Hope *et al.*, 1997).

Physical examination

General appearance

Prior to taking a history or undertaking a physical examination the health care professional must observe the patient's general condition and prioritize care. If the condition is not under control, an urgent medical opinion is required to prevent further distress. Observe the patient's colour, checking for central cyanosis especially around the lips and mucous membranes of the mouth. This could be a new problem and suggestive of poor gas exchange within the lungs and indicative of pulmonary oedema or other respiratory diseases. Central cyanosis could also be a sign of impaired cardiac function. In the less acute situation you may observe the face for signs of hypercholesterolaemia in the form of xanthelasma (yellow fatty deposits at the inner side of the eyelid) and corneal arcus (cholesterol deposits on the edge of the corneas) (Walsh *et al.*, 1999). Observe the hands for peripheral cyanosis, checking for colour and warmth, either on an introductory handshake or when taking the pulse. It is also an opportunity to look for nicotine stains and splinter haemorrhages. Respiratory function should be observed for signs of dyspnoea on exertion, watching carefully as the patient takes off outer clothing or moves around the consulting room.

Pulse and blood pressure

The radial pulse should be measured for a full minute and the rate and rhythm should be recorded. Tachycardia is defined as >100 and bradycardia is defined as <60 (Bickley, 1999). Any irregularities should be noted along with the force of the pulse. If the pulse is irregular or an abnormality is detected at the time of the consultation then it may be worth undertaking an ECG.

Blood pressure (BP) should be taken either with a sphygmomanometer or a digital analogue machine. It is vital if an electronic version is used that it is recognized as being reliable and is calibrated. Likewise, the sphygmomanometer should be in good working order, calibrated and the tubing should be of an appropriate length. The appropriate cuff size should be used ensuring that the bladder covers two thirds of the upper arm. The patient should be sitting down quietly for 3 minutes prior to taking the reading. It is important that the arm is well supported and straight and ensure that clothes do not constrict the top of the arm. The cuff should be level with the heart and the sphygmomanometer in a position level with the practitioner's eye so as not to distort the reading. The brachial pulse should be isolated and the cuff inflated 30 mmHg above where the pulse disappears. The stethoscope should then be placed over the brachial pulse site, taking care not to press too hard as this can distort the artery, producing false sounds. Ensure that the stethoscope does not touch any clothing or the rubber tubes of the cuff as it may cause friction sounds and therefore reduce the accuracy of the reading. The cuff should be deflated slowly at 2–3 mmHg and the blood pressure measurement should be recorded to the nearest 2 mmHg. The sounds heard with the stethoscope while taking the blood pressure are called Korotkov sounds. The systolic BP is measured at Korotkov phase I when the first clear tapping sounds which continue in repetition appear. The diastolic is recorded when the sounds disappear (phase V).

On the first visit the BP should be taken in both arms and recorded. If there is a difference the higher reading should be taken as the blood pressure reading. If the patient is anxious or agitated this should be noted. It is vital to record any cardiovascular medication that the patient may be taking. Two readings should be taken with a minute interval between readings. Blood pressure and pulse rate measurements are often carried out in haste, however, it cannot be stressed enough how important it is to undertake this essential skill with competency and with well-maintained and calibrated equipment.

Peripheral pulses

In a full cardiovascular assessment, all pulses should be checked. In the feet the dorsalis pedis and the posterior tibial pulses will be weak or absent in the presence of peripheral vascular disease. Check the toes for colour and warmth. If examination reveals poor pulses then popliteal and femoral pulses must be checked. There is the possibility of detecting popliteal or femoral aneurysms (Walsh *et al.*, 1999). If peripheral vascular disease is suspected then undertaking a Doppler assessment is vital to ascertain the severity of the condition. Ask the patient if they experience any pain in their calves when walking and if so how far do they have to walk before it comes on and for how long they have to rest before it is relieved.

Body mass index

Weight and height should be recorded and the body mass index (BMI) calculated.

BMI = weight (kg) divided by height (m^2).

A skilled practitioner will extend the clinical examination to include a full chest examination, measurement of the jugular venous pressure (JVP) and auscultation of heart sounds.

Heart sounds

The aim of auscultation is to detect abnormalities in the heart beat. The normal 'lub dub' sound represents the closure of the heart valves. The first heart sound (S1) is the tricuspid and bicuspid valves closing. The aortic and pulmonary valves open in silence but when they close at the end of systole, and the ventricles are beginning to fill with blood, the second heart sound (S2) can be heard. The third heart sound, usually faint, is due to the ventricles filling with blood under the effect of gravity. The

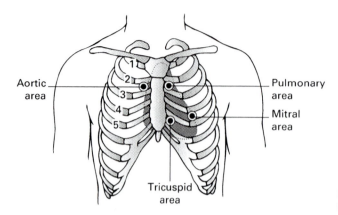

Figure 11.4 Sites for auscultation of heart sounds

emptying of the atria, expelling the last small amount of blood at the end of diastole may produce a faint fourth heart sound (S4). S3 and S4 may not be heard. Abnormal heart sounds, for example murmurs and clicks, may be due to a

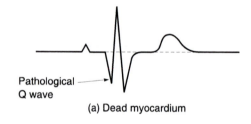

Pathological Q wave

(a) Dead myocardium

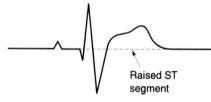

Raised ST segment

(b) Acutely damaged myocardium

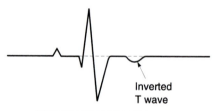

Inverted T wave

(c) Myocardial ischaemia
Note: There are a range of other causes for T wave inversion

Figure 11.5 Ischaemic ECG changes (reproduced with kind permission from Walsh *et al.*, 1999)

variety of causes (Figure 11.4). It is important to relate what is heard to the overall clinical history of the patient.

Investigations

Electrocardiogram (ECG)

The ECG will aid the diagnosis of heart disease by recording the rhythm and electrical activity of the heart. A resting ECG should always be undertaken, however, the results may be normal in those patients who present with a history of angina. Always use the ECG as an investigation to aid the diagnosis of heart disease in conjunction with a detailed examination and information gained from the clinical history. When a patient is suspected of having an acute myocardial infarction then an ECG will be recorded over a number of days to monitor the changes and measure the degree of myocardial damage. On day one following a myocardial infarction the Q wave will become more prominent and ST elevation will develop. By days 3–4 there will be T wave inversion. Angina may be detected if ST depression or T wave inversion is recorded. A resting ECG could indicate whether a patient has had a previous myocardial ischaemia. Figure 11.5 demonstrates the ischaemic ECG changes.

ECG is vital in identifying and diagnosing arrhythmias, however, it may be very difficult to catch on a single ECG recording and therefore 24-hour ambulatory ECG monitoring is utilized.

Exercise ECG is very helpful in diagnosing myocardial ischaemia. The patient is exercised, either by treadmill or exercise bike, following an agreed protocol and an objective assessment is made. The most common protocol used is the Bruce protocol whereby the angle and the speed of the treadmill or exercise bike is increased every 3 minutes. The ECG is observed for ST depression changes indicating myocardial ischaemia.

Other investigations

Coronary angiography is undertaken to investigate the functional ability of the valves, severity of atherosclerosis in the coronary arteries and the contractability and pressure within the heart. This procedure is usually reserved for patients for whom angioplasty or coronary artery bypass grafts (CABG) are being considered. An echocardiogram is used to identify the potential cause of the heart failure and detect valvular defects and ventricular dysfunction. Radionuclide tests, which include thallium/myoview scans, are also very useful in confirming a diagnosis of CHD, especially if the patient cannot undertake an exercise ECG. A chest X-ray is indicated in heart failure to detect cardiomegaly, pulmonary oedema or other causes of breathlessness.

Clinical biochemistry

The recommended investigations are outlined in Table 11.4.

Cardiovascular medications

It is imperative that reference is made to a current edition of the British National Formulary for up to date therapeutic recommendations, dosages, contra-indications and side effects.

Antiplatelet drugs

Antiplatelet drugs are used to reduce the risk of a further cardiac event in patients who have had a major cardiac event (APTC, 1994a). Aspirin has been shown to reduce the incidence of pulmonary embolism and venous thrombosis

Table 11.4 Clinical biochemistry key investigations*

	Investigation	Rationale
Stable angina	Haemoglobin (Hb). Plasma glucose. Total cholesterol and HDL cholesterol	Exclude anaemia and diabetes. Estimation of cardiovascular risk factor
Heart failure	Hb. Renal function	Exclude anaemia. Exclude renal/hepatic disease
Arrhythmias	Renal function. Urea and electrolytes. Thyroid function tests	Exclude thyroid disease. Monitor electrolyte balance
Hypertension	Creatinine. Urea and electrolytes. TC cholesterol and HDL cholesterol. Urinalysis for blood glucose and protein	Assess renal function. Estimation of cardiovascular risk factor
Diuretic therapy	Urea and electrolytes. Glucose	Monitor electrolyte balance and glucose control
Hyperlipidaemia	Full lipid profile. Liver function tests prior to starting statin therapy and then 1–3 months after starting treatment. Thereafter every 6 months to a year	Monitor lipid profile. Assess liver function prior to starting statins and monitor thereafter

* How frequent these investigations are undertaken will depend on local guidelines, previous results and the patient's overall health. Unless stated they are done on an annual basis.

in medical patients and in postoperative cardiac surgical patients (APTC, 1994b). The long-term use of aspirin in patients who have no history of vascular disease is not recommended. The daily recommended dose is 75–300 mg daily. Aspirin is contraindicated in the patient who has asthma, an active peptic ulcer, haemophilia or other bleeding disorders.

It should be noted that in the event of a patient presenting with unstable angina or an acute myocardial infarction, they should be given 300 mg to chew while waiting for medical assistance. The patient should be advised to take aspirin with or after food to reduce the risk of peptic ulceration or indigestion.

Other antiplatelet drugs include clopidogrel, ticlopidine, dipyridamole. There are others that can be used in specific circumstances.

Anticoagulants

This group of drugs includes warfarin and heparin. Warfarin therapy has been proven to reduce the risk of a further cardiovascular or cerebral event (Smith *et al.*, 1990; EAFT, 1993). Its use is indicated in patients who have had mechanical valve replacement, a deep venous thrombosis, pulmonary embolism or have atrial fibrillation. Warfarin is preferred over aspirin post-MI if there have been complications like heart failure, left ventricular thrombus or atrial fibrillation (Cairn *et al.*, 1998). It is vital that the patient's international normalized ratio (INR) is monitored. The patient should seek advice from a pharmacist prior to taking any over the counter medication.

Warfarin should be taken at the same time each day. The patient should be warned that they will bruise easily and if cut they will bleed for longer than usual. Alcohol is permitted but it should be in moderation. A diet rich in vitamin K should be avoided, for example broccoli, spinach and cod liver oil. The main side effect to be aware of is haemorrhaging.

Nitrates

These include glyceryl trinitrate (GTN) (tablets, sprays and patches), isosorbide mononitrate and isosorbide dinitrate and they are indicated in patients who have angina. Nitrates work by dilating the coronary arteries, increasing the blood flow to the myocardium. By increasing blood perfusion to the heart muscle myocardial ischaemia is relieved. Nitrates cause blood vessels to dilate throughout the body and this reduces venous return to the heart and filling pressure in the heart (preload) is reduced. The dilation of the arteriolar vessels causes a drop in resistance and therefore afterload pressure in the heart is reduced. This all leads to an over-all reduction in myocardial oxygen demand. The main side effects include flushing, pounding headache, postural hypotension, dizziness and nausea.

It is imperative that patients know how to use GTN tablets or spray appropriately because, all too often, they have received inadequate education to enable them to benefit fully from the drug.

The following advice should be given to patients taking GTN tablets or spray:

> GTN tablets or spray are used to relieve pain in an angina attack. It can also be taken before doing anything that is known to cause angina. The tablet or spray should be placed under the tongue and allowed to dissolve. No fluid should be taken with the GTN tablet or spray. If the mouth is dry, take a glass of water prior to taking the GTN tablet to moisten the mouth. It is important that the patient sits down when taking the medication but if that is not possible they should lean against a wall. Patients who experience headaches with GTN use should be advised that they can remove the tablet, if it has not totally dissolved, once the chest pain has gone.

GTN tablets or spray takes 2–3 minutes to take effect and lasts for approximately 30 minutes. Assessing angina control can be aided by asking the following questions:

- How frequent are the angina attacks?
- Does less effort bring them on?
- How severe are the attacks?
- How effective is the medication?
- How much medication is needed to relieve the angina?

Medication should be stored in the original container and carried with the patient at all times. The spray needs to be replaced every 2 years and the tablets 8 weeks after the bottle has been opened. GTN tablets or spray can be purchased from a pharmacist without a doctor's prescription.

When angina starts the patient should initiate the following steps:

- Use GTN tablets or spray and rest for 5 minutes
- If the pain is still present take a further dose of GTN tablets or spray and rest for a further 5 minutes
- If the pain continues take another GTN tablet or spray. If the pain is still present 15 minutes from onset seek medical assistance immediately – call emergency services.

If the pain is more severe than normal and is accompanied by sweating, nausea and/or shortness of breath the patient should ring emergency servies. They should be advised to take GTN tablets or spray while waiting for the ambulance along with chewing aspirin 300 mg (unless contraindicated).

Long-acting nitrates (isosorbide mononitrate and isosorbide dinitrate) can be used as part of the patient's regular anti-anginal therapy. However, it is important to note that patients on long-acting nitrates can develop tolerance, which will reduce the therapeutic effects of the nitrates. A regimen that gives a nitrate-free period for 6–8 h avoids the risk of tolerance. For example, 0800 h and 1400 h for isosorbide mononitrate and 0800 h, 1400 h and 1800 h for isosorbide dinitrate (BNF, 2000).

Beta-blockers

These include atenolol, propanolol, bisoprolol, acebutolol, betaxolol, metoprolol, carvedilol, celiprolol, labetolol, nadolol, oxprenolol, pindolol, sotal and timolol. The mode of action is to reduce the effect of adrenaline on the heart. Beta-blockers are used in the medical management of patients with angina, post-MI, hypertension and arrhythmias. They have been proven to reduce mortality rate in post-MI patients (Yusaf *et al.*, 1985). It has also been reported that their use can reduce mortality in patients with mild to moderate heart failure (Lockhart *et al.*, 2000). Beta-blockers are contraindicated in patients with asthma, COPD and severe heart failure. The value of beta-blockers to diabetic patients has been proven (Kendall *et al.*, 1995), however, they should be used with caution in this group of patients as they mask the symptoms of hypoglycaemia. The side effects of beta-blockers include lethargy, nausea, diarrhoea, skin rashes, sexual dysfunction, nightmares, cold hands and feet and dyspnoea.

Angiotensin-converting enzyme inhibitors (ACE-inhibitors)

These include captopril, enalapril and lisinopril. The use of these drugs post-MI has been shown to reduce the incidence of both heart failure and mortality (HOPE, 2000). They are also effective in the management of heart failure and hypertension.

Renin is produced by the kidneys in response to changes in blood pressure. It reacts in the circulation and becomes angiotensin which, in turn, is converted into angiotensin II by the angiotensin-converting enzyme (ACE). Angiotensin II is a powerful chemical causing vasoconstriction thereby increasing blood pressure and is also involved in fluid retention. ACE inhibitors work by blocking the production of the angiotensin-converting enzyme (ACE) thereby preventing the conversion of angiotensin I to angiotensin II. When the patient is commenced on this drug they should be monitored very carefully. ACE inhibitors are sometimes combined with diuretics and digoxin in heart failure (BNF, 2000). It is important to monitor renal function and urea and electrolytes. The side effects of ACE inhibitors include postural hypotension and persistent dry cough.

Angiotensin II receptor antagonists

These have similar properties to ACE inhibitors. However they do not inhibit the breakdown of bradykinin and other kinins. This appears to prevent the persistent dry cough associated with ACE inhibitors.

Calcium antagonists (otherwise known as calcium-channel blockers)

These drugs act by interfering with the inward movement of calcium ions through the cell membranes. There are three types of calcium antagonists:

Type 1 (phenylalkylamines) – act mainly on the conducting pathways of the heart reducing the heart rate, an example is verapamil.

Type 2 (dihydropyridines) – work mostly on the atrial smooth muscle and therefore relieve angina and blood pressure, an example is nifedipine.

Type 3 (benzothiazepines) – a combination of both of the above, an example is diltiazem.

Calcium antagonists are recommended for the management of angina and hypertension (Fox *et al.*, 1996; Heidenreich *et al.*, 1999). The side effects include flushing, headaches, dizziness, faintness, swelling of the ankles and gastrointestinal disturbances. *Note*, grapefruit juice increases the plasma concentrations of dihydropyridine calcium antagonists (with the exception of amlodipine) and verapamil (BNF, 2000).

Potassium-channel activators

These are indicated in the patients with angina and nicorandil is currently the only potassium-channel activator available. It works by opening up the potassium channels across the cell membranes allowing potassium ions to pass freely and relax the muscles. It works in an opposite way to calcium channel antagonists. Side effects include initial headache, flushing, indigestion or dizziness.

Diuretics

This class of drug includes thiazides, loop diuretics and potassium sparing diuretics. Their use is indicated in hypertension and heart failure. Thiazides, which include bendrofluazide and chlorthalidone, work by inhibiting the reabsorption of sodium at the beginning of the distal convoluted renal tubule. Thiazides can cause impotence, which should resolve when the drug is stopped. Loop diuretics, which include frusemide and bumetanide, work in a similar way to thiazides but at the ascending limb of the loop of Henlé and they tend to be more potent. Both these drugs work within 1 to 2 h of oral administration. They both have an extensive range of side effects, which include electrolyte, metabolic and gastrointestinal disturbances. Hypokalaemia can be a problem and the options include either taking a potassium

supplement or using a potassium sparing diuretic like spirolactone or amiloride.

Cardiac glycosides

Digoxin is indicated in heart failure and supraventricular fibrillaton, especially atrial fibrillation. It works by increasing the force of the myocardial contraction and reduces the conductivity in the atrioventricular node (BNF, 2000). The patient should be monitored for digoxin toxicity, particularly in the elderly. Digoxin plasma concentration monitoring should take place at least 6 h after the patient has taken the dose. The side effects of toxicity include nausea, vomiting, loss of appetite and heart rate abnormalities.

Lipid lowering drugs

Statins

Statin therapy has been proven to reduce morbidity and mortality rates from CHD (Scandinavian Simvastatin Survival Study Group, 1994). Their use is indicated in hyperlipidaemia and they include atorvastatin, simvastatin, fluvastatin and pravastatin.

Statins work in the liver and inhibit the enzyme 3-hydroxy-3-methlglutaryl coenzyme (HMG-CoA), which prevents acetyl CoA being converted into cholesterol. This leads to a decrease in cholesterol production, increased numbers of chemical receptors on the surface of liver cells and increase in LDL clearance. Triglycerides are also lowered and HDL raised.

Liver functions tests should be carried out prior to commencing a statin and repeated within 1–3 months and thereafter every 6–12 months. Side effects include altered liver function tests, myositis, rash and sometimes nausea and vomiting or altered bowel function. It is also important to monitor for muscle side effects like myalgia and myopathy.

Other lipid lowering drugs

Fibrates
These include ciprofibrate, fenofibrate, gemifibrozil and bezafibrate. Their main action is in reducing raised triglyceride levels in the blood. They also reduce LDL cholesterol and raise

HDL cholesterol. Side effects include gastro-intestinal disturbances and pruritus.

Management

The management of the patient with CHD will be dependent on the severity of the disease. Treatment options include medical management and/or surgical intervention. This could be percutaneous transluminal coronary angioplasty (PTCA), intracoronary stents and/or surgical revascularization (coronary artery bypass graft surgery). Irrespective of which option is chosen, the management of CHD risk factors has to continue, to reduce the risk of a further cardiac event.

It is essential to establish a good working partnership with the patient, their family and carers. Making any change can be difficult and the patient may feel uncomfortable and anxious. It is important to stress that feelings of fear and anxiety are normal and you need to offer reassurance and support. The key to making changes that are sustainable is to be consistent in the information that is given to the patient by all the professionals in the team. There are numerous frameworks available to assist professionals to be structured in their approach to change management. The key is to *elicit* the patient's thoughts, beliefs and readiness to change. The professional then needs to *explain* the reason why the change is important, demonstrating why a particular lifestyle choice has a negative impact on the person's health. This is followed by *negotiating* a plan of action and agreeing goals. Vital to the success is the *support* offered to the patient (Scholfield, 1996). This process of change is ongoing and professionals must be prepared to return to the same issues on numerous occasions. The key is not to become disillusioned but remain motivated in assisting the patient to make positive changes, no matter how small they may be.

The cycle of change outlined by Prochaska and DiClemente (1986) is a useful tool to help professionals focus on where patients are in the willingness to change (Figure 11.6).

Smoking

Smoking cessation has been covered within Chapter 8.

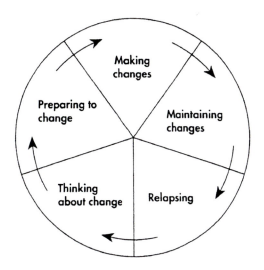

Figure 11.6 Cycle of change (adapted from Prochaska and DiClemente, 1986)

Diet

Current recommendations advocate a Mediterranean diet, low in saturated fat and rich in fresh fruit, vegetables, fibre and fish (especially oily fish) (De Lorgeril *et al.*, 1999). A low fat diet reduces the incidence of CHD (NHS Centre for Review and Dissemination, 1998a). The key is to explore with the patient different ways in which their diet can be adapted to incorporate these recommendations. Food should be enjoyable and if it becomes a chore then the person's quality of life can be affected and they are less likely to maintain the dietary changes over a sustainable period. Initial assessment of eating patterns can be aided by the patient keeping a food diary, which can be used to highlight areas where their diet can be improved. If the patient cannot reduce their cholesterol to <5 mmol/l (LDL3 mmol/l) or by 30%, whichever is the greater, then pharmaceutical intervention may be considered.

Diabetes

Type 2 men have a two to fourfold greater annual risk of CHD (British Heart Foundation, 2000a). The effective management of diabetes is covered in Chapter 6. It is vital that all the risk factors outlined in this chapter are addressed with patients who have diabetes.

Exercise

Patients should be encouraged to take a moderate amount of exercise, at least three times a week for 20 minutes and optimal of 5 times a week for 30 minutes. If the patient has undergone a cardiac rehabilitation programme then they will have gained confidence in their ability to exercise within sensible parameters without compromising their health. They should still be able to hold a conversation and never be in a situation where they are too breathless to talk.

Health professionals should liaise with local cardiac rehabilitation teams to ensure that a consistent approach is adopted when advising patients of exercise regimens. Exercise is contraindicated if the patient has certain conditions. These include:

- an uncontrolled cardiac condition
- uncontrolled diabetes
- the existence of any acute systemic disease
- a recent embolism or deep vein thrombosis
- recent episode of thrombophlebitis
- the existence of any acute systemic disease.

Blood pressure

Hypertension is defined as a systolic pressure >140 mmHg and diastolic >90 mmHg. The target for blood pressure (BP) control is for a systolic pressure of <140 mmHg and a diastolic of <85 mmHg. If the patient has diabetes then the target is for systolic <40 mmHg and diastolic <80 mmHg (Wood *et al.*, 1998; Ramsay *et al.*, 1999). All patients should have their risk factors assessed and be offered lifestyle advice.

If the diastolic BP is >100 mmHg and/or the systolic is >200, unless an emergency, then this should be confirmed over 1–2 weeks and treatment should be considered.

If the diastolic BP is >100 mmHg and/or the systolic is >160 then this should be confirmed over 3–4 weeks. If there are other cardiovascular complications then treatment should be considered. If there are no other complications then it should be confirmed over 4–12 weeks and treatment considered.

If the systolic BP is between 140 and 159 mmHg and/or the diastolic BP is between 85 and 99 mmHg and the patient has diabetes, cardiovascular complications or target organ damage then treatment should be considered.

If these are absent then the BP should be monitored yearly along with all other modifiable risk factors (Ramsay *et al.*, 1999).

Secondary causes of hypertension should be investigated. These include renal disease, primary hypothyroidism or drug induced (for example corticosteroids).

Alcohol

Current recommendations for alcohol consumption are 3–4 units per day for men and 2–3 units per day for women (DoH, 2000). A useful screening tool to use when you suspect that a patient's alcohol intake may be high is the CAGE guide (Mayfield *et al.*, 1974, as cited in Bickley, 1999). The series of questions should explore the following themes:

- Cutdown: does the patient ever feel the need to cut down?
- Annoyed: do they ever get annoyed if their drinking habits are criticized or questioned?
- Guilty: do they ever feel guilty about their drinking habits?
- Eye-opener: do they ever feel the need for a drink first thing in the morning?

The key is to work with the patient and refer to the appropriate professional if there is a serious problem with alcohol consumption.

Stress

Effective stress management could reduce the rate of MI or premature death from CHD. However, research studies have been small and the results were not consistent. This leads to an element of uncertainty and the call for more rigorous research trials to be undertaken (BMJ, 2000).

Relaxation techniques are an integral part of cardiac rehabilitation and assist the patient to reduce anxiety levels and gain confidence in dealing with events that can trigger anxiety. Many forms of physical activity, for example yoga, walking and swimming can be very effective at reducing stress levels. The use of relaxation tapes and breathing exercises should be encouraged. It may be appropriate to refer the patient, family member or carer to a stress counsellor if the patient needs more support.

Cardiac rehabilitation

Cardiac rehabilitation reduces the risk of another major cardiac event (Oldridge *et al.*, 1988; O'Connor *et al.*, 1989).

Cardiac rehabilitation is defined by the WHO (1993) as:

the sum of activities required to influence favourably the underlying cause of the disease, as well as the best possible physical, mental and social conditions, so that they (people) may, by their own efforts preserve or resume when lost, as normal a place as possible in the community. Rehabilitation cannot be regarded as an isolated form or stage of therapy but must be integrated within secondary prevention services of which it forms only one facet.

The key components of a cardiac rehabilitation include secondary prevention, a programme of exercise, relaxation and stress management, education and support to make the psychological and social adjustments following a significant cardiac event (NHS Centre for Review and Dissemination, 1998b). Identifying the psychological needs of the patient, family and carers is vital. Failure to recognize and acknowledge problems in this area could impede a patient's physical recovery. The key is to adopt a patient-centred approach, holistically assessing the social, cultural, physical psychological and vocational needs to ensure that optimum health is achieved. This cardiac rehabilitation process should start as soon as the patient is diagnosed with CHD or as soon as possible after an acute cardiac event (WHO, 1993).

The success of a cardiac rehabilitation programme is the ability of primary and secondary services to work in collaboration to meet the needs of the patient. Health professionals need to look at innovative ways of working together across professional boundaries and develop clear communication pathways to enhance the sharing of information. Brannen (2000) demonstrates the vital role that cardiac liaison nurses have in bridging the gap between primary and secondary care. This was achieved by introducing an educational programme to promote the effective use of The Heart Manual (Lewin *et al.*, 1992). Integrated care is discussed in more detail in Chapter 2.

The British Association of Cardiac Rehabilitation (BACR) (Coates *et al.*, 1995) outline four phases of cardiac rehabilitation.

Phase one – inpatient stay

This should start as soon as someone is admitted to hospital (DoH, 2000). Individualized management plans should be written to meet the identified needs of the patient, family and carer.

Phase two – immediate post-discharge

Assessment of risk is further explored and strategies are put in place to assist the patient to make the lifestyle changes that will reduce their cardiac risk. Continuing support and education are vital from the health care team. The patient and family should be encouraged to become involved in local support groups.

Phase three – intermediate post-discharge

The outpatient rehabilitation programme continues the work in phase two but incorporates a structured exercise programme. Ongoing advice is given on health promotion, psychological problems, lifestyle modification and vocational issues.

Phase four – long-term maintenance

The primary health care team (PHCT) continues the long-term follow up of patients within a structured approach to secondary prevention of CHD. Ongoing health and social issues should be managed by the PHCT with referral to a specialist for further medical management, psychological help or assistance with lifestyle. Certain factors can increase the risk of a poor outcome from cardiac rehabilitation (Noy, 1998), these include:

- history of anxiety or depression
- a low educational level
- environment of social and economic deprivation
- isolated within the community
- poor support.

Each patient is an individual and therefore the health care team need to be sensitive to each query as it arises. Several key areas need special attention in relation to advice given post-MI and CABG.

Driving

Patients should be advised not to drive for at least 4 weeks after a myocardial infarction, coronary artery bypass grafting or after an episode of unstable angina. Following PTCA, driving should be avoided for one week. Generally the Driver and Vehicle Licensing Centre (DVLA) do not need to be informed for an ordinary licence but the patient's insurance company should be advised. Holders of Heavy Goods Vehicle (HGV) licences must inform the DVLA and to continue to hold their licence they will have to prove they can undertake exercise for 9 minutes of a full Bruce protocol from 1 month onwards post-MI. This has to be undertaken free of anti-anginal medication for 48 h prior to the test (Lockhart *et al.*, 2000). Driving should be avoided in any condition like arrhythmias, systemic embolism, dizziness or episodes of syncope. Once arrhythmias are under control and stable for 4 weeks then driving can be resumed.

If a pacemaker has been inserted, driving should be avoided for 1 week and the DVLA should be notified. If the patient has an implantable cardioverter defibrillator then the DVLA have to be informed and driving may be permitted after 6 months. It is recommended that the patient avoids driving if they have any uncontrolled symptom which is compromising their cardiovascular system (British Heart Foundation, 2000b).

Advice of when to return to work

Patients whose recovery following a MI has been uneventful can return to work within 6 weeks as a rough guide, if the job is non-manual. However, if it is manual then a 12-week period off work is recommended. Following CABG, it is generally recommended to have 8 weeks off for a non-manual job and at least 12 weeks for a manual job. This will allow the healing process to be completed.

Advice on when to resume sex

As a guide if the patient can briskly climb up and down two flights of stairs without having anginal symptoms or being unduly out of breath, then they can have sex without compromising their health. It is best to avoid sex for at least 2 h after a heavy meal or after a hot bath. Ensure the room is warm. If sexual intercourse does bring on angina then the patient could try using their GTN tablet or spray prior to the intercourse to prevent the attack. Following CABG it may be advisable, initially, to avoid positions that put undue pressure on the sternal wound.

Travel advice

Patients should always inform their insurance company of any cardiac condition and should not be afraid to shop around for the best price. It is recommended that following an MI the patient should wait 2–3 weeks. If, however, it is a long haul flight then they should wait 3–6 months. It is always advisable to contact the airline directly for guidance.

Structured care

To be able to achieve the National Service Framework standards, outlined in Table 11.5 (DoH, 2000), it is essential that a systematic approach to care is adopted, which utilizes the skills of the whole multidisciplinary team. Adopting an integrated approach can enhance the quality of the care provided to the patient. Nurse-led clinics have been proven to be effective in managing CHD and improving the patient's quality of life (Imperial Cancer Research Fund OXCHECK Study Group, 1995; Fullard, 1998).

All professionals need to feel confident and competent to provide education, advice and care to patients with CHD. Evidence-based practice should incorporate a system of audit and review which will inform practice and facilitate the continuing development of the service based on information retrieved through feedback and evaluations. These are outlined in detail within the chapter on clinical governance.

Table 11.5 The National Service Framework for Coronary Heart Disease (DoH, 2000).
12 Service Standards

Reducing heart disease in the population

1   The NHS and partner agencies should develop, implement and monitor policies that reduce the prevalence of coronary risk factors in the population, and reduce inequalities in risks of developing heart disease

2   The NHS and partner agencies should contribute to a reduction in the prevalence of smoking in the local population

Preventing CHD in high-risk patients

3   General practitioners and primary care teams should identify all people with established cardiovascular disease and offer them comprehensive advice and appropriate treatment to reduce their risks

4   General practitioners and primary healthcare teams should identify all people at significant risk of cardiovascular disease but who have not developed symptoms and offer them advice and treatment to reduce their risks

Heart attack and other acute coronary syndromes

5   People with symptoms of a possible heart attack should receive help from an individual equipped with and appropriately trained in the use of a defibrillator within eight minutes of calling for help, to maximize the benefits of resuscitation should it be necessary

6   People thought to be suffering from a heart attack should be assessed professionally and, if indicated receive aspirin. Thrombolysis should be given within 60 minutes of calling for professional help

7   NHS trusts should put in place agreed protocols/systems of care so that people admitted to hospital with proven heart attacks are appropriately assessed and offered treatments of proven clinical and cost effectiveness to reduce their risk of disability and death

Stable angina

8   People with symptoms of angina or suspected angina should receive appropriate investigation and treatment to relieve their pain and reduce their risk of coronary events

Revascularization

9   People with angina that is increasing in frequency or severity should be referred to a cardiologist urgently or, for those at greatest risk, as an emergency

10   NHS trusts should put in place hospital-wide systems of care so that patients with suspected or confirmed coronary heart disease receive timely and appropriate investigation and treatment to relieve their symptoms and reduce their risk of subsequent coronary events

Heart failure

11   Doctors should arrange for people with suspected heart failure to be offered appropriate investigations that will confirm or refute the diagnosis. For those in whom heart failure is confirmed, its cause should be identified – treatments most likely to both relieve their symptoms and reduce their risk of death should be offered

12   NHS trusts should put in place agreed protocols/systems of care so that, prior to leaving hospital, people admitted to hospital suffering form coronary heart disease have been invited to participate in a multidisciplinary programme of secondary prevention and cardiac rehabilitation/The aim of the programme will be to reduce their risk of subsequent cardiac problems and to promote their return to a full and normal life

An example of a way in which to achieve some of the goals of the NSF is provided by The Primary Care Team, The Medical Centre, Shipston-on-Stour, Warwickshire. The team devised a protocol which demonstrates a comprehensive approach meeting standards 3 and 4 of the NSF (DoH, 2000). It is advocated that care should be shared between the patient's doctor and a nurse-run clinic. The indications for recall, home visiting and referral are all meticulously outlined within the protocol. Table 11.6 summarizes the stages of the protocol.

Conclusion

The impact of a diagnosis of CHD can have a devastating effect on an individual, their family and carers. Health care professionals have a responsibility to improve the quality of life of patients in their care. This means not only addressing the clinical management of CHD, but being sensitive to the psychological, social and spiritual needs of the patient. Every patient is unique, with different perceptions about the nature of CHD and what it will mean to them and their families. A holistic approach to care that identifies and recognizes the patient's needs will enhance the relationship between the health care practitioner and the patient.

The ultimate aim of care should be to improve the quality and parity of health and social service provision throughout the country irrespective of age, gender, race, culture, religion, disability or sexual orientation (DoH, 1997).

Useful addresses

For England and Wales

British Heart Foundation
14 Fizhardinge Street
London
W1H 4DH
Tel: 44 (0) 208 987 9419;
Fax: 44 (0) 208 486 1273

Family Heart Association
7 North Road
Maidenhead
SL6 1PL
Tel: 44 (0) 1628 628638

For Scotland

British Heart Foundation
4 Shoe Place
Edinburgh
EH6 6UU
Tel: 44 (0) 131 555 5891; Fax: 44 (0) 131 225 3258

Table 11.6 Summary of the stages of the protocol for the structured approach of CHD prevention and management (DoH, 2000)

Stage 1	*Priority 1*: the identification of patients with established CHD and the development of a disease register *Priority 2*: the identification of high-risk patients with diabetes or hypertension. If their risk was >30% then they would be managed in the same way as secondary prevention patients *Priority 3*: opportunistic screening of the rest of the practice population identifying and recording modifiable and non-modifiable risk factors
Stage 2	Assessment of all patients in priority 1 and 2 and those with a family history of CHD. All modifiable risk factors should be identified and managed appropriately
Stage 3	Assessment of cardiovascular risk in primary prevention patients
Stage 4	Lifestyle advice to all patients
Stage 5	Management of risk factors

It is recommended that the full protocol is referred to for detailed information.

References

Antiplatelet Trialist Collaboration (APTC) (1994a) Collaborative overview of randomised trails of antiplatelet therapy – I: Prevention of death, myocardial infarction, and stroke by prolonged antiplatelet therapy in various categories. *British Medical Journal* **308**, 81–106

Antiplatelet Trialist Collaboration (APTC) (1994b) Collaborative overview of randomised trails of antiplatelet therapy – II: Maintenance of vascular graft or arterial patency by antiplatelet therapy. *British Medical Journal* **308**, 159–168

Armstrong G E (1997) Lifestyle management: exercise. In: (Lindsay G M, Gaw A, eds) (1997). *Coronary Heart Disease: A Handbook for the Health Care Team.* Churchill Livingstone, Edinburgh

Bickley L (1999) *Bate's Guide to Physical Examination and History Taking*, 7th edn. J B Lippincott & Co, Philadelphia

BMJ (2000) Issue 3. *British Medical Journal* Publishing Group, London

Boon N A, Fox K A A, Bloomfield P (1999) Diseases of the cardiovascular system. In: (Haslett C, Chilvers R, Hunter J A A, Boon N A, eds) *Davidson's Principles and Practice of Medicine*, 18th edn. Churchill Livingstone, Edinburgh

Brannen J (2000) Cardiac rehabilitation: getting it right. *Primary Health Care* **10** (7), 25–28

British Heart Foundation (2000a) *Coronary Heart Disease Statistics*. BHF, London

British Heart Foundation (2000b) *Fact file: Driving and the Heart*. BHF, London

British National Formulary (2000) British Medical Association/Royal Pharmaceutical Society of Great Britain, London

Cairn J A, Theroux P, Lewis H D *et al.* (1998) Antithrombotic agents in coronary heart disease. *Chest* **114**, 611S–633S

Coates A, Mcgee H, Stokes H, Thompson D (1995) *BACR Guidelines for Cardiac Rehabilitation*. Blackwell Science, Oxford

Dawber T R, Meadows G F, Moore F E (1951) Epidemiological approaches to heart disease; the Framington Study. *American Journal of Public Health* **41**, 279–286

De Lorgeril M, Salen P, Martin J *et al.* (1999) Mediterranean diet, traditional risk factors, and the rate of cardiovascular complications after myocardial infarctions. Final report of the Lyon Diet Heart Study. *Circulation* **99,** 779–785

Department of Health (1996) *Strategy Statement of Physical Activity*, London, as cited in British Heart Foundation (2000a)

Department of Health (1997) *The New NHS: Modern, Dependable*. HMSO, London

Department of Health (1998) *Smoking Kills*: White paper on Tobacco. HMSO, London

Department of Health (1999) *Saving Lives: Our Healthier Nation*. HMSO, London

Department of Health (2000) *National Service Framework for Coronary Heart Disease: Modern Standards and Service Models*. HMSO, London

European Atrial Fibrillation Trial (EAFT) (1993) Study Group. Secondary prevention in non-rheumatic atrial fibrillation after transient ischaemic attack. *Lancet* **342**, 1255–1262

Fox K L, Mulcahy D, Findlay I *et al.* on behalf of the TIBET study Group (The Total Ischaemic Burden European Trial (TIBET) (1996) Effects of atenolol, nifedipine SR and their combination on the exercise test and the total ischaemic burden in 608 patients with stable angina. *European Heart Journal* **17**, 96–103

Fullard E M (1998) Organisation of secondary prevention of coronary heart disease in primary care: the nurse' perspective. *Coronary Health Care* **2**, 193–201

Heidenreich P A, MacDonald K M, Hasttie T *et al.* (1999) Meta-analysis of trials comparing beta-blockers, calcium antagonists and nitrates in stable angina. *Journal of the American Medical Association* **281**, 1927–1936

HOPE, The Heart Outcomes Prevention Evaluation Investigators (2000) Effects of an angiotensin-converting enzyme inhibitor, ramipril, on cardiovascular events in high-risk patients. *New England Journal Medicine* **342**, 1445–1453

Hope R A, Longmore J M, Hodgetts T J, Ramrakha P A (1997) *Oxford Handbook of Clinical Medicine*, 3rd edn. Oxford University Press, Oxford

Imperial Cancer Research Fund OXCHECK Study Group (1995) Effectiveness of health checks conducted by nurses in primary care: final results of the OXCHECK study. *British Medical Journal* **310**, 1099–1104

Kendall, *et al.* (1995) Cited in: (Lockhart L, McMeeken K, Mark J, Cross S, Tait G, Isles C, eds) (2000) Secondary prevention after myocardial infaction: reducing the risk of further cardiovascular events. *Coronary Health Care* **4,** 82–92

Lewin B, Robertson I H, Cay E L, Irving J B, Campbell M (1992) Effects of self help post myocardial infaction rehabilitation on psychological adjustment and use of health services. *Lancet* **329**, 1036–1040

Lindsay G M (1997) Risk factor assessment. In: (Lindsay G M, Gaw A, eds) *Coronary Heart Disease: A Handbook for the Health Care Team*. Churchill Livingstone, Edinburgh

Lockhart L, McMeeken K, Mark J, Cross S, Tait G, Isles C (2000) Secondary prevention after myocardial infaction: reducing the risk of further cardiovascular events. *Coronary Health Care* **4**, 82–92

Lorimer R A (1997) Coronary heart disease: pathology, epidemiology and diagnosis. In: (Lindsay G M, Gaw A, eds) *Coronary Heart Disease: A Handbook for the Health Care Team*. Churchill Livingstone, Edinburgh

McCaffery M, Beebe A, Latham J (eds) (1994) *Pain Clinical Manual for Nursing Practice*. Mosby, London

Mayfield, D, McLead, G, Hall P (1974) The CAGE questionnaire. *American Journal of Psychiatry* **131**, 1121

Morton P G (1993) *Health Assessment in Nursing*, 2nd edn. FA Davis, Philadelphia

NHS Centre for Review and Dissemination (1998a) Cholesterol and coronary heart disease: screening and treatment. *Effective Health Care Bulletin* **4** (1), 1–15

NHS Centre for Review and Dissemination (1998b) Cardiac Rehabilitation. *Effective Health Care Bulletin* **4** (4), 1–11

Noy, K (1998) Cardiac rehabilitation: structure, effectiveness and the future. *British Journal of Nursing* **7** (17), 1033–1040

O'Connor G T, Buring G E,Yusuf S *et al.* (1989) An overview of randomised trails of rehabilitation with exercise after myocardial infarction. *Circulation* **80**, 234–244

Oldridge N B, Guyatt G H, Fisher M E, Rimm A A (1988) Cardiac rehabilitation after myocardial infarction: combined experience of randomised clinical trials. *Journal of the American Medical Association* **260**, 945–50

Oparil S (1996) Cardiovascular risk reduction in women. *Journal of Women's Health* **5** (1), 23–32

Prochaska J O, DiClemente C C (1986) Towards a comprehensive model of change. In: (Miller W R, Heather N, eds)

Treating Addictive Behaviour: Processes of Change. Plenum Press

Ramsay L E, Williams B, Johnstone G D *et al.* (1999) British Hypertension Society guidelines for hypertension management 1999: summary. *British Medical Journal* **319**, 30–35

Sacks F, Pfeffer M A, Moye L A *et al.* (1996) The effect of pravastatin on coronary events after myocardial infarction in patients with average cholesterol levels. *New England Journal of Medicine* **335**, 1001–1009

Scandinavian Simvastatin Survival Study Group (1994) Randomised trial of cholesterol lowering in 4444 patients with coronary heart disease: the Scandinavian Simvastatin Survival Study (4S). *Lancet* **344**, 1383–1389

Scholfield T (1996) Individual interventions and behaviours. In: (Lawrence M, Neil A, Fowler G, eds) *Prevention of Cardiovascular Disease: an Evidence-based Approach*. Oxford University Press, Oxford

Smith P, Arnesen H, Holme I (1990) The effect of warfarin on mortality and reinfarction after myocardial infarction. *New England Journal of Medicine* **333**, 1301–1307

Tortora G, Grabowski S (2000) *Principles of Anatomy and Physiology*, 9th edn. Addison Wesley

Tunstall-Pedoe H, Kuulasmaa K, Mahonen H, Ruokokoski E, Amouyel P (1999) Contribution of trends in survival and coronary event rates to change in coronary heart disease mortality: 10 year results from 37 MONICA Project populations. *Lancet* **353**, 1547–1557

US Department of Health and Human Services (1990) *The Health Benefits of Smoking Cessation: a report of the surgeon general*. US DHSS, Maryland

Walsh M, Crumbie A, Reveley S (1999) *Nurse Practitioners: Clinical Skills and Professional Issues*. Butterworth-Heinemann, Oxford

Wild S, McKeigue P (1997) Cross sectional analysis of mortality by country of birth in England and Wales, 1970–92. *British Medical Journal* **314**, 705–710

Wood D, Durrington P, Poulter N *et al.* (1998) on behalf of the Societies. Joint British recommendations on prevention of coronary heart disease in clinical practice. *Heart* **80** (suppl. 2), S1–S29

Yusaf S, *et al.* (1985) Beta blockade during and after myocardial infarction: an overview of the randomised trials. *Progress in Cardiovascular Disease*. **27**, 335

Chapter

12

Thyroid disease

Una Hake and Barbara Maudsley

Patient's perspective

Initially I was so afraid of what my symptoms could be and I feared the worst. I just felt so awful and out of control. Finding out that I had an overactive thyroid gland came as a great relief but I expected to feel well again very quickly. This did not happen and during those long months off work I became depressed and worried that I would never be completely well again. The other aspect that kept me awake at night was anxiety about my eyesight. I couldn't get rid of the nagging, maybe irrational fear, that I would go blind. On reflection it seems impossible for an educated man to have these ideas, but that's what really happened.

After some months of treatment I was beginning to feel much better and more optimistic, I was also sleeping better. But it was still difficult for me to come to terms with the fact that it was an ongoing condition that would require treatment and attending the surgery probably for the rest of my life. I doubt that I have yet made the adjustment from someone who was perfectly healthy to someone now dependent on medication and help from the medical profession.

Introduction

The thyroid gland has a wide ranging impact upon many of the organs and tissues of the body. An overactive or underactive thyroid results in widespread manifestations and frequently requires long-term management. Patients with thyroid problems often have to live with long-term medication and face regular monitoring of their condition. They therefore face the same permanent alterations to their life-style as some patients who live with longterm illness. This chapter aims to provide an overview of the various types of thyroid disease and to consider how the health care professional might assess a patient with such a condition. Treatment options will be discussed and useful contacts for patients and health care professionals will be provided.

Prevalence

The 'average' general practitioner with a list of 2500 patients may expect to see two or three new patients with thyroid disease each year (Hasler and Schofield, 1990).

Physiology

Figure 12.1 provides an overview of the regulation of thyroid hormone secretion in the body. The hypothalamus secretes thyrotrophin releasing hormone (TRH), a tripeptide which stimulates production of thyroid stimulating hormone (TSH), a polypeptide from the anterior lobe of the pituitary gland. TSH stimulates the thyroid gland to increase the release of thyroxine (T4) and triiodothyronine (T3). The thyroid gland produces mainly T4, some of which is converted to T3 in the blood or tissues; 85% of T3 is produced in this way, 15% is secreted from the thyroid gland. T3 is primarily responsible for the observed effects of the thyroid hormones. Most T3 and T4 in the plasma is protein bound, to thyroxine-binding globin (TBG). It is

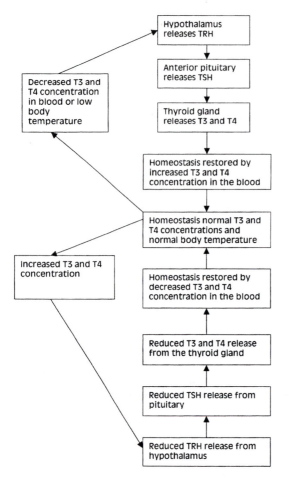

Figure 12.1 Regulation of thyroid hormones

Table 12.1 The effects of the thyroid hormones on peripheral tissues (Martini, 1995)

Elevate consumption of oxygen and energy causing a rise in body temperature

Heart rate and force of contraction are elevated causing a rise in blood pressure

Sensitivity to sympathetic stimulation is increased

Sensitivity of respiratory centres to changes in oxygen and carbon dioxide are maintained

Red blood cell formation is stimulated

Other endocrine tissue activity is increased

Turnover of minerals in bones is increased

It is clear that an alteration in the production of thyroid hormones will have far reaching effects on the body. The conditions resulting from abnormal thyroxine production can be broadly split into two main areas – hyperthyroidism (or overactive thyroid) and hypothyroidism (or underactive thyroid).

Pathophysiology

Hyperthyroidism (thyrotoxicosis)

This condition occurs when too much thyroxine is produced and it is also known as thyrotoxicosis, exophthalmic goitre, toxic goitre or Graves' disease (Walsh, 1997). The excess of thyroid hormone abnormally speeds up many of the body's functions resulting in an increase in metabolic rate, a flushed skin, a rise in heart rate and blood pressure, restlessness, irritability and fatigue. Approximately 1 in 1000 females and 1 in 10 000 males develop this condition and it is rare in children (Hope *et al.*, 1996). The exact cause of hyperthyroidism is not known although it is thought to be an autoimmune response.

Graves' disease is the most common form of hyperthyroidism and it is associated with insulin-dependent diabetes mellitus and pernicious anaemia. It occurs at any age, but most often in females between the ages of 20 and 40 years. Often there is a family history, which may indicate a genetic influence. It is an autoimmune disease, develops antibodies to its own tissue, i.e. thyroid tissue and this causes the problem. In Graves' disease, one type of antibody attaches to the cells that make up the thyroid gland and stimulates the production of

the unbound portion that is active. In addition to stimulating the production of T3 and T4, TSH increases the extraction of iodine from the blood in the thyroid gland and increases the size and number of the thyroid cells. Clearly, this all results in an increase in the circulating levels of thyroid hormones. As the thyroid hormones rise, a negative feedback system results in a reduction of the secretion of TSH by the pituitary.

Thyroid hormones readily cross cell membranes and bind to receptors in the nucleus, on the surface of the mitochondria and in the cytoplasm. The effects are widespread; the body's metabolic functions are kept going at the correct pace and this is essential for growth and cognition. The effects of the thyroid hormones are listed in Table 12.1.

large amounts of thyroxine. In Graves' disease exophthalmos, discomfort and watering of the eyes occurs.

Toxic adenoma describes the presence of a hyperactive nodule which is often solitary. It affects people who are usually 30–50 years of age. The nodule produces increased levels of T3 and T4 and, on scanning, the nodule is 'hot', usually benign and the rest of the gland is suppressed.

Subacute thyroiditis usually occurs in the postpartum period. It is often associated with a painful goitre. A raised erythrocyte sedimentation rate is usually found and it is thought to be linked to a viral cause. This condition is usually self-limiting.

The commonest *iatrogenic* cause of hyperthyroidism is an intentional increase in the patient's ingestion of thyroxine tablets. A patient may choose to increase their own dose of thyroxine either because they forget to take it for a few days or because they do not generally take it at all or they want to take some before visiting their doctor. Another reason is because they feel it helps them to lose weight.

Other causes include toxic multinodular goitre, choriocarcinoma and ovarian or testicular teratoma containing thyroid tissue.

Symptoms of hyperthyroidism

The symptoms of hyperthyroidism include:

- Weight loss and increased appetite
- Dislike of hot weather
- Sweating
- Restlessness, irritability, frenetic activity and insomnia
- Tremor of the hands
- Frequent stools
- Menstrual changes, light periods, oligomenorrhoea or amenorrhoea
- Emotional instability
- Shortness of breath, palpitations
- Itch
- Infertility may be the presenting problem
- Loss of libido, impotence.

Signs of hyperthyroidism

- Raised pulse with a steep rise on physical exertion
- Atrial fibrillation
- Warm peripheries

- Fine tremor
- Lid lag
- Thyroid enlargement and/or nodules
- Thyroid bruit
- Exophthalmus
- Brisk reflexes

Most people will not have all the symptoms but a combination of two or more may be present. The onset of thyroid disease is often insidious with the symptoms usually developing over weeks or months (Hopcroft and Forte, 1999).

Hypothyroidism

This condition occurs when the thyroid gland fails to produce enough thyroxine. This abnormally slows down many of the body's activities. Hypothyroidism is relatively common, approximately 2 in 100 females and 1 in 1000 males are affected, and this tends to run in families. Hypothyroidism can occur at any age, but the incidence is higher in the elderly. The deficiency of thyroxine may be primary, due to a disorder of the thyroid itself, or secondary, due to a disorder of the pituitary or hypothalamus. If this condition occurs congenitally in childhood, the result may be cretinism. In cretinism, the child fails to achieve normal physical or mental and development. In the adult, hypothyroidism causes myxoedema, which refers to the collection of symptoms associated with hypothyroidism (see Symptoms of hypothyroidism listed below).

Primary hypothyroidism accounts for 95% of all cases of hypothyroidism in adults (Walsh, 1997). Autoimmune thyroid disease is the most common and this is referred to as Hashimoto's thyroiditis. This is associated with insulin-dependent diabetes mellitus, Addison's disease and pernicious anaemia. Secondary hypothyroidism may also be due to destruction of the thyroid tissue following surgery. A less common cause is iodine deficiency, which causes enlargement of the thyroid gland and a goitre. This condition was once common in inland areas distant from the sea where a natural supply of iodine in the soil and water was deficient. Nowadays, this has been almost eliminated by the addition of iodine to table salt. A further cause of primary hypothyroidism is the use of antithyroid drugs such as thiocarbamides, sulphonylureas, amiodarone and lithium.

Hypothyroidism can also develop following thyroidectomy or radioactive iodine treatment where an excess of thyroid tissue has been destroyed and the remaining gland is unable to produce enough thyroid hormone to meet the needs of the body. Dyshormonogenesis can also occur. This is a genetic cause which is autosomal recessive.

The primary cause of goitrous hypothyroidism is Hashimoto's thyroiditis. This is an autoimmune disease in which there is lymphocyte and plasma cell infiltration. Hashimoto's thyroiditis affects women between 60 and 70 years of age and they are often euthyroid. A raised auto-antibody titre is often present and antibodies to hepatitis C virus are also common and may act as a trigger for Hashimoto's thyroiditis.

Symptoms of hypothyroidism

The symptoms of hypothyroidism tend to develop insidiously and include:

- Lethargy
- Tiredness
- Weight gain
- Aches and pains
- Constipation
- Feeling cold
- Dry skin and hair
- Depression
- Menorrhagia, amenorrhoea, metorrhagia
- Hoarse voice
- Memory loss and confusion
- Loss of libido, infertility.

Signs of hypothyroidism

- Toad-like face
- Non-pitting oedema
- Bradycardia
- Goitre
- Congestive cardiac failure
- Dementia
- Slow reflexes
- Loss of eyebrows (outer $\frac{1}{3}$rd)

Physical examination

The physical examination in a patient with suspected thyroid disease should include a general inspection and an assessment of the cardiovascular system, the respiratory system, the eyes and the nervous system as well as an abdominal examination to exclude teratoma. In particular, it is important to check the patient's vision and their reflexes, which are likely to be sluggish in a patient with hypothyroidism and brisk in a patient with hyperthyroidism. Assessment of the thyroid gland begins with an examination of the neck. It is important to note, however, that the thyroid may be enlarged and the patient may not show any signs of thyroid disease and conversely the thyroid gland may be normal (or not palpable) and the patient may show signs of either an underactive or overactive thyroid. A diagram of the thyroid gland can be found in Figure 12.2 (Bates, 1999).

Inspection

Observe the neck noting any obvious swelling and whether or not this is symmetrical. Note any scars, skin changes, difficulty in swallowing or breathing. Give the patient a glass of water and observe the neck during swallowing, observing any abnormalities. By asking the patient to swallow, the thyroid cartilage, thyroid gland and cricoid will all rise and it should be possible to note symmetry of movement (MacLeod, 1979).

Palpation

Stand behind the patient and palpate the thyroid gland including the isthmus and lateral lobes for size, shape (smooth or nodular), tenderness and mobility. The examiner places the fingers of both hands on the patient's neck so that the index fingers are just below the cricoid and by asking the patient to swallow it may be possible to palpate the glandular tissue as it rises and then falls back to the resting position. Feel for cervical and supraclavicular nodes (Walsh *et al.*, 1999). If a swelling at the front of the neck is an enlarged thyroid it will always move on swallowing.

Percussion

If there are any signs of retrosternal enlargement of the thyroid gland it may be useful to percuss gently at the base of the neck over the chest and elicit a dull sound.

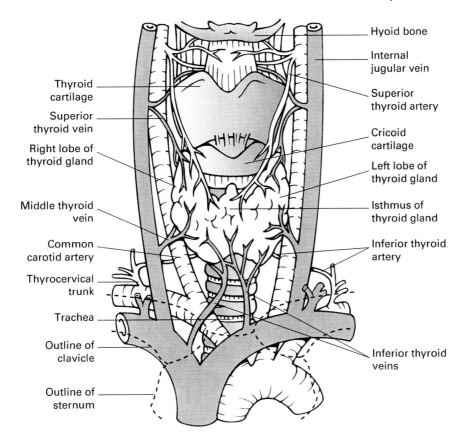

Figure 12.2 Location and anatomy of the thyroid

Auscultation

Listen with the stethoscope over the gland. If a bruit is heard this is due to the increased vascularity of the gland and it may suggest hyperthyroidism. If the thyroid gland is enlarged (goitre) it would be useful to find out the following:

1. Is the thyroid smooth or nodular?
2. Is the patient euthyroid, thyrotoxic or hypothyroid?
3. If the thyroid is nodular, is there a single or multiple nodules?
4. Palpable cervical lymph nodes.
5. Are the carotids displaced (benign goitre) or not (possibly a thyroid)?

An interpretation of findings on examination of the thyroid gland can be found in Table 12.2.

Eye examination

Examination of the patient who may have a thyroid disorder should include an eye examination. Check for lid lag by asking the patient to close their eyes and test the patient's visual fields, visual acuity and eye movements.

Tests and investigations

In some patients you may choose to screen for thyroid disease in the absence of other signs and symptoms. This may be justified in the following circumstances:

- Suspected congenital hypothyroidism newborns are tested
- On carbimazole, amiodarone or lithium

Table 12.2 Interpretation of findings on examination of the thyroid gland

If there is a *smooth non-toxic goitre* then the possible causes are:

1   endemic (related to iodine deficiency)
2   congenital
3   thyroiditis
4   physiological
5   autoimmune (including Hashimoto's thyroiditis)

A smooth toxi goitre. Grave's disease

A multinodular goitre is usually euthyroid but hyperthyroidism may develop

The single thyroid nodule is a common surgical problem, 10% of which will be malignant

Single nodules are usually caused by cysts, adenoma, discreet nodule in a multinodular goitre and malignancy

- After neck irradiation
- Postpartum thyroiditis
- Hypercholesterolaemia
- Depression
- Infertility
- Antepartum haemorrhage
- Diabetes mellitus Type 1
- Dementia
- Autoimmunity (e.g. Addison's disease)
- Turner's syndrome
- Obesity
- Menorrhagia
- Carpal tunnel syndrome
- Poor growth in children
- Women over the age of 40 years with non-specific complaints.

In the patient who has presented with signs and symptoms of thyroid disease, the following tests and investigations will form part of your assessment. Assess the blood pressure and pulse because the thyroid hormones affect heart rate and contraction. Blood tests should include thyroid function tests, full blood count, erythrocyte sedimentation rate, biochemical profile, lipids and thyroid autoantibodies.

Blood tests

Thyroid function tests

O'Reilly (2000) estimates that 9–10 million thyroid function tests are carried out in England and Wales each year. The results take a great deal of expertise to interpret, however, in general TSH will be reduced <0.01 mu/l in hyperthyroidism and raised to >2.0 mu/l in thyroid failure. Free T4 and T3 will be raised in hyperthyroidism. Subclinical alterations in biochemical norms have been found to be associated with the onset of depressive states (Eales, 2000) and Hanna *et al.* (1999) point out that patients who receive thyroxine treatment may have thyroxine concentrations above the normal but remain clinically euthyroid. It is important therefore to combine thorough history taking and physical examination skills with the results of investigations before arriving at a therapeutic decision. Experience has shown that thyroid function tests are not totally reliable and biochemical assessments cannot deliver the diagnostic accuracy expected of them (O'Reilly, 2000). It remains important therefore to treat the patient and not the laboratory result.

Full blood count

A full blood count is carried out to exclude anaemia, which may be normochromic normocytic in hyperthyroidism and normochromic macrocytic in hypothyroidism.

Erythrocyte sedimentation rate

Erythrocyte sedimentation rate may be raised in thyroiditis.

Biochemical profile

There may be an abnormal liver function test and CK, AST, LDH may be raised due to abnormal muscle membranes. Measurement of serum electrolyte levels may reveal hyponatraemia due to inappropriate antidiuretic hormone (ADH) secretion (Guyton, 1996). In altered parathyroid function calcium levels may be changed.

Thyroid autoantibodies

Thyroid autoantibodies may be raised in Hashimoto's disease.

Lipids

Increased thyroid hormone decreases the quantity of cholesterol, phospholipids and triglycerides even though it increases the free fatty acids. Decreased thyroid secretion greatly increases the concentration of cholesterol, phospholipids and triglycerides resulting in fatty deposits in the liver. This large increase in circulating blood lipids in prolonged hypothyroidism is often associated with severe arteriosclerosis (Guyton, 1996).

Electrocardiogram

An electrocardiogram taken before therapy is valuable as changes may be strongly suggestive of hypothyroidism.

Ultrasound

If a goitre is present, ultrasound distinguishes between cystic 'hot', probably benign and solid, possibly malignant 'cold' nodules.

Thyroid test

A 131 Uptake test using radioactive iodine is carried out. If the patient is hyperthyroid, there is diffuse uptake. The lesions may be solitary or multinodular. Thyroid scanning can also help to determine the extent of retrosternal goitre and to detect ectopic thyroid tissue and thyroid metastases (this will involve a body scan).

Advice and treatment

The effects of thyroid disease are far ranging and can result in the patient feeling extremely unwell, as can be seen in the patient's perspective presented at the beginning of this chapter. It may be necessary to spend some time explaining thyroid disease to the patient and providing them with contact numbers to seek further information should they choose to pursue it. It is likely that the patient's self-image will have altered as they have experienced either the slowing down of all of their body functions over a number of months or they have experienced increasing restlessness and irritability. In either case, the health care professional needs to provide support and advice to the patient to help them manage and understand their condition. In many situations treatment with medication will correct the disorder, however, the patient will have to learn how to self-manage the medication regimen and how to be alert to changes in health.

Hyperthyroidism

In hyperthyroid disease the patient may be extremely restless and irritable. In either the hospital or community the environment needs to be managed to minimize the patient's anxiety. Family and friends can be encouraged to reduce the amount of stress the patient is experiencing by limiting visitors and other stressors. Due to the increased metabolic rate the patient may have lost weight and will need careful dietary advice. A high protein, high carbohydrate, high calorie diet should be encouraged and you might want to consider recommending decaffeinated drinks. Due to sweating, the patient will need to increase fluid intake. In the absence of cardiac or renal problems the patient with hyperthyroidism may need 3–4 l of fluid daily (Walsh, 1997).

There are several ways in which the patient's sexual patterns might be altered. In women the menstrual cycle may slow down or even stop and men may become impotent. Libido may be reduced and this can have a devastating effect on the patient and his or her partner. This is a difficult area for patients to address in consultations and so you may have to introduce the subject during the history taking process. You could consider using an opening line such as: 'Many people who have problem with their thyroid gland also find that they experience changes in their sexual patterns, have you noticed anything like this?' You may also want to enquire about the patient's last menstrual period, the regularity of the periods and whether there has been a change in the pattern of menstruation in the preceding months. It is important to explain the cause of these changes to the patient to help them come to an understanding of the problem and be reassured that, with treatment, the problems should abate.

Medications

Antithyroid drugs are the mainstay of treatment in hyperthyroidism. In addition to treating hyperthyroidism they are used to prepare patients for thyroidectomy and for long-term management.

Carbimazole and propylthiouracil

The most common treatment is carbimazole. Propylthiouracil is used in patients with a sensitivity reaction to carbimazole. Both drugs act primarily by interfering with the synthesis of thyroid hormones (Khot and Polmear, 1994).

The Committee of Safety of Medicines (CSM) states that carbimazole can cause bone marrow suppression, which induces neutropenia and agranulocytosis. It is important therefore that the patient should be asked to report any symptoms of infection, especially sore throat, and a white blood cell count should be performed if there is clinical evidence of infection. Carbimazole should be stopped promptly if there is clinical or laboratory evidence of neutropenia.

The dose of carbimazole is 20–60 mg daily and it is maintained at this dose until the patient becomes euthyroid which usually takes 4–8 weeks. The dose is then progressively reduced to 5–15 mg daily often for up to 18 months. Rashes are common and then, if necessary, propylthiouracil can be substituted. Further information relating to this can be found in the British National Formulary (2000).

Antithyroid drugs need to be given only once daily, despite having a short half-life, because of their prolonged effect on the thyroid. A relapse is common with the above 'low dose' regimen and the 'block and replace' regimen is becoming more frequently used. An example of this would be carbimazole 40 mg orally daily until hypersecretion has stopped then T4 (thyroxine) is added in, for example 50–150 µg daily by mouth. This two-drug regimen is continued for one year. About half of those with Graves' disease will have a lasting remission. The advantage of 'block and replace' is that hypersecretion is better controlled and follow up is less onerous for the patients (McGregor, 1996).

Propanolol

Propanolol is a beta-blocker which is used for the rapid relief of thyrotoxic symptoms and may be used in conjunction with antithyroid drugs or as an adjunct to radioactive iodine. Thyroid function tests are not altered by beta-blockers. Side effects of propanolol include bradycardia, heart failure, bronchospasm, hypotension, fatigue and gastrointestinal disturbances. For a full review of the side effects and contraindications see the British National Formulary (2000) and the Drugs and Therapeutics Bulletin (1998).

Surgery

It may be necessary to manage hyperthyroidism with surgery involving partial thyroidectomy. This would be indicated if the patient was experiencing pressure symptoms, which may occur with retrosternal goitre, hyperthyroidism, carcinoma or for cosmetic reasons. Surgical intervention does, however, come with some risks including recurrent laryngeal nerve palsy, damage to parathyroid glands and haemorrhage. The patient may become hypothyroid or hyperthyroid following surgery.

Radioiodine

Radioactive sodium iodine (iodine-131) solution is used for the treatment of thyrotoxicosis, particularly where there has been relapse after medical therapy or compliance. In patients with cardiac disease and in those who relapse after thyroidectomy, radioactive sodium iodine can also be useful (BNF, 2000). The patients almost always ultimately become hypothyroid and will need thyroxine (Hope *et al.*, 1996).

Decisions on treatment rest on local expertise and the patient's age. In general treatment with carbimazole is the first line of treatment, however, surgery may be the treatment of choice in a young patient and radioactive iodine in an elderly patient.

Hypothyroidism

In hypothyroidism the patient may have slowed down dramatically both at home and at work. Their family and colleagues need to be made aware that their condition is reversible with treatment, but in the meantime they need support and tolerance as they have to recover from the effects of thyroid deficiency. Initially improvement is slow and small changes need to be emphasised. Some may need extra clothing and bedding to prevent hypothermia. Dry skin should be treated with emollients and the avoidance of soap. The diet should be low in calories and high in fibre to reduce constipation. Although there may be an alteration in the lipid profile this is due to the lack of thyroxine. Once replacement is complete the profile usually returns to normal without changing dietary habits.

Medication

Thyroxine sodium is the treatment of choice for maintenance therapy in the patient with an underactive thyroid. The initial dose should not exceed 100 µg taken daily preferably before breakfast; 25–50 µg of thyroxine is used in the elderly or those with cardiac disease. The dose is increased at intervals of 4 weeks, checking thyroid function tests before increasing or decreasing the dose. The usual maintenance dose is 100–200 µg daily as a single dose. It is important to note that thyroxine's half-life is 7 days. The side effects of thyroxine usually occur at excessive doses and include arrhythmias, anginal pain, tachycardia, palpitations, restlessness, diarrhoea and vomiting. See the British National Formulary (2000) for a full overview of the side effects and contraindications. Treatment is usually life-long and should be monitored yearly using standard blood tests of full blood count, thyroid function tests and fasting serum lipids.

Thyroid eye disease

Thyroid eye disease is a clinical diagnosis which may be made in the presence or absence of thyroid autoantibodies. It occurs when there is retro-orbital inflammation and lymphocyte infiltration, which causes swelling of the contents of the orbit. The usual procedure is referral to specialist ophthalmologist.

History

The patient will present with a history of decreased visual acuity, double vision, discomfort and/or protrusion of the eyes. Decreasing acuity may mean optic nerve compression. If there is evidence of decreased visual acuity refer the patient onto an ophthalmologist immediately as decompression of the optic nerve may be necessary. If the eye cannot protrude for anatomical reasons, optic nerve compression may be all the more likely. However, nerve damage does not necessarily occur with protrusion.

Signs

Signs of thyroid eye disease are commonly exopthalmos and lid lag but also include proptosis/exophthalmos, conjunctival oedema, corneal ulceration, papilloedema, optic atrophy, lid lag, lid retraction, loss of colour vision, ophthalmoplegia (especially of upward gaze) from muscle tethering and fibrosis.

Investigations

Rose Bengal eye drops are used for locating damaged areas of the cornea due to disease. Rose Bengal is more efficient than fluorescein for the diagnosis of conjunctival epithelial damage. It stings excessively unless a local anaesthetic is instilled beforehand.

Management

Hypromellose eye drops 0.25% for lubrication as often as is needed. There is no upper limit to dose frequency or volume instilled. Lateral tarsorraphy, systemic steroids and 5% guanethidine eye drops may reduce lid retraction. Surgical decompression uses space in the ethmoidal, sphenoidal and maxillary sinuses. Orbital radiotherapy, cytotoxic drugs, and plasmapheresis have proved to be less reliable in managing this condition. Diplopia may be managed with a Fresnel prism stuck to one lens of a pair of spectacles, this allows for reasonably easy alteration as the exophthalmos changes (McGregor, 1996). It is important to note that eye disease may pre-date other signs of Graves' disease, and does not always respond to treatment of thyroid status. Furthermore, it may develop for the first time following treatment of hyperthyroidism, and often becomes worse after treatment.

Differential diagnoses

In order to reach a differential diagnosis it is important to exclude the following because often the patient presents complaining of a lump in the neck. These include reactive lymphadenitis due to local infection, prominent normal lymph nodes, goitre, sebaceous cyst and thyroglossal cyst. Less common diagnoses include brachial cyst, pharyngeal pouch, cervical rib, actinomycosis, primary lymphoma or secondary neoplastic metastases. Rare potential diagnoses include tuberculosis of cervical lymph nodes, thyroid carcinoma, carotid body tumour or aneurysm, sarcoidosis, cystic hygroma (Hopcroft and Forte, 1999). Differential diagnosis in:

Hyperthyroid

- anxiety state
- mania

Hypothyroid

- diabetes
- addisons
- pernicuous anaemia
- depression
- senility

In some situations you may come across important findings during the history taking process or on the physical examination. A neck lump fixed to the skin without a punctum requires urgent referral to exclude a tumour, dysphasia with a neck lump is a serious symptom unless associated with a transient sore throat and endoscopy may be necessary. Beware of a hard swelling developing rapidly in the thyroid, in this case carcinoma must be excluded. A neoplastic type lymph node enlargement without cause needs urgent referral.

Case study

The patient who provided the perspective on living with thyroid disease at the beginning of this chapter, consented to a taped interview about his experiences of the condition. The following is a summary of the interview and we include it here to provide an insight into the challenges of living with the disease and the effect it can have upon the whole of the patient's life.

David is a 41-year-old married man with two children aged 10 and 3 years. He is employed as a business development area manager for a finance company. His alcohol intake is approximately 20 units per week, and he smokes 25 cigarettes per day. He is usually fit and well with no other medical conditions or hospital admissions. There is no family history of thyroid disease, although his mother did have maturity onset diabetes mellitus.

On returning from a holiday in Spain he arrived at the surgery complaining of tremor, rapid pulse, weight loss (6 kg), frequency of bowel movements, up to four times a day. He had also experienced an intolerance to the heat on holiday, together with increased sweating and he was experiencing generalized aches and pains. On examination he had a fine tremor. The thyroid was not enlarged, and there was slight bilateral exophthalmos. He had a tachycardia of 103 and was in sinus rhythm. Blood pressure was normal at 136/70 mmHg.

A provisional diagnosis of hyperthyroidism was made at the first consultation based on clinical signs and symptoms. Blood test results confirmed the diagnosis of hyperthyroid disease a few days later. He was commenced on carbimazole 20 mg daily, and propanolol 10 mg three times a day. He was seen by the endocrinologist 6 weeks later. A 'block and replace' regimen was used.

Blood result readings taken at monthly intervals:

	July	August	September	October
TSH (mu/l)	<0.1 (0.47–4.5)	<0.1	<0.1	<0.1
T4 (pmol/l)	>100 (9.7–25.7)	55.9	16.4	8.2
T3 (pmpl/l)	8.4 (3.7–6.9)	21.3	8.4	7.1

Full blood count and biochemical profile were normal. Thyroid antibodies to thyroid peroxidase – 1396.0 H Elisa Unit (0.0–50.0).

After having a review by the consultant endocrinologist David's 'block and replace' regimen was prescribed at carbimazole 20 mg twice daily and once the thyroid gland had been suppressed he was to add thyroxine 100 μg daily and be reviewed in clinic in 2 months time.

David's immediate reaction to his diagnosis and treatment was initially one of relief but his main concerns were, 'will this ever get right, will it recur and will it affect my work?' Fortunately he works for a large company who can easily absorb his workload and absence from work. Nevertheless David's anxiety remained high at this time and he experienced difficulty sleeping. This was probably a combination of physiological and psychological causes.

When he returned to the clinic, he was experiencing eye problems. Both eyes were sticky, aching, with blurred and double vision if he looked quickly to the side. There was no proptosis, but some soft tissue swelling of the upper and lower lids. There was no conjunctival oedema, his visual acuity was 6/9 in the right eye and 6/5 in the left eye. He undoubtedly had Graves' ophthalmopathy. Those at greater risk of reduced visual acuity are those for whom proptosis does not develop. He was commenced on prednisolone 30 mg daily, and continued on carbimazole 20 mg twice daily.

At about this time David was given written information about his disease in the form of a leaflet from The British Thyroid Foundation, and he himself purchased The British Medical Association booklet called *Thyroid Disorders* (Toft, 1999) from a local chemist. He found this most informative, and this helped him to understand his symptoms and treatments. He also discovered a group for people with thyroid problems. Unfortunately the nearest meeting being 30 miles (48 km) away, was too far for him to attend, but it did make him feel less isolated.

During the following months, David's physical condition improved. His weight increased, his bowel habits returned to normal, and the sweating and tremor resolved. His eye symptoms did not respond quite so quickly. It is well documented that despite suppression of the thyroid gland, eye symptoms commonly do not revert to normal as would be expected. He still has diplopia particularly when looking upwards and laterally. Oral prednisolone was gradually reduced, despite persisting eye problems. Suppression of the overactive gland was complete and David did have to start on thyroxine tablets as suppression with carbimazole became excessive. He became hypothyroid, with the following results: TSH 3.8, T4 5.6, T3 3.7. Gradually his eye symptoms became less. He occasionally uses hypromellose eye drops, as his eyes become very dry, being more painful when walking on windy days.

David's treatment is ongoing, and will probably be life-long. In total he was off work for 9 months, eventually returning to work on a part-time basis 2 days per week. On the positive side he has stopped smoking, and reduced his alcohol intake. One of David's main concerns is a fear of missing his tablets. He is worried that his symptoms will recur. He is therefore very compliant in taking his medication, which is really good considering that this will be a life-long exercise. He recognizes his condition is quite rare, and his knowledge and understanding of his thyroid disease is good. In his words he says 'that it controls metabolism, thought processes, energy levels, the whole body'.

Overall David felt that his illness had not affected his family life. Although he did comment that his wife appeared quite stressed on occasions. She in turn commented about David's mood swings, sometimes irrational anxieties. He was encouraged by a slow improvement in his general well-being, and was managing to work from home. David's parents and brother have been very anxious throughout the illness. In the beginning they had no knowledge of thyroid disease, but with David's help they gradually learnt more about it. They were keen to have blood tests despite not having any symptoms and fortunately all of the tests were normal.

David continues to remain reasonably well controlled. He attends clinic regularly and so is well monitored. It is also an opportunity to discuss any worries or concerns that he might have.

Conclusion

The effect of thyroid disease on the individual varies from the minor cosmetic to major systemic disease. Over- and underactivity of the thyroid gland may lead to serious social and medical consequences. For example a patient with thyrotoxicosis may appear as a fussy neurotic complainer, while the undiagnosed patient with hypothyroidism may lose their job because of 'lack of drive' or even end up in a psychiatric unit because of lethargy, forgetfulness and confusion. Once a diagnosis has been established it is important to have an effective system in place for follow up, monitoring and ongoing support. Health care professionals have a major role to play in working with patients to manage this long-term chronic condition. It is important to retain a holistic perspective including the psychosocial effects of the patient's condition.

The authors would like to acknowledge Dr Michael Howse, General Practitioner, Kendal, for his advice and support.

Useful contacts

The British Thyroid Foundation
PO Box 97
Clifford
Wetherby
West Yorkshire
LS23 6XD
Reg. Charity No. 1006391

Thyroid Eye Disease Association (TED)
Solstice, Sea Road
Winchelsea Beach
East Sussex
TN36 4LH
Tel. No. 0179 7222 338

References

Bates B (1991) *A Guide to Physical Examination and History Taking*, 5th edn. J B Lippincott Company, Philadelphia

British National Formulary 39 (2000) *British National Formulary*. British Medical Association, London

Drugs and Therapeutics Bulletin (1998) Managing subclinical hypothyroidism. **36**, No. 1, pp 1–3

Eales M (2000) Thyroid function testing means different things to different people. *British Medical Journal* **321**, 1080

Guyton A C (1996) *Textbook of Medical Physiology*. Saunders Company, London

Hanna F W F, Lazarus J H, Scanlon M F (1999) Controversial aspects of thyroid disease. *British Medical Journal* **319**, 894–899

Hasler J, Schofield T (1990) *Continuing Care. Management of Chronic Disease*. Oxford University Press, Oxford

Hopcroft K, Forte V (1999) *Symptom Sorter*. Radcliffe Medical Press Ltd, Oxford

Hope R A, Longmore J M, Hodgetts T J, Ramrakha P S (1996) *Oxford Handbook of Clinical Medicine*. Oxford University Press, New York

Khot A, Polmear A (1994) *Practical General Practice – Guidelines for Logical Management*. Butterworth-Heinemann, London

MacLeod J (1979) *Clinical Examination*. Churchill Livingstone, Edinburgh

Martini F (1995) *Fundamentals of Anatomy and Physiology*, 3rd edn. Prentice Hall, New Jersey

McGregor A M (1996) *Oxford Textbook of Medicine*. Oxford University Press, London

O'Reilly D S (2000) Thyroid function tests – time for a reassessment. *British Medical Journal* **320**, 1332–1334

Souhami and Moxham (1995)

Toft A (1999) *Understanding Thyroid Disorders*, 2nd edn. British Medical Association, Banbury

Walsh M (ed.) (1997) *Watson's Clinical Nursing and Related Science*, 5th edn. Baillière, Tindall, London

Walsh M, Crumbie A, Reveley S (1999) *Nurse Practitioners. Clinical Skills and Professional Issues*. Butterworth-Heinemann, Woburn

13

Dermatology

Jean Sargeant

Introduction and patient's perspective

Dermatological conditions account for many consultations both in primary and secondary care. A holistic approach is an important part of caring for patients with chronic skin conditions. This chapter aims to give a brief overview of the basic principles of dermatology, the common conditions seen and how to recognize them. It will explain how to examine the skin for dermatological conditions. The correct use of terminology to identify lesions and rashes is imperative if the health care professional is to have credibility in both diagnosis and referral to other agencies. A working knowledge of therapeutic intervention is also important and will be included. This chapter should be used in conjunction with dermatology textbooks and journals.

The psychological, physical and emotional well-being of the patient during ill health and its impact on family and partners is acutely important in the management of people with skin conditions. Skin rashes and lesions are often highly visible and may have an enormous psychosocial impact. It is estimated that psychological distress affects up to 30% of patients attending hospital outpatient clinics for skin conditions (Gawkrodger, 1997).

The following account gives a mother's perspective of living with a child who has eczema. The name of the child has been changed to ensure confidentiality.

I have an 8-year-old daughter who has suffered from eczema since she was 3 months old. It was minimal at first until she was 2 years old when it became much worse, until she was six. She had to wear 'wet wraps', which covered her whole body, except her head. We used steroid tablets, creams, bath oils, emollients and medication at night to make her sleep, but they didn't work.

Nicola was bathed up to three times a day and often this continued throughout the night. Her bandages were changed every 2 hours through the night, which left both Nicola and myself feeling very tired and miserable, so much so that I needed to take antidepressant medication. At night I would lie next to her and count how many times she scratched each part of her body and hope it would get less. Eventually I would turn over and try to ignore her because I knew there was nothing else I could do to help her. All of the bedding was changed daily and all clothing was washed separately.

Nicola couldn't do the things other children did, for example swimming was out because the chlorine in the water dried her skin. She was unable to go to parties because she became too hot when playing the games and this would make her scratch until she bled. School trips were out because someone needed to be there to apply cream to her skin. Even shopping in a warm supermarket would start the scratching. Holidays needed to be in this country, as many times we needed to return home for antibiotics from her GP, for infected eczema.

Just when you think there is no light at the end of the tunnel and you have both shed many tears, things begin to improve. Nicola's skin is wonderful (for now), she still gets the odd flare or reaction to something but we don't need wet wraps now.

We are even chancing a holiday abroad this year!

Epidemiology

Skin problems are extremely common and account for approximately 10% of general practice consultations and 6% of hospital outpatient appointments. Referrals from primary care in just over one year amount to 1% of the UK population. Occupational health is also an issue, as skin problems are the biggest single industrial cause of absence from work and the most common form of occupational disease (Gawkrodger, 1997).

The prevalence of skin disease will vary with the age, sex, race and occupation of patients within the practice population. A sparsely populated rural area will produce different dermatological conditions to that of a densely populated industrial area. The practice with a large elderly population may see more skin malignancies, conversely the younger practice population may have more consultations for eczema and acne.

Affluence as well as poverty seems to be a factor. The current trend of taking holidays abroad to hot climates creates its own problem. Fair-skinned people who expose themselves to short periods of strong sunlight increase their risk of skin malignancies. It would appear that eczema is more prevalent in British schoolchildren in social classes one and two than those in lower classes (Williams *et al.*, 1994).

Pathophysiology

In order to manage skin diseases effectively, it is first necessary to have an understanding of the structure and function of skin.

Structure

Figure 13.1 is a diagram of the structure of the skin and it shows the difference in texture of skin with and without hair.

The skin accounts for approximately 16% of our body weight and is the largest of our permanently visible organs. It consists of three layers: the epidermis, dermis and the appendages.

The epidermis consists of stratified squamous epithelium, which is divided into two layers. The superficial layer is devoid of blood vessels, the cells have no nuclei and the cytoplasm has been converted into keratin, which renders the skin waterproof. The cells are dead and are constantly being shed and replaced by the deeper layer. These basal cells are rounded and have a nucleus, which gradually flattens as they approach the surface. Melanocytes make up 5–10% of these cells (Gawkrodger, 1997) and produce melanin pigment. This pigment gives protection to the basal epidermal cells by absorbing UV radiation, which causes abnormal cell division, leading to skin malignancy. This explains why fair-skinned people, who have less pigment in their skin than dark-skinned people, are more at risk of skin cancer when exposed to strong sunlight. Thin skin covers the body and limbs and is approximately 0.8 mm thick and four layers deep. Thick skin is found on the palms of the hands and soles of the feet, is thought to be five layers deep and may measure up to six times more in depth than thin skin (Martini, 1995).

The dermis consists of fibrous and connective tissue and has an extensive blood supply called the cutaneous plexus. It also contains sensory nerve fibres, hair follicles and sebaceous glands. Up to 70% of the dermis is collagen, which gives the skin its elasticity and suppleness.

Appendages consist of hair, nails and sweat glands and are formed by tubular folding of the epidermis into the dermis. Hair projects from almost all of the body's skin surface, with the exception of the sides and soles of the feet, parts of the external genitalia, palms of the hands and sides of the fingers and toes. There are approximately 5 million hairs on the human body (Martini, 1995), only 100 000 of which are on the head. There are two types of hair. Vellus hair can be found over most of the body and has the appearance of the soft fuzz of a peach skin. Terminal hair is coarser and found, for example on the head, eyebrows and eyelashes.

Nails are hard keratin plates, which originate as thickening of the epidermis at the nail root, close to the periosteum of the bone and protect the distal ends of fingertips and toes.

Sweat is a colourless liquid which is made up of approximately 99% water and electrolytes, (mostly sodium chloride). Sweat is constantly produced by the eccrine glands and usually evaporates very quickly from the skin without

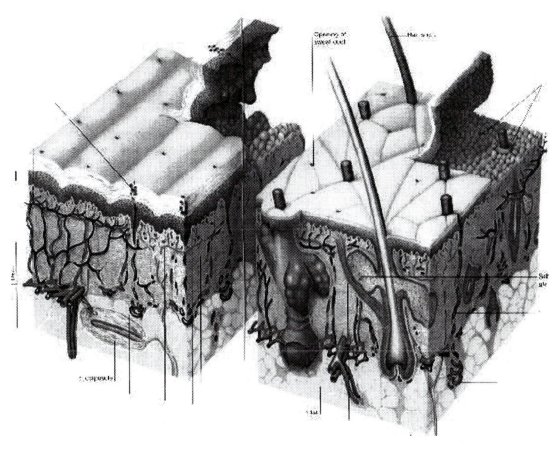

Figure 13.1 Structure of the skin (reproduced by kind permission of Gawkgodger)

being noticed. It is controlled by the sympathetic nervous system and this form of sweat production is called insensible perspiration. When the amount of sweat increases and becomes visible, for example in times of stress, the condition is known as sensible perspiration.

Appocrine glands begin to secrete at puberty and are connected to hair follicles. They produce a thick, white, sticky, potentially odorous solution and can be found in the axilla and surrounding the anogenital region, navel and nipples. Sebaceous glands produce oil (sebum), which lubricates the skin and slows down water loss, while also keeping hair supple. They are more prominent on the face and scalp, absent on the hands and feet and are very sensitive to hormonal change.

Function of skin

The functions of the skin can be summarized as:

- Protection of the internal organs
- Temperature control
- Excretion of body waste
- Sensation – contains the end organs of the sensory nerve fibres, therefore allows the feelings of touch, pressure, pain and temperature
- Development of hair and nails
- Secretion of sebum
- Allow synthesis of vitamin D3, by the action of sunlight, to be converted into calcitriol.

Terminology

The diagnosis of skin diseases is dependent on the accurate description of skin lesions, therefore the same terminology should be used between health care professionals to ensure consistency. The word *lesion* is used to describe an area with changed colour, elevation or texture that is surrounded by normal skin (Ashton, 1998). Listed below is a selection of the most common terminology in general usage. There are two main groups of lesions, primary and secondary.

Primary lesions

A *primary lesion* may develop on previously normal skin, for instance a freckle or mole, but always without any preceding skin change. Listed below are some of the common terms used for describing primary skin lesions (Bates, 1995).

Macule – small flat lesion, that is not palpable and only recognizable by its localized area of colour change, for example a freckle or petechia.

Palpable, elevated solid masses

Papule – a raised, therefore palpable, lesion, described as being a solid mass and less than 5 mm in diameter.

Nodule – as above but can affect any layer of the skin and measures greater than 5 mm in diameter, often feels deeper and more solid than a papule.

Tumour – a nodule, greater than 5 mm.

Plaque – flat collection of coalescing papules, greater than 2 cm in diameter but rarely larger than 5 mm in height, for example psoriasis.

Wheal – an irregular, transient area of oedema of the dermal layer of skin, which may be either white or red in colour, for example an insect bite.

Superficial skin elevations, with free fluid in the cavity between the skin layers

Vesicle – small blister within 5 mm, forming fluid in the dermis or epidermis, for example herpes simplex.

Bulla – blisters larger than 5 mm in diameter, filled with serous fluid.

Pustule – a blister filled with pus, larger lesions are called abscesses.

Secondary lesions

A secondary lesion is a lesion that has changed from its primary state. An example of this is a crust, which is a secondary lesion and it has changed from its primary state as a vesicle. A primary lesion which is scratched, becomes a secondary lesion as it has progressed from its primary state.

Crust – commonly known as a scab, this is the secondary change in a vesicle or pustule, as the epidermal surface is disturbed and the resulting fluid, which has escaped, hardens over the surface of the lesion.

Erosion – epidermal depression with moist area, for example a ruptured vesicle.

Ulcer – as above, although involving the dermis and subcutaneous tissue, often due to vascular insufficiency.

Fissure – a crack in skin, which may extend as far as the dermis, often found in athlete's foot.

Folliculitis – superficial inflammation and pus in the hair follicle, often caused by *Staphylococcus aureus* and may be aggravated by the use of ointments to the skin. Can be a problem with eczema, and it may be worth considering creams rather than ointment.

Millia – these are commonly known as whiteheads and are small cysts, often the size of a pinhead and commonly found on the face.

Comedone – commonly known as a blackhead, it is a mixture of shed keratin cells, dried sebum and bacteria, forming a plug in a hair follicle.

Cyst – arises from the hair follicle, producing a sac, with a collection of cream-cheese-like substance, which forms a spherical bulge on the skin surface.

Erythema – redness that blanches under pressure, associated with inflammation.

Telangiectasia – caused by visible dilatation of the dermal blood vessels, often apparent on the face.

Petechiae – haemorrhagic spots, which do not lose their colour when pressed against a glass, measuring approximately 1–2 mm in circumference, usually rusty purple in colour. These lesions are serious and are associated with severe pyrexia, for example meningitis, however, they may also be due to a clotting disorder.

Scale – exfoliating epidermis, for example dandruff. The layers should be scraped to see if they divide easily, as in a diagnosis of psoriasis.

Hyperkeratosis – overproduction of the keratin layer, without flaking.

Scar – dermal damage replaced by connective tissue, may be pink or white, but does not extend past the borders of the original injury.

Keloid – scar tissue, which extends beyond the margin of the original injury.

Atrophy – translucent skin, which may be depressed and wrinkled, as a result of epidermal or dermal thinning, often showing blood vessels beneath. This condition may be noticeable in patients who have used potent steroid ointments and creams over a prolonged period.

Alopecia – loss of hair. This can be more specifically described as alopecia totalis which is the description given to total scalp hair loss or alopecia versalis which describes total body hair loss.

Lesion arrangements and shape

The shape in which a lesion is formed is important in the diagnosis of skin disease, therefore, here are some common names and descriptions, which apply to both primary and secondary lesions.

Annular – used to describe a circular lesion in which the rim is different to that of the centre.

Geographic – this is a lesion with an irregular shape, rather like an outline of a country on a map.

Verrucous – wart-like.

Linear – these lesions are either single, or a cluster of long thin lines.

Koebner phenomenon – this condition occurs when a lesion develops at the site of trauma, such as a linear scar or scratch, within which, for example a line of warts or psoriasis may develop.

Target – these lesions are concentric, usually coloured red or pink and due to inflammation.

Serpiginous – as the description suggests, snake-like.

Discrete – these are lesions which are separated by normal skin.

Disseminated – describes discrete lesions which have become widespread.

Generalized – is the terminology used for a rash which covers most of the body.

Unilateral – is a lesion which does not pass the centre line of the body, for example a dermatomal rash such as herpes zoster.

Taking a structured dermatological history

When a patient presents with a skin lesion, it is tempting to go directly to the site of the lesion to inspect the problem. This temptation should be avoided, as care taken to collate a comprehensive history, will not only save time, but will reduce the risk of misdiagnosis.

Allow the patient time to describe the symptoms they are experiencing. While listening to the patient, the nurse gets a picture of the presenting problem but, of equal importance, is more easily able to establish, by the patient's voice and body language, the psychological impact it has on their lives. When the patient has given their account, it is useful to discuss the problem further by carrying out a symptom analysis of the problem. A useful tool is the PQRST method described by Morton (1993) as discussed below.

Provocation/palliation

It is necessary to explore the cause of the skin problem, which is often not immediately apparent. The health care professional will need to adopt a sensitive, but rigorous, open questioning approach. The use of medication, whether prescribed, borrowed or bought over the counter may be a contributory factor. It is important to ascertain the mode of distribution, either ingested or applied topically. It may be obvious to the patient, for example, that their rash has developed following a course of penicillin, however, the patient who presents with sunburn, may not be aware that the oral medication they have been taking for their fungal toenails, increases photosensitivity. It is also important to note what makes the problem worse; for example, the use of detergents may exacerbate contact dermatitis, while an antihistamine cream may make an itchy rash worse. The patient may notice that their rash tingles when exposed to a change in temperature, which could give a clue to a diagnosis of herpes zoster. The rash may be transient, it is therefore necessary to discover what makes it improve, for example the urticarial rash, which could last 24 hours, may have a shorter duration if an antihistamine tablet is ingested. An emollient may give instant relief to the discomfort of dry skin.

Quality

These questions are designed to gain an accurate description of the lesion, for example you might want to ask the patient 'can you describe it to me?' It is important to ascertain if the lesion is exuding and if so what kind of exudate. It may be the cream-cheese consistency of a sebaceous cyst, or an erythematous lesion exuding pus. A lesion that repeatedly heals, forms a crust, then breaks down, should alert the health professional to a possible malignancy. Lesions that are transient may develop in different places and may last less than 24 h, giving a possible diagnosis of urticaria. You might also want to ask the patient 'how does it feel?' The sensation of the lesion may also give clues to its origin. A very itchy rash could be scabies, while a rash that tingles may be herpes zoster, alternatively a lesion that gives the sensation of heat, may be infected.

Region

The patient may be reluctant to disrobe to show a rash or lesion and may therefore, only show one lesion and neglect to mention that other areas of the body are affected. It is important to ascertain the site and distribution of the whole lesion, which will once again assist with diagnosis and therefore you may need to encourage some patients to remove clothing so you can assess the whole of the skin.

Severity

If the patient has pain it may be useful to use a scale of 0–10 to assess its severity. Zero would represent no pain at all and 10 would represent the most severe pain imaginable. It is also important to ask the patient how they are feeling, for example do they feel systemically unwell, or pyrexial, which may be a sign of viral or bacterial infection.

The degree to which the rash or lesion affects the patient's daily activity needs assessment. The child with eczema may be restricted from living life to the full by well-meaning parents who overprotect him, in a bid to reduce exacerbation of the rash. The young man with psoriasis may be embarrassed by his appearance, which may have a huge impact on his ability to interact with his peers. The patient with contact dermatitis may be reluctant to admit that the cause of her rash is due to the chemicals she uses in her job as a hairdresser, as it may affect her livelihood. It is also useful to enquire if the lesion or rash causes the patient to lose sleep, for instance scabies is intensely itchy at night. A child, who awakes frequently in the night due to the itch of eczema, can cause stress to the whole family unit. A patient with a lesion causing concern, may be awake at night worrying about the possibility of malignancy.

Time

The duration of the rash or lesion is significant. A lesion that has been quiescent for a number of years and suddenly begins to grow over a few weeks is cause for concern. The picture will be clearer if the patient is able to distinguish between a pigmented lesion, which is increasing in diameter or becoming raised. A malignant melanoma may initially increase in diameter *before* becoming raised, where a benign naevi may become raised as it matures. A rash that has been present over a number of weeks may have lesions at different stages in development. Careful inspection of all lesions is important and may give a clue to diagnosis. It is important to discuss, if the patient can remember, when the skin was last normal and also what were the first symptoms of the problem, for example itch, or erythema.

After you have carried out a symptom analysis of the patient's skin disorder there are some other important areas to cover in the history taking process.

Environmental factors

The problem could possibly be caused by something at home, for instance fabric conditioner or shampoo, detergents, soap or perfume. Do not be reassured if the patient says they have not used a different soap powder, it may be the same 'new improved' product which causes the rash. It is important to enquire whether there has been a new pet in the family or if any of the animals are infested with lice. Contact with plants or sunlight may also be a clue to diagnosis. A farm worker may have an outbreak of ringworm in his dairy herd, which may help to diagnose his own skin lesion.

Medication

A careful check should be made of all current medication, whether ingested or applied topically. Rashes may be a side effect of medication, for instance a reaction to penicillin or non-steroidal anti-inflammatory drugs. The patient may have been using the same oral medication over a long period of time, but may suddenly develop a drug-induced rash. Antihistamine creams often exacerbate a problem and the prolonged use of steroid cream may thin the skin or cause perioral acne. The type of topical agent, for example whether it is a cream or an ointment, may be important. The agents used in a cream or an ointment may be a causative factor. Be aware that the medication used may be borrowed from medication prescribed to others, or bought 'over the counter' from a pharmacy.

Past history

It is possible that the lesions are similar to those previously treated successfully. If the rash looks eczematous it will help to ascertain if the patient had eczema as a child or if there is evidence of asthma, hay fever or eczema in the family. When a malignant skin lesion is a likely diagnosis, it will be necessary to ask if the patient has lived in a hot climate or been exposed to long periods of sunlight while abroad. The diagnosis of skin malignancies is dealt with elsewhere in this text. Systemic illness may also give clues to skin conditions, for example pernicious anaemia and thyroid disease may be a linked to vitiligo.

While exploring the patient's past history it is necessary to obtain details of previous allergies, drug-induced rashes or exposure to chemicals. It may also be necessary tactfully to discuss personal hygiene. The problem may not be lack of hygiene, but washing too often. The consulta-

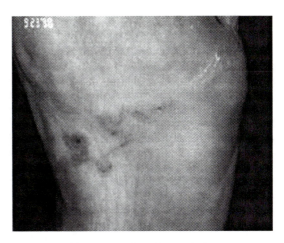

Figure 13.2 Serpiginous lesion

tion may also require the need tactfully to discuss sexual health issues, for example if a rash associated with gonorrhoea is suspected.

Family history

A family history, which includes hereditary problems such as eczema, psoriasis or malignant melanoma, may be important to note. This should not detract from a thorough examination of the presenting lesion. It is also useful to discuss if the rash or lesion is of short duration and whether anyone else in the family is suffering from the same problem. A viral illness may affect others and could give a clue about the presence of the coxsackie virus for example.

Social history

Social factors such as overcrowding and inadequate housing may also affect lesions and rashes, for example poor hygiene and a house with inadequate sanitation may predispose the child with herpes simplex on the lip to impetigo. Travelling abroad can produce its own problems, as demonstrated in Figure 13.2.

This photograph shows a serpiginous lesion in a patient who presented in surgery after a tropical holiday. The diagnosis was of a cutaneous larvae migrans, a worm that burrows under the skin. The patient complained of a sensation of something crawling beneath the skin.

Examination of the skin

Examination of the skin can be distressing for a patient if they are required to disrobe. The patient may not be expecting to be asked to take off their clothes if, for example, they present with a lesion on their thigh, so a tactful explanation with an assurance of privacy will be required. As the examination involves the whole body, it should be performed with sensitivity, and steps taken to ensure that the patient is prepared both physically and emotionally. As previously discussed, skin lesions or rashes such as psoriasis or unsightly birthmarks may have a huge psychological effect. If the health professional has taken a comprehensive history, he or she should have a greater awareness of the impact that the rash or lesion has on the patient.

Examination should be performed in a warm, well-lit room. While daylight is preferable, it is recognized that this is not always possible. Artificial light may mask jaundiced skin. A magnifying light may be useful. Lesions and rashes often evolve over time. A sketch of the rash or lesion, noting its position and distribution, is useful to refer to at a later date. The process of examination should be systematic using both inspection and palpation. Do not be afraid to touch the skin, the patient will often be reassured by this. The skin may give an indication of systemic disease and therefore should not be viewed in isolation. If the lesion is on the face, it may be necessary to request that the patient removes make up.

Examination should begin by general inspection of the whole body, noting the distribution of the rash or lesion. The distribution of a rash can aid diagnosis, for example a rash that develops unilaterally, following the pattern of a dermatome, is likely to be shingles. An itchy rash, which develops in skin flexures, may have a diagnosis of atopic eczema. A rash developing on the extensors is more likely to be psoriasis.

Inspection and palpation of the skin

Colour

The patient may notice their skin colour has changed, but may not divulge the information unless asked. It should be assessed for pallor, redness, cyanosis and jaundice. The latter is more difficult to assess, as the patient with a failing sun-tanned skin may look slightly jaundiced. The lips, hard palate and sclera give good indication of suspected jaundice. Pressing a glass to the lips will aid diagnosis. The pallor of anaemia is most easily seen in the conjunctiva, fingernails and mucous membrane of the mouth. These areas will also be affected by central cyanosis, the diagnosis for which could be lung or congenital heart disease. However, do not be fooled, a cold examination room may also have the same effect!

Moisture

Dry skin may be a sign of hypothyroidism or atopy, while oily skin may have a disposition to acne. Anxiety may be a cause of perspiration.

Temperature

The back of the hand should be used to assess skin temperature. Pyrexia may be of viral or bacterial origin or due to hyperthyroidism; conversely cool skin may be caused by hypothyroidism. Note any localized areas of redness and assess for heat.

Texture

This assessment is to ascertain if the skin is smooth or rough, thick or thin.

Mobility and turgor

The ease with which a fold of skin is lifted, will assess its mobility. The rate at which it returns back to normal is called turgor and is used to assess hydration of the skin.

Bruising

Consider any bruising of the skin; assess its age and distribution.

Nails

Note the shape and colour, look for signs of clubbing, the causes of which are varied. The nails should be smooth. Roughened pitted nails could be indicative of psoriasis.

Hair

The hair should be assessed for quality, quantity and distribution. An excess of facial and body hair on a young woman may be an indication of polycystic ovarian syndrome.

Lesion

As previously discussed it is important that lesions are not viewed in isolation. If the history warrants it, examination of the lymphatic system may be required. The lymph glands should be assessed for texture (smooth or rough), tenderness (which may indicate infection) and tethering (lesions that are fixed to the surrounding structures are indicative of malignant disease). An abdominal examination to assess for liver and spleen enlargement may also be necessary where malignancy is suspected.

Figure 13.3 shows the correct technique for examination of the lymph glands. The popliteal, inguinal and abdominal glands should also be examined. The glands of the anterior triangle should be examined from behind, using one hand at a time (Figure 13.3a,b) while the posterior glands should be examined from the front (Figure 13.3c).

Description of the lesion

An accurate description of a rash or lesion is imperative. A lesion, as previously discussed, may change over time, so it is important to be able to describe the primary lesion. The description should include:

Site and distribution of the lesion. Symmetrical lesions affect both sides of the body and are usually endogenous, for example eczema, psoriasis or acne (Figure 13.4). Asymmetrical lesions, affecting one side of the body, are usually due to external factors, such as bacterial or fungal lesions. A rash that follows a dermatome is often shingles.

Colour is important, for instance a red lesion caused by dilated blood vessels which blanch under pressure, is called erythema. White lesions are caused by lack of pigment. A bruise can be determined by its changing colours, from purple through to brown, as it ages.

Shape and size need to be accurately recorded as, with time, it may change. The border of a lesion is important and will aid diagnosis. A lesion with a poorly defined border, which merges into other skin, is characteristic of eczema. A lesion with a raised scaling edge and central clearing is indicative of ringworm. It is important to note that a lesion with a raised, pearlized border and depressed centre indicates a basal cell carcinoma.

Surface and texture need to be assessed, to see if the lesion is flat or raised, smooth or rough. Palpation is extremely important and should be performed first with the fingertips. Deeper palpation should be executed using thumb and index finger. The lesion may lie on the surface of the epidermis or include the deeper subcutaneous tissue. A squamous cell carcinoma will be depressed at its surface but thickened at its base, which could be missed if not correctly

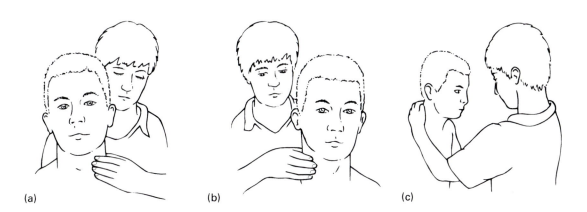

(a)   (b)   (c)

Figure 13.3 Examination of lymph glands

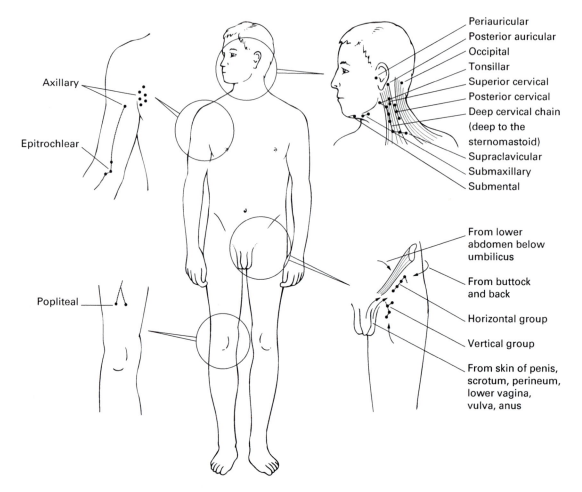

Figure 13.4 Distribution of lymph nodes

palpated. Ashton and Leppard (1992) define lesions as:

- Soft – feels like the lips
- Normal – feels like the cheeks
- Firm – feels like the tip of the nose
- Hard – feels like the forehead.

Secondary lesions may be present, depending on the duration of the problem. It is important for the health care professional to ascertain which lesions are primary and secondary presentations, to reduce diagnostic doubt.

Referral letter

The referral letter should encompass all information relating to the clinical findings. Documentation of the use of past and current medication is particularly important. This should include the name of the drug, the amount used and its duration of treatment. A photograph of the lesion will also be helpful and many practices now have cameras for this purpose. The use of the internet may be common practice in the future, to achieve prompt diagnosis of lesions, by scanning photographs and sending them via e-mail. The consultant will also wish to know what is expected from the referral, for example a diagnosis, reassurance, treatment or advice. The patient should also be fully aware of why they are being referred, approximately how long their referral will take and advised of realistic expectations from the consultation.

Common conditions

Atopic eczema

Definition

Eczema is defined as an itchy, scaling, erythematous rash with poorly defined edges.

Aetiology

This condition usually presents in infancy and may affect the whole body, including the face. Two-thirds of infants presenting with eczema will have a family history of atopy. Twelve to 15% of infants will be affected by eczema, many in the first few months of life and 60% of those will have developed the problem by the age of 6 months. Seventy-five per cent of children will be in remission by approximately 15 years of age. In infancy, the rash may be widespread over the body and face, including the napkin area. As the child gets older the rash may contain itself to the flexures of the skin, for example behind the knees and inner aspects of the elbows. Eczema causes intense pruritus, which often produces secondary excoriation and infection.

It is useful to remember the four 'w's which may affect eczema: water, wool, worry and the weather.

Psychosocial impact

Eczema is highly visible and may have a profound emotional impact on the patient, parents of children with eczema, extended family and friends. A child with eczema may have disturbed nights, usually from the intense pruritus, which may keep other members of the family awake. Longer consultation appointments to parents of children with eczema will be necessary. Parents need a careful explanation of the aetiology of the disease and the treatments used to combat it, while also being aware that, although eczema may go into remission with age, there is, at present, no cure.

Management

The fingernails should be kept short. This will reduce lichenification with scratching. Treatment options include steroid creams, ointments and wet wraps (see Medication). Many referrals to secondary care are caused by exacerbations due to the difficulties associated with compliance with medication.

Eczema can be exacerbated by many factors such as the use of biological washing powders and scented fabric conditioners. The use of soap, which dries the skin and bubble baths, should be avoided. Water also dries the skin, however, bathing should not be discouraged, but instead it should be used in conjunction with emollients and bath additives. The weather may also give rise to problems as some patients find their eczema is worse in warm weather, as it increases pruritus, and others may find the extra layers of clothing worn in the winter months exacerbate their problem. Perioral eczema is often worse in teething babies in cold weather, due to excess salivation.

Cotton clothing should be worn next to the skin and woollen clothing avoided in those patients who have a reaction to lanolin. Food allergies are often cited as a cause of exacerbation of eczema. If a patient decides to try an exclusion diet to manage the condition, the advice of a dietician will be essential.

Nappy rash may be either fungal, eczematous or both, it will be helpful, where possible, for the child's nappy to be removed as often as possible, to help to alleviate the problem. Plastic pants and disposable nappies occlude the skin and potentiate the affect of steroid creams, which should be taken into consideration, prior to application.

Adult atopic eczema

Atopic eczema most often occurs in children, however, it may continue into adulthood. Adults with eczema may require counselling about choosing a suitable occupation, which will not exacerbate the problem. The majority of adults may be symptom free, however, they may have eruptions on the hands if exposed to irritants to which they are more susceptible. This may prove difficult to resolve and there may be exacerbations periodically. It is thought that stress may be a factor. A diagnosis may be difficult, especially if the adult cannot remember the eczema of their childhood, however, a history of sibling atopy may provide the answer. Adult eczema is more likely to develop in cold weather and is prelevant in patients who have their hands frequently immersed in water, which degreases the skin. People who work in occupations such as nursing or domestic work are more commonly affected. The rash may commence under a wedding ring or may be worse between the fingers, where the skin has not been dried effectively. It may be possible to use potent steroids on the palms of the hands but milder steroids on the back. It is worth noting that lanolin is often an irritant to patients with eczema and creams containing the substance should be avoided. In susceptible patients, woollen clothing should not be worn next to the skin.

Seborrhoeic eczema

Definition

This condition is recognized by excess dandruff and it affects the nasal flares, ears and eyebrows. This condition is commonly known as cradle cap in children and mainly affects the scalp and eyebrows of infants.

Management

Seborrhoeic eczema in adults may be fungally infected and may require combined antifungal and low-dose steroids to resolve. Infants are treated with olive oil, to soften the scales of cradle cap overnight, and then the scalp should be washed daily with a mild baby shampoo and thoroughly rinsed.

Stasis eczema

Definition

This condition is commonly seen in elderly patients who have venous insufficiency. It is a gravitational eczema, which commonly affects sites such as the area over the medial malleolus.

Management

Stasis eczema may merely require the use of regular emollients. In severe cases the treatment may include mild to moderate topical steroid treatment and four layer bandaging. The use of a Doppler, to assess arterial pressure, is essential prior to commencing this treatment, as arterial insufficiency may also be present. The use of four layer bandaging is a specialist technique and should only be performed by health care professionals who are trained in its management.

Pompholyx

Definition

This is a severe form of hand eczema, the cause of which is not always known. It produces recurrent groups of erythema, vesicles and lichenification on the palms of the hands.

Management

When examining the patient with pompholyx, it is advisable to look at the feet for further lesions. The use of a potent steroid ointment, twice daily, will be required. In extreme cases, it may be necessary to occlude the hands overnight, with plastic gloves. The use of plastic potentiates the effect of the steroid ointment and should only be used as a last resort.

Postpartum eczema

Definition

Women in the puerperium are occasionally affected by hand eczema. It is thought that this may be due to the reduction in both oestrogen and cortisol levels, although the increase in washing, with small babies, may be also be a factor.

Management

The use of cotton gloves beneath rubber gloves will help to alleviate the problem and the use of a potent steroid at night will relieve itching.

Complications of eczema

The following problems frequently cause complications in the management of eczema:

Staphylococcus aureus is a bacterial infection, which is estimated to be present in 90% of infected eczema (Hicks, 2001). Dry cracked skin creates a medium for the introduction of infection. Paradoxically, occlusion of the skin with ointments produces a warm moist atmosphere for colonization by bacteria.

Eczema herpeticum is caused by the herpes simplex virus and may be mistaken for a secondary bacterial infection within an eczematous rash. The condition is potentially serious and will require oral antiviral medication.

Molluscum contagiosum affects mostly children and young adults and is a viral (poxvirus) skin infection. The condition is often a complication of eczema. Lesions are umbilicated, pearly pink/white in colour and are spread by physical contact. Each lesion measures approximately 2–4 mm and is oval shaped, with a punctum. Many lesions will resolve spontaneously within 9–12 months, however, it is thought they may resolve more quickly if the surface of each individual lesion is disturbed. The lesions can occur anywhere, but are most commonly found on the trunk, neck and face. A group of lesions seen on the side of the trunk may typically develop on the inner aspect of the upper arm, by direct contact.

Management

An explanation to parent and child, regarding the duration of the lesions and how to prevent spread of the condition to other siblings, combined with reassurance that the condition is not serious, is important. Precautions for the prevention of spread of infection include bathing separately and the use of personal towels and flannels. Patients with a severe problem may need referral to a dermatologist for removal of the lesions.

Treatment

It is essential to consult the most recent Formulary for guidance on the use of treatments.

Emollients

It is most important, when considering therapy, not to underestimate the use of emollients and bath oils. These therapies are essential in the management of eczema, to hydrate the skin. Some emollients contain lanolin, which may cause an exacerbation of the rash in susceptible patients. Emollients may be used for washing as a soap substitute and moisturizer and they may be used as often as required. Cream-based products are less effective than ointments, but may be more cosmetically acceptable.

Topical steroids should never be used in isolation. Many patients are under the mistaken impression that the use of a steroid cream negates the need for an emollient. It is important to provide the patient with a careful explanation to ensure they understand the nature of their treatment regimen. Topical steroid treatments should never be used as moisturizers and the routine use of combined steroid and antibiotic creams should be avoided. Ointment preparations are more effective than creams, because they stay on the skin for longer, however, patients often dislike their greasy preparation. It may be necessary to consider changing to creams, in place of ointments, where recurrent skin infection is a problem. The use of repeat prescriptions for steroid preparations should be avoided. If steroid medication is required for children, the use of hydrocortisone 1% is suitable in the short term, however, stronger steroid preparations require a second opinion. The use of mildly potent steroid cream (hydrocortisone 1%) to the face should be avoided in children, however, if necessary, may be used in adults sparingly, avoiding the eyelids, where it is more readily systemically absorbed. As previously discussed, topical potent steroids may cause thinning of the skin with inappropriate long-term use, therefore they should be used with caution.

Zinc paste bandages are often used to help to alleviate the problem of persistent eczema, especially where scratching is a problem. The bandages are often used in conjunction with 'wet wraps'. These are mildly elasticated bandages (Tubifast), used to keep dressings in place, where adhesive tape would be inadvisable. The wet wraps are placed in warm water, then applied either over the top of zinc paste bandages and/or steroid cream and emollient.

A further application of dry Tubifast is then applied.

Oral antihistamine may be appropriate for short-term use, to relieve itching. Modern non-sedating antihistamines are ineffective in relieving the itch of eczema, however, preparations such as chlorpheniramine are beneficial in some cases. Patients should be warned that these medications can cause drowsiness and therefore affect their ability to drive and operate machinery. The use of topical antihistamines should be avoided.

Antibiotic treatment, both in primary and secondary care, should be used with caution to help to avoid global resistance, although clinically significant infection should be treated. Infection is common in eczema and should be suspected where the condition worsens despite adequate treatment. There are many antibiotic creams available for mild infection, however, systemic antibiotics are often necessary to eradicate the problem. The use of flucloxacillin is the preferred antibiotic of choice for skin infections or erythromycin for those patients who react to penicillin.

Assessing quantities for topical medication

Topical medication is measured by fingertip units. This is a useful way of explaining to patients how much medication is required. It is also helpful when assessing prescribing requirements. One fingertip unit is the amount that covers the index terminal phalanx and it is equal to 0.5 g of cream or ointment. The adult face and neck requires 1 g of ointment, the hand 0.5 g, the arm 1.5 g, the foot 1 g, the leg 3 g and the torso front and back require 6 g. The amount of steroid creams and ointments will vary according to the age of the patient, the duration of the treatment and potency of the steroid.

Review

The regimen of contacts with the health care professional will vary according to the severity of the eczematous condition. Parents will require extensive support and reassurance when their child is initially diagnosed with eczema. They will require longer consultations, which will need to incorporate a detailed explanation of the aetiology of the disease and the way in which they can help their child. Initially consultations may need to be weekly to allow parents to gain the necessary skills in dealing with the condition. Both children and adults should not be given repeat prescriptions for steroid preparations. The use of steroid medication needs to be carefully monitored to avoid side effects. The patient should be seen weekly while using the medication to monitor its progress. When the skin is quiescent a 6-monthly appointment may be valuable to monitor progress and help the patient to maintain some control over their condition.

Contact dermatitis

Aetiology

The terms *dermatitis* and *eczema* are often used interchangeably. The word *dermatitis* should be used with care as there may be a link with the patient's employment and this could lead to medico-legal complications. Contact dermatitis is often difficult to diagnose as it may involve multiple agents. It is exogenous and is often prevalent in patients who have a history of atopy.

Psychosocial impact

Occupational dermatitis may affect the patient's livelihood and have a drastic impact on the family unit. Avoiding irritants or allergens can be impossible in the workplace and if the condition becomes chronic the patient may need to consider a change of occupation.

Definition

The rash of contact dermatitis is itchy, scaling and erythematous, with poorly defined edges.

Management

Taking a thorough history, which includes enquiries about medication, cosmetics, hobbies and occupation, will be required to alert the health care professional to contact dermatitis. Referral for patch testing is an option although this may prove to be difficult if the condition has several causes. A diagnostic clue may be taken from the distribution of the rash. The wrist is a common presentation, for example

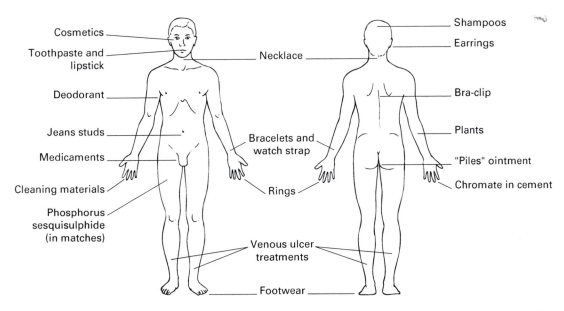

Figure 13.5 Clues for irritants in contact dermatitis (reproduced with kind permission from Gawkrodger, 1997)

and if it is confined to one wrist this should alert the health professional to a nickel allergy from a watch strap. Figure 13.5 provides an overview of the distribution clues for contact dermatitis.

Avoidance of the irritant or allergen is the best form of treatment, although this is not always possible. The use of steroid medication is the treatment of choice for relief from this condition, however, the use of emollients will help to relieve the dry skin.

Review appointment

Contact dermatitis will require regular weekly appointments in the acute phase. The purpose of the appointments will be to monitor the appropriate use of topical steroid medication and condition of the lesion. An appointment will also allow the health care professional to deliver appropriate health education and occupational health advice where appropriate.

Acne vulgaris

Aetiology

This condition affects male and female adolescents in equal numbers and commonly presents between the ages of 12 and 16 years, although it may also develop later in life. The condition affects over 80% of adolescents and is the most common skin condition. Acne accounts for one in seven consultations in primary care.

Definition

Distribution of the rash is usually the face, back, shoulders and chest and will consist of a mixture of comedones, pustules, whiteheads and papules. These areas are rich in sebaceous glands and the condition arises from increased sebum secretion, bacteria, hyperkeratosis and a sensitivity to the androgen hormones, which are unstable in puberty.

Psychosocial impact

Acne vulgaris can be a visible, disfiguring and psychologically distressing condition and appears at a time in a young person's life when many feel vulnerable and self-conscious. Young people are often embarrassed or even become clinically depressed about their skin. Acne may be worse in females premenstrually. The patient with acne may find it difficult to discuss the impact it is having on their lives, it is therefore imperative that the patient feels as comfortable as possible during the consultation.

Acne is a self-limiting illness but may take many years to resolve.

Management

Contrary to popular belief, the condition is not affected by diet or poor hygiene. It is often helpful to explain to the patient that the comedones noted on their skin are not due to dirt but are made of melanin. The aim of acne treatment is to prevent scarring. Reducing the severity of the acne has the added benefit of increasing the patient's self-esteem.

Treatment

Treatment of acne varies with severity and it is useful to enquire about previous medication. There are over the counter treatments available but many may cause the skin to become irritated and cause an exacerbation of the condition. In mild to moderate acne there are a number of topical solutions that may be helpful. Benzoyl peroxide can be applied topically twice daily, but may cause irritation. An antibiotic lotion may be of benefit when infection is present. Topical clindamycin is one option that may be beneficial in mild to moderate acne. Patients need to be made aware that initially, experimentation will be necessary until a product is found that is suitable to their needs. The use of oral antibiotics for moderate to severe acne is the next line of treatment. This is often oxytetracycline 500 mg twice daily and patients should be warned of their contraindication in pregnancy. The oral contraceptive pill may be affected if patients develop diarrhoea while taking antibiotics. If contraception is required with females, it may be useful to consider an anti-androgenic contraceptive pill such as Dianette. This would reduce acne while also giving contraceptive protection. Severe acne may require a dermatological opinion. Delay in referring acne that is failing to resolve may cause scarring. The treatment of choice at this stage will most probably be isotretinoin. This medication is used when conventional oral antibiotic therapy has failed. Patients should be carefully counselled before treatment. The drug is teratogenic therefore females must use a reliable method of contraception for one month prior to, during and after treatment. Blood lipids and liver function tests should be closely monitored. Treatment usually lasts approximately 4–6 months.

Review appointments

Monthly review is recommended while taking oral therapy to assess progress.

Acne rosacea

Definition

Acne rosacea affects both men and women and is more common in middle age. The cause of the condition is unknown. Rosacea affects the cheeks, forehead, nose and chin and has a characteristic butterfly appearance on the face. The condition has pustules, telangiectasia and papules over erythema, however, it is devoid of comedones and the secretion of sebum is normal.

Psychosocial impact

This condition is distressing for the patient and requires a careful explanation of diagnosis, management and treatment with realistic outcome measures.

Management

Topical metronidazole is the drug of choice for mild rosacea. If unsuccessful the use of tetracycline for 2–3 months treatment is recommended. Prolonged treatment may be required if the condition persists.

Review appointments

Monthly appointments are recommended while the rash is actively being treated.

Psoriasis

Aetiology

Psoriasis affects approximately 2% of the population, affecting both sexes equally. It is estimated that only 12% of patients access healthcare regarding their psoriasis (Savin, 1998). The condition commonly affects patients between the ages of 20 and 30 years of age, but can present at any age. It is unusual in children younger

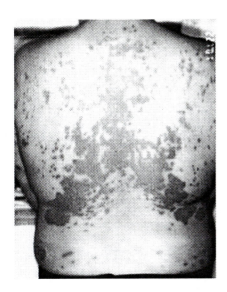

Figure 13.6 Psoriasis

than 7 years of age. There is a family history of psoriasis in approximately 30% of presenting patients.

Definition

Psoriasis is defined as erythematous, non-itchy, well-demarcated, plaques with a characteristic silvery scale (Figure 13.6). The lesion, when scratched will produce large amounts of dry skin and increase the silvery appearance. They are usually symmetrical and affect the elbows, knees and pre-tibial areas, but can affect any part of the body, including the scalp and nails.

Psychosocial impact

This condition can have a devastating psychological affect. Many patients are too embarrassed to access healthcare facilities. The condition is incurable. Patients who can access help often get support from a self-help group. Many patients become disillusioned with their medication regimen and this can lead to problems with compliance with treatment.

Management

Management of the psychological effect of the condition is equally as important as the medication. Treatment of psoriasis varies with the severity of the condition and there are many products available. Patients with moderate to severe psoriasis should be referred for specialist treatment.

Impetigo

Aetiology

Impetigo has reduced in incidence with improvements in social circumstances. It commonly affects children and is usually caused by *Staphylococcus aureus* bacteria entering via a break in the epidermal layer. The bacterium may be present in the nose, axilla and perineum and intermittently will affect up to 20% of the population (Gawkrodger, 1995). Bullous impetigo is seen in adults and children (Figure 13.7).

Definition

This condition is an infection of the epidermis. It is characterized by fine vesicles that burst to form golden crusts. The infection is most commonly present on the face and hands. It is extremely infectious and is usually a primary condition. However, it may present as a secondary infection of skin conditions, such as eczema or head lice. Bullous impetigo may affect any part of the skin and the bullae can measure up to 2 cm. The lesions in bullous impetigo spread rapidly.

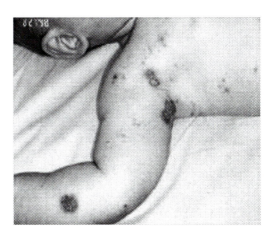

Figure 13.7 Impetigo

Psychosocial impact

Parents of children who develop this infection will require a careful explanation of the impact it may have on the family unit. Impetigo is still viewed by many as a disease of poor hygiene and parents may be distressed by the stigma attached to the condition. If the condition is visible and extensive the child may need to be excluded from school.

Management

The golden crusting lesions should be carefully removed using wet soaks. Parents should be advised that the infected child requires their own towels and flannels. Medication depends on the severity of the problem. Severely infected lesions or bullous impetigo will require systemic antibiotics. The antibiotic of choice for skin infection is flucloxacillin or erythromycin when penicillin is not appropriate. Topical lesions will require an antibiotic cream such as mupirocin.

Review appointment

The frequency of consultations required will depend on the severity of the infection. Systemic antibiotic medication will require review 1 week after treatment commences to assess progress. The infection will normally resolve during this time. Topical treatment will also require weekly assessment until resolved. A second consultation will provide the ideal opportunity tactfully to deliver health education advice on skin hygiene if required.

Folliculitis

Definition

This condition affects the hair follicles and is often seen in the beards of men, or in women who remove body hair by waxing. It is an acute infection and is characterized by erythema and pus originating in the hair follicle. The cause is usually the bacterium *Staphylococcus aureus.*

Management

The condition is usually treated in the same way as impetigo, as it often has the same bacterial infection.

Review appointment

This will again depend on the severity of the condition, however, the same regimen of appointments will be required as for impetigo. Health education regarding hair removal methods may be necessary.

Skin malignancy

The incidence of malignant melanoma is rapidly increasing and therefore is worthy of mention in this chapter.

Malignant melanoma

Aetiology

The incidence of malignant melanoma is rising by 7% annually and is twice as likely to affect young women than men. While still rare it is estimated that 18% of cases occur in patients between the ages of 15 and 40. Fifty per cent of lesions will develop from previous naevi, however, the rest will develop from normal skin. Prognosis is dependent on the thickness of the melanoma. The Breslow test is used to determine the depth of the tumour. This is the measurement of the tumour from its granular layer to the deepest melanocyte. The lesion spreads initially along the junction between the epidermis and dermis before becoming raised. At this point it has usually grown deeper into the dermal layer and has infiltrated blood and lymphatic systems, increasing the likelihood of metastatic spread.

Definition

The lesion is a malignant tumour of melanocytes and is commonly found on the back of males and the lower leg in women, but may occur elsewhere.

Patients who are at risk from this condition are those who have:

- A family history of melanoma
- A history of severe sunburn in childhood
- Fair skin (red heads are particularly susceptible) with a tendency to freckle
- Sunbathers
- Have multiple benign moles.

Management

Any lesion suspected of being malignant should be immediately referred for a dermatological opinion. Lesions that should alert the health care professional to the potential for a malignancy include those which have:

- a recent increase in size or shape with an irregular outline
- a variation in colour
- bleeding, scaling, crusting or exuding
- new lesions.

Health education is imperative in the prevention of malignant skin disease. Ideally this should commence with advice to parents regarding the protection of infants from the sun. Patients should be encouraged to report any moles that have the features described above.

Conclusion

This chapter has given a brief overview of the basic principles of working with patients who have a skin condition. In all patients with skin conditions it is necessary to take a holistic view to consider the psychosocial impact of the condition on the patient and their family members. As with the majority of chronic illness, the patient's life is likely to be affected in profound and individual ways. It is the role of the health care professional to understand the impact of the illness on the patient and to work with them and their families to develop the most appropriate treatment and management regimen for their particular situation.

Useful contacts

The Psoriasis Association
Milton House
7 Milton Street
Northampton
NN2 7JG
Tel 01604 711129

National Eczema Society
Hill House
Highgate Hill
London
N19 5NA
Tel 0207 281 3553
Eczema Information line 0870 241 3604
www.eczema.org

Acne Support Group
PO Box 230
Hayes
NB4 0UT

The British Red Cross camouflage service is available via a referral from your doctor or consultant. Further information about the service can be obtained from local branch headquarters.

References

Ashton R (1998) The art of describing skin lesions. *Dermatology in Practice*. March/April pp. 11–14

Ashton R, Leppard B (1992) *Differential Diagnosis in Dermatology*. Radcliffe Medical Press Limited, Oxford

Bates B (1995) *A Guide to Physical Examination and History Taking*, 6th edn. J B Lippincott & Co, Philadelphia

Gawkrodger D J (1997) *Dermatology*. Churchill Livingstone, Edinburgh

Hicks R (2001) Infected eczema. *Practice Nurse* **21**, 31–38

Jackson A (1998) Is this mole alright? *The Practitioner* **242**, 254–264

Martini F (1995) *Fundamental of Anatomy and Physiology*, 3rd edn. Prentice Hall, New Jersey

Morton P G (1993) *Health Assessment in Nursing* 2nd edn. F A Davis & Co, Philadelphia

Savin J (1998) GP care of psoriatic patients. *Dermatology in Practice*. October, No. 3

Walsh M, Crumbie A, Reveley S (1999) *Nurse Practitioners Clinical Skills and Professional Issues*. Butterworth Heinemann, Oxford

Williams H C, Strachan D P, Hay R J (1994) Childhood eczema: disease of the advantaged? *British Medical Journal* **308**, 1132–1135

Index

Printed in the United Kingdom by
Lightning Source UK Ltd., Milton Keynes
139243UK00001BA/4/A